Manual of Gynecardiology

Angela H.E.M. Maas • C. Noel Bairey Merz
Editors

Manual of Gynecardiology

Female-Specific Cardiology

Springer

Editors
Angela H.E.M. Maas
Department of Cardiology
Women's Cardiac Health Program
Radboud University Medical Center
Nijmegen
The Netherlands

C. Noel Bairey Merz
Director Barbra Streisand Women's Heart Center, Linda Joy Pollin Women's Heart Health Program, Director
Preventive Cardiac Center
Cedars-Sinai
Los Angeles, USA

ISBN 978-3-319-54959-0 ISBN 978-3-319-54960-6 (eBook)
DOI 10.1007/978-3-319-54960-6

Library of Congress Control Number: 2017942963

Printed on acid-free paper

This Springer imprint is published by Springer Nature
The registered company is Springer International Publishing AG
The registered company address is: Gewerbestrasse 11, 6330 Cham, Switzerland

Preface

In the past 25 years, we have made notable progress in our understanding of women's heart disease and women's hearts. Groundbreaking studies have informed us so much more about the novel risk factors that can impact women's likelihood for cardiovascular disease (CVD).

Ongoing work is aimed at achieving wide-scale understanding and usage of these risk factors, which include adverse pregnancy outcomes, estrogen deficiency, and premature menopause, in medical guidelines for diagnosing and treating women. Even so, we still have a job to do in educating women, including young women, about heart disease risk—and in educating their physicians. Meanwhile, CVD death rates are declining in all age groups except one—women 35–54 years.

Investigation advocacy campaigns are needed to translate these findings into clinical practice and care. Healthcare provider education regarding sex- and gender differences in CVD and clinical trials testing sex- and gender-based therapies are needed. We need to continue to advocate for women's heart disease as a specific research topic in education and funding agencies.

The *Manual of Gynecardiology* gives an update on our current knowledge in cardiology care for women and provides practice tools for cardiologists, trainees, and nurse practitioners. Women with signs and symptoms of ischemic heart disease are still too often evaluated and treated along the male standard, leading to uncertain diagnoses and inappropriate treatment. This especially accounts for younger females under 65 years of age, who have more often nonobstructive coronary artery disease and vascular dysfunction rather than focal obstructive disease. Considering women's health along a horizontal life approach can be helpful to distinguish low- and high-risk women from each other.

We hope that this book adds to the knowledge of all those who aim to improve cardiology care in women.

Nijmegen, The Netherlands — Angela H.E.M. Maas, M.D., Ph.D., F.E.S.C.
Los Angeles, CA — C. Noel Bairey Merz, M.D., F.A.C.C., F.A.H.A.

Contents

Chapter 1
Cardiovascular Disease Risk in Women: What Makes It Different from Men

Angela H.E.M. Maas and C. Noel Bairey Merz

Abstract Sex-related differences in ischemic heart disease (IHD) and other manifestations of cardiovascular disease are currently not taken into account in the various existing risk scores. This often leads to an underestimation of the actual CVD risk in women. Traditional risk factors, female-specific risk factors and non-traditional risk variables are discussed in this chapter with their meaning in order to identify the high risk woman.

Keywords Diabetes mellitus • Dyslipidemia • Estrogen • Female-specific risk factors • Gestational diabetes • Hypertensive pregnancy disorders (HPD) • Ischemic heart disease (IHD) • Lifestyle • Medication adherence • Menarche menopause • Migraine • Miscarriages • Polycystic ovary syndrome • Preeclampsia • Premature CVD • Non-traditional risk variables • Sex-hormones • Risk scores • Statins • Traditional risk factors

Introduction

Clinical manifestations of cardiovascular diseases (CVD) develop on average 7–10 years later in women than in men and are the major cause of death worldwide (www.who.int). With the modernization of life-style over the past decades, CVD morbidity and mortality is anticipated to further increase in the coming years with a shift towards younger age at first events [1–4]. Overweight, obesity, cigarette smoking, unhealthy food and lack of physical exercise have become the greatest

---

A.H.E.M. Maas, M.D., Ph.D. (✉)
Department of Cardiology, Women's Cardiac Health Program,
Radboud University Medical Center, Nijmegen, The Netherlands
e-mail: angela.maas@radboudumc.nl

C. N. Bairey Merz, M.D.
Director Barbra Streisand Women's Heart Center, Linda Joy Pollin Women's Heart Health Program, Director Preventive Cardiac Center, Cedars-Sinai, Los Angeles, USA
e-mail: noel.baireymerz@cshs.org

A.H.E.M. Maas, C.N. Bairey Merz (eds.), *Manual of Gynecardiology*,
DOI 10.1007/978-3-319-54960-6_1

threats to our health, already starting at young age. The proportion of total deaths attributable to CVD in Europe is greater for women (51%) than for men (42%) [5]. The majority of first manifestations of CVD events nowadays are different from the endpoints acute coronary syndromes (ACS) and stroke that are mostly used in observational studies and randomized trials [6]. Heart failure (HF), transient ischemic attack (TIA), stable angina, atrial flutter/fibrillation and peripheral arterial disease (PAD) are now the most common first manifestations of CVD [7]. In men below 60 years of age an ACS occurs 3–4 times more often than in women, while the earliest clinical signs of CVD in similar aged females are dominated by TIA's [6, 8]. At older age, HF and strokes are the most common expressions of CVD in both men and women. These sex-related differences in clinical manifestations of CVD should be leading in determining optimal individual prevention strategies for both men and women within every age category. This is even more crucial for younger women because the absolute 10 years risk assessment for fatal CVD events under-estimates their overall cardiovascular risk [9]. The later onset of ischemic heart disease (IHD) in women compared to men is often attributed to sex-differences in hormonal status during the fertile period of life [10], although observational data and estrogen trials do not support this [11, 12]. This leads to the persistent erroneous assumption among cardiologists and other health care providers that women are 'protected' against CVD [13, 14]. In combination with the low awareness in women themselves, they still remain undervalued and undertreated in primary and secondary prevention [4, 15–17]. Even when having had a premature ACS, both women and their doctors keep on underestimating their actual risk [4, 18]. In this chapter we will focus on the traditional and non-traditional female-specific risk factors in women and provide useful tools to better identify women at increased risk for premature CVD.

Women and Lifestyle Factors

In the EUROASPIRE I-IV studies an important increase was shown in the prevalence of obesity and diabetes in women, next to a rise and subsequent stagnation in the number of young female smokers [19, 20]. Smoking has a particularly harmful effect at younger age with a 60% increased risk for IHD in women when compared to men [21]. The higher relative risk for an ACS in young females smokers (<55) dilutes at older age when the classical traditional CVD risk factors predominate. Smoking induces (premature) atherosclerosis through endothelial dysfunction, inflammation and LDL-cholesterol oxidation, with a shift towards a higher pro-coagulant state in the circulation [22]. This explains the lack of obstructive CAD in young female smokers when having an ACS. They often have their menopause about 2 years earlier than non-smokers and this importantly contributes to premature manifestations of IHD [23–25]. Current smoking is also one of the key modifiable risk factors in women for other types of CVD, such as PAD, aortic diseases and strokes [26–30]. Passive (second hand) smoking is also more harmful for women than men, increasing the risk for an ACS by 40%, when having lived with a smoker for more than 30 years [31].

Table 1.1 Risk factor goals and target levels for important cardiovascular risk factors

Smoking	No exposure to tobacco in any form
Diet	Low in saturated fat with a focus on wholegrain products, vegetables, fruit and fish
Physical activity	At least 150 min/week moderate aerobic PA (30 min for 5 days/week) or 75 min/week of vigorous aerobic PA (15 min for 5 days/week) or a combination thereof.
Body weight	BMI 20–25 kg/m^2, waist circumference <94 cm (men) or <80 cm (women)
Blood pressure	<140/90 mmHg (lower in most patients with DM, younger age groups and in very high risk patients)
Lipids primary targets LDL-C HDL-C Triglycerides	**Very high risk:** < 1.8 mmol/L (<70 mg/dL) **High risk:** < 2.6 mmol/L (<100 mg/dL) **Low to moderate risk:** < 3.0 mmol/L (<115/mg/dL) No target, but >1.0 mmol/L (>40 mg/dL) in men and >1.2 mmol/L (>45 mg/dL) in women No target, but <1.7 mmol/L (<150 mg/dL) indicates lower risk and higher levels indicate a need to look for other RF.
Diabetes	HbA1c <7% (<53 mmol/mol)

Adapted from: Piepoli MF et al. 2016 European guidelines on cardiovascular disease prevention in clinical practice [42]

In large population-based studies overweight and obesity in adolescence have shown to be strong predictors of CVD mortality in adulthood [32]. The percentage of obese women across the US and Europe equals that in men, whereas its impact on the development of CVD is greater in women [33–35]. This is expected to worsen even more among the expanding ethnic heterogeneous populations within Europe. Central obesity often leads to the metabolic syndrome (MetS) which has a higher relative risk for insulin resistance, dyslipidemia and hypertension in women than in men [36]. Physical inactivity and sedentary lifestyle habits are also directly related to an increased CVD risk in postmenopausal women [37]. Active lifestyle counseling, culturally sensitive to education level and socio-economic status (SES) are needed to impact adverse lifestyle habits, for which women and especially immigrants are in disadvantage [38].

There are currently several US/ESC guidelines for healthy life-style advise in general and for women in particular [17, 39–41]. In Table 1.1 most important life-style advise and risk factor goals from the latest 2016 updated ESC guidelines CVD prevention are summarized [42].

Genetic Predisposition: Strong Risk Factor for Premature CVD in Women

Systematic collection of family history of premature CVD death (<60 years) to routine cardiovascular risk assessment is an important additive tool in improving risk estimation [43–45]. Coronary artery calcium (CAC) scores are higher in families with premature CAD and especially in women [46, 47]. In patients with premature ACS, a positive family history has been shown to be associated with greater severity of CAD at angiography [48]. The risk increases with younger age of events/death and the number of affected first relative(s) [44, 49, 50]. It is therefore important to assess family history more detailed than only in a binary yes or no. Several studies have shown that a positive family risk is an even stronger risk factor for women than for men [47, 51]. Also, women with repeated pregnancy losses and hypertensive pregnancy disorders more often have an increased family risk for CVD compared to women after normal pregnancies [52–55]. Patient A, with premature symptomatic hypertension illustrates the importance of a positive family risk and a previously complicated obstetric history.

Patient A : Woman 51 years, second opinion

Medical history:
4× miscarriage
Menopause 45 years
Hypothyroidism since 5 years
Total cholesterol 5.7 mmol/l, LDL-C 3.2 mmol/L, TG 1.8 mmol/l

Patient history:
Since 2 years she has symptoms of tiredness, dizzyness and recurrent chest pain.
This occurs during cycling, climbing of the stairs and vacuuming, but also for hours at rest.
She has lost her energy and has severe symptoms of sweating. Often heart pounding at night, fluid retention in her ankles and nycturia 4×. She stopped smoking 6 years ago.
Family risk: P CABG at 55 years, having hypertension, M previous VTE, S HELLP syndrome, Fr hypertension.

Physical exam:
BMI 26 kg/m$_2$, RR 170/10$_3$ mmHg and 160/100 mmHg. Soft systolic ejection murmur, normal pulmonary sounds. No peripheral edema.

ECG at rest : SR 75/min, ST-T segment abnormalities inferior and anterolateral.
Abnormal.

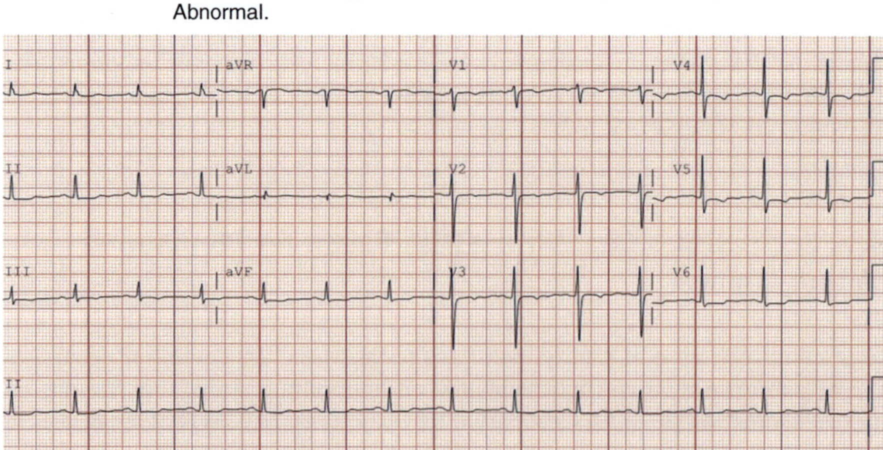

CAG was performed elsewhere after a submaximal, non-conclusive X-test

CAG: normal, also no signs of non-obstructive coronary artery disease (NOCAD).

Discussion:
It was first concluded elsewhere that she may have exercise-induced astma, but she had no relief from her symptoms with bronchodilators.
After adequate treatment for her family-related hypertension however, with a combination of an angiotensin-II antagonist and low dose b-blocker, her symptoms disappeared and she gradually regained her energy.

Conclusion: young woman at elevated family risk with recurrent symptoms due to shear stress/endothelial dysfunction caused by premature hypertension

Gender-Shift in Prevalence of Traditional Risk Factors During Life-Course

At younger age men have a more adverse CVD risk profile, while after 65 years of age women have relatively more clustering of risk factors [16, 41, 56]. There is apparently an important gender-shift in CVD risk between 45 and 65 years of age when women have their menopause transition. It is therefore crucial not only to consider risk factors in relation to sex, gender and ethnicity, but also to the phase in life of the individual patient. Moreover, different interactions exist between women and men among the various CVD risk factors during our lifecycle [57]. This is not taken into account in the large number of prediction models that are currently available [58] . The 2013 ACC/AHA prevention guidelines atherosclerotic cardiovascular disease (ASCVD) now use the contemporary risk algorithm for improved prediction in an increasingly ethnically heterogeneous population [59]. In women, many traditional risk factors (dyslipidemia, hypertension, insulin resistance) change in an adverse direction between 50 and 60 years of age, making it necessary to reconsider these factors when they are in their late fifties/early sixties. Table 1.2 illustrates important gender differences in weighting of traditional risk factors during middle-age.

Table 1.2 Sex differences related to traditional CVD risk factors

Risk factor	Women	Men
Age-threshold increased CVD risk	≥55 years	≥45 years
Family risk premature CVD	First degree <65 years	First degree <55 years
Smoking	2× elevated RR ACS < 55 years	Most important RF < 50 years
Total Cholesterol	10% increase after menopause	Stable after 50 years
HDL-cholesterol	≥1,2 mmol/L	≥1.0 mmol/L
LDL-cholesterol	14% higher after menopause	No change after 50 years
Diabetes mellitus	1.5–2.0× higher RR mortality risk than in men Independent RF for HFpEF	CVD mortality <lower than in women

ACS acute coronary syndromes, *CVD* cardiovascular disease, *RF* risk factor, *RR* relative risk, *HFpEF* heart failure with preserved ejection fraction
References: Verschuren [67]; Prescott [21]; Dallongeville [19]; Huxley 2006

Cardiovascular Risk Age and 'lifetime' Risk for Cardiovascular Disease

Young women (<55 years) at increased risk for CVD have a low absolute risk for a relatively short-term cardiovascular event in risk charts such as the SCORE, which is commonly used in Europe. This may lead to serious undertreatment of lifetime risk and irreversible longterm cardiovascular damage. In 2007 a relative risk chart has been developed to compare the actual risk with the 'ideal' risk of that age, e.g. higher relative risk (RR) in young female smokers than in non-smokers [60]. This has been changed into the more appropriate 'cardiovascular risk age' in the 2012 and 2016 updated version of the ESC CVD prevention guidelines [41, 42]. The *risk age* of a person with several cardiovascular risk factors is the age of a person with the same level of risk but with 'ideal levels' of risk factors. Thus, a high-risk 40 year old woman, such as a heavy smoker, may have a risk age of ≥60 years. This illustrates the likely reduction in life expectancy for a young person with a low absolute but high RR of CVD if preventive measures are not adopted. Risk age is automatically calculated in the latest revision of HeartScore (www.HeartScore.org). An important improvement of the 2016 ESC SCORE charts is a better recognition of disease risk in younger age-groups, in women and in diabetics [42].

For women it may also be important to focus on 30-years 'lifetime' risk of all manifestations of CVD and not solely on 10 years risk of IHD [60, 61]. At older age, the risk of strokes and heart failure is higher than for ACS. Adding signs of subclinical atherosclerosis by using the CAC score to risk factor assessment, significantly improves risk prediction, which is especially important for younger women [42, 62–65]. In the UK National Institute for Health and Care Excellence (UK–NICE) guidelines measurement of the CAC score in intermediate risk patients has now been added to the guidelines in patients with symptoms of angina [66].

Dyslipidemia and Statin Use in Women

Low HDL- cholesterol is a stronger CVD risk factor in women than men, with values that remain stable or decline somewhat during menopause transition [67]. In contrast, between 45 and 60 years of age, total cholesterol and LDL cholesterol levels rise about 10–14% in women, while there is no significant change in men [68–70]. Figure 1.1 outlines the change in total cholesterol levels (male/female) with ageing derived from a Dutch population-based cohort [67]. In Fig. 1.2 pre-and postmenopausal lipid values are depicted. While the beneficial effects of secondary prevention with statins in women are beyond any doubt [71], their efficacy in primary prevention is controversial [72–75]. This is caused by an under-representation of women in clinical trials, a lack of sex-specific analyses and a too young age at inclusion of participating women. In the MEGA-study it

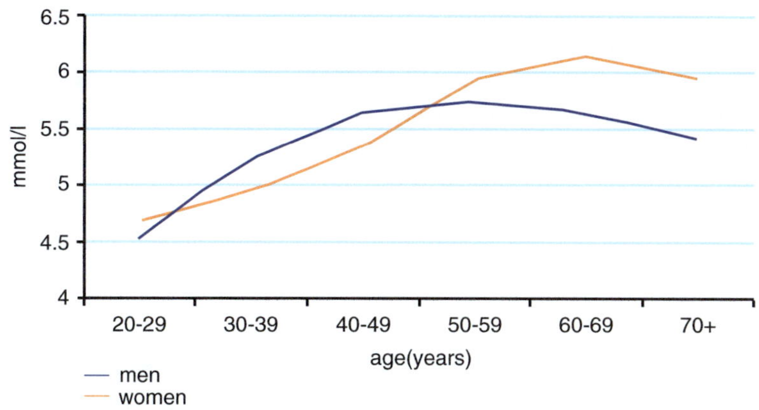

Fig. 1.1 Age/gender related changes in total cholesterol levels. Doetinchem-cohort and REGENBOOG-project [67]

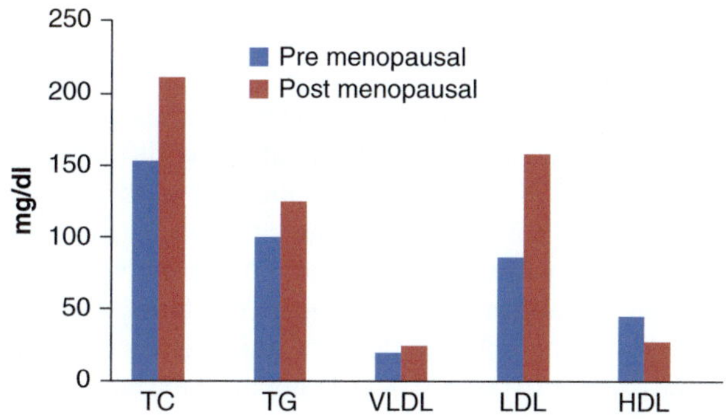

Fig. 1.2 Lipidprofile in pre- and postmenopausal women. Source: Reddy KS et al. 2013 [69]

was shown in 5300 women that primary prevention with a statin for mild hypercholesterolemia (Total cholesterol 5,7–7,0 mmol/L) is useful upward of 55–60 years of age, when CVD risk increases and more combined risk factors are present [76]. This has also been an important consideration in the JUPITER-trial, which included 11.001 men ≥50 years and 6801 women ≥60 years at intermediate CVD risk [71, 77]. In a recent meta-analysis of the Cholesterol Treatment Trialists' (CTT) Collaboration database, no difference was found in the effectiveness of statins in men and women at an equivalent risk of CVD [78]. This is in agreement with the current ESC guidelines CVD prevention, which are less strict than the 2013 ACC/AHA guidelines for the prevention of dyslipidemias [41, 79–81]. According to the UK-NICE guidelines, the majority of men over 50 years and more than half of all women over 60 years, having a 10% CVD risk over 10 years, will qualify for statin use in primary prevention [82].

Reported side-effects of statins vary among populations, ranging from 5 to 25%, and mainly consist of muscle symptoms such as myopathy, myalgia and weakness

[83–85]. Discontinuation of medication occurs more often in real life than in clinical trials [86]. The majority of patients report statin-associated muscle-related adverse effects within the first 3 months of initiating therapy [87] . Women report more adverse symptoms than men, which is a serious reason for their lower adherence to therapy [88–91]. It may be difficult however to ascertain whether symptoms of muscle pain are indeed related to statin use or to other causes [92]. Fatigue, fibromyalgia and arthrosis-related (inflammatory) symptoms are quite common in middle-aged women [93, 94]. A contributing mechanism to explain the increased susceptibility for side effects of statins in women is their interaction with CYP3A4 inhibitors [95]. Besides, other causative factors for myopathy are related to certain genetic variants and an interaction with mitochondrial function [96–98]. The negative publicity in the lay press has led to the biased expectation that statin use is harmful [99]. Early statin discontinuation in patients with an appropriate indication for it use increases the risk of ACS and cardiac death [85, 100]. Therefore, healthcare providers should re-challenge more often with other statins whenever possible, or perhaps start with a lower dose, while putting the side-effects on muscle into perspective by appropriate counseling and shared decision making [101, 102]. According to the advice of the European Atherosclerosis Society (EAS) intake on alternating days or twice a week may also be a pragmatic option [103]. Noteworthy is that the attitude towards chronic medication use and preferences for complementary and alternative medicines may be different among both genders [104]. Although PCSK9 inhibitors (monoclonal antibodies) are very effective in reducing LDL-cholesterol in statin-intolerant patients, its (expensive) use is at first being restricted to patients with primary hypercholesterolemia or mixed dyslipidemias who are not adequately controlled with statins. Long term efficacy and safety data are not yet available and the cost-effectiveness of these new agents in patients with heterozygous FH or ASCVD do not meet the currently generally acceptable criteria [105, 106].

Treatment of Hypertension in Women

Blood pressure levels show important gender differences during lifetime and the long-term consequences of hypertension for the development of atrial fibrillation, left ventricular hypertrophy and heart failure with preserved ejection fraction (HFpEF), which are worse for women than for men [107]. Hypertensive women develop more vascular and myocardial stiffness than men at old age, and more often have isolated systolic hypertension, reflecting aortic stiffness [108, 109]. The diameter of the aorta increases with age, more in men than women, wherefore gender-specific and age-adjusted normal values are needed [110]. In developed countries 30% of adult individuals have hypertension and this number is even higher in low-middle income countries, reaching up to 53% of all women [111, 112].

For every 20 mmHg SBP and 10 mm Hg DBP increase in BP, there is a doubling of mortality both from IHD and stroke for subjects aged 40–89 years [113]. In the EUROASPIRE III study women were less well treated for their hypertension than men and considering the results of EUROASPIRE IV, which again demonstrated that blood pressure is often not optimally controlled, there is still room for improvement [19, 20]. Although younger women are at lower absolute cardiovascular risk than elderly women, this should not impede the detection and effective management of hypertension within each age category. After the results of the Systolic Blood Pressure Intervention Trial (SPRINT) –trial it is expected that treatment goals for hypertension will become more strict and age-dependent [114, 115]. Many symptoms may accompany elevated blood pressure, such as headaches, palpitations, tiredness and chest pain, for which physicians should be alert (see patient A and Chap. 5).

Diabetes Mellitus: Mind the Consequences in Women

With the rise in the number of low physical activity and overweight/obese individuals, the prevalence of type II diabetes (T2DM) is increasing. Treatment of T2DM in women used to be less optimal than in men, but disparities in care are getting smaller [19, 116–118]. After adjustment for their higher clustering of risk factors, women with T2DM still have a twofold increased CVD risk than men [119–122]. They also have more signs of inflammation and more unfavorable changes in coagulation and endothelial function leading to a greater cardiometabolic risk factor load [123, 124]. In addition, the pattern of IHD and the occurrence of vascular and myocardial stiffening with ageing also shows important gender differences that affect outcomes negatively [125]. Diabetic women have a more diffuse and non-obstructive pattern of coronary artery disease (NOCAD) than men, with higher rates of coronary microvascular dysfunction (CMD) which is more difficult to diagnose and to treat than focal obstructive CAD in the epicardial coronary arteries. Hypertension and T2DM are strongly and inversely related risk factors for CVD in postmenopausal women [126]. Moreover, T2DM is an independent risk factor for the development of HFpEF in women, which often remains unrecognized in clinical practice [127, 128]. An echocardiography study in patients with T2DM over 60 years of age showed that 28% of women and 18% of men had previously unknown signs of HFpEF [128]. Both type I and type II diabetes promote inflammation which affects both genders differently and also show differences among pre- and postmenopausal women [129–133]. Adverse outcomes of pregnancy are associated with both types of diabetes and there is evidence to suggest that women with diabetes undergo earlier menopause than women without diabetes [134, 135]. The 2013 ESC guidelines on diabetes, pre-diabetes and CVD extensively describe very relevant aspects of this subject, but are importantly lacking a gender-specific viewpoint [136]. Longterm follow-up data from the Rancho Bernardo study showed that women with diabetes and angina had a three-to four-fold greater risk of dying from CHD than women who had diabetes without angina, independent of covariates [137, 138]. There were no independent associations found in men. In 2015 the AHA has released a scientific statement on the current knowledge of gender differences in the ASCVD consequences of diabetes, with a stronger relative mortality risk in women than in men [139]. This also concerns stroke and PAD [138, 139]. There is growing evidence that the MetS and diabetes are also associated with an increased prevalence of breast cancer in women with more adverse outcomes [140, 141].

In asymptomatic patients (male/female) with T2DM a high coronary artery calcium score (CAC) has been shown to be an important predictor of adverse CVD events [142]. As women with T2DM often have a diffuse pattern of CAD with concomitant coronary vascular dysfunction and HFpEF in the elderly, symptom recognition of IHD can be difficult. Patient B is an example of a high risk T2DM female patient (family, gestational diabetes, early menopause, premature hypertension) with recurrent angina symptoms which were poorly recognized as being related to CMD.

Patient B: Second opnion, woman 58 years

Medical history:
- astma since youth
- 2× GDM (insuline dependent)
- menopause at 42 years
- hypertension 45 years
- T2DM (diet)
- recurrent diverticulitis
- cholecystectomy at 55 years
- CAG 2 and 4 years ago: no abnormalities

Patient history:

Since 1 year she has recurrent symptoms of chest pain with radiation to the jaws, left arm and shoulders. These symptoms can be induced by exercise, but also often occur at rest and in the early morning in bed. Relief by nitroglycerine sublingual most of the time, but not always. She has lost condition, has more dyspnea at exertion than before. She has T2DM (diet) since several years. She cannot lose any weight. Stopped smoking 35 years ago. Intolerance for B-blockers.

Family risk: P at 50 years 2× PCI, M hypertension, a stroke and T2DM at older age.

Med: Acetylsalicylic acid 38 mg, pantoprazol 40 mg, irbesartan/HCT 300/12.5 mg, simvastatin 40 mg

Physical examination: BMI 33.8 kg/m$_2$,
RR 140/87 mmHg, 165/100 mmHg, auscultation normal

ECHO: normal, EF 61 %, no signs of LVH, or diastolic dysfunction

Discussion: diagnosis (per exclusionem) coronary microvascular dysfunction (CMD) and hypertension in woman with T2DM and elevated CVD risk.
Advise to add diltiazem 2dd 120 mg to her medication.
Blood pressure normalizes with a reduction of anginal symptoms and improvement of her physical condition. She still has stable symptoms of chest pain from time to time.

Several studies have compared the effectiveness of PCI versus coronary artery bypass surgery (CABG) in patients with T2DM and multi-vessel CAD [143–146]. In all studies it was found that CABG provides better longterm outcomes in male *and female* diabetic patients. Although women with diabetes are less likely to be referred for CABG, this is a class I therapeutic recommendation in diabetic patients (male/female) with stable IHD [147].

Female-Specific Risk Factors: Tools to Identify Young Women at Higher Risk

Sex-specific factors related to hormonal and reproductive status are known to relate to CVD risk. It is unclear yet, to which extent and within which stage(s) of life these female-specific risk factors are relevant to CVD risk estimation in women. When considering all age-groups together, reproductive and pregnancy related disorders do not seem to be relevant in 10 years risk estimation [148, 149]. However, when focusing on younger patients (<55 years) evidence is increasing that assessment of female-specific risk factors may indeed add to identify women at higher risk [51, 150, 151]. This is especially important as young women are considered to be at low risk, until a first premature event has occurred. Reproductive and pregnancy-related factors may predispose to earlier signs of endothelial dysfunction, vascular inflammation and atherosclerosis [152–154] . This is less relevant for the older female population, having a higher prevalence of traditional risk factors with more advanced and more easily detectable atherosclerosis. It is to be expected that a combination of genetic risk together with (several) female-specific reproductive and non-traditional risk factors related to inflammatory diseases are more predictive in identifying women at high risk for premature CVD, than one or two single factors alone [150]. In Fig. 1.3 several female-specific risk variables and non-traditional risk factors to identify potentially high risk women are depicted, see also the patient cases in this chapter. The justified weighting of these various risk variables remains to be further investigated.

Age at Menarche

Over the past decades there has been a shift in age at menarche (first menstrual period) from ≥12 years towards younger ages. Early age at menarche (8–12 years) has been associated with increased body mass index (BMI), higher risk of MetS, T2DM and more CVD risk factors in adolescent girls and in young women studied up to age 40 year [155–159]. The association of age at menarche and CVD risk is only partly mediated by adiposity [160]. In a recent large study a more U-shaped association was found between age of menarche and IHD [161]. As late menopause is protective for CVD, the timing of estrogen exposure in the reproductive years

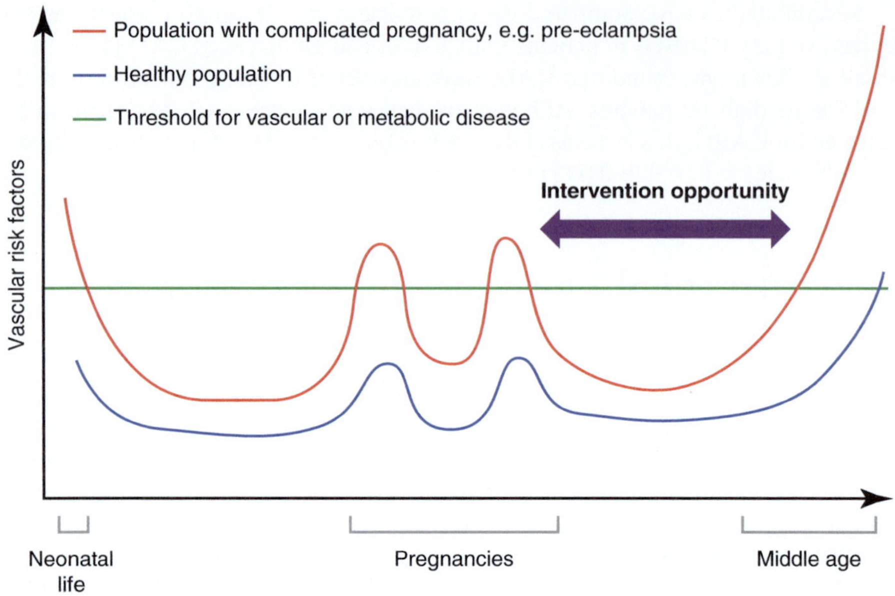

Fig. 1.3 Vascular damage after hypertensive pregnancy disorders. Adapted from Sattar & Greer 2002 [192]

may be more important than the total number of years of estrogen exposure [162]. In more than fifty percent of women the onset of menarche is caused by a combination of environmental and genetic factors of which more than 30 genetic loci have been identified [163–165]. Sufficient data are currently lacking to determine the value of age at menopause in individual risk prediction.

Polycystic Ovary Syndrome (PCOS)

Polycystic ovary syndrome (PCOS) is a complex disorder characterized by oligomenorrhea, amenorrhea, hyperandrogenism, and polycystic appearance of the ovaries [166]. It is the most common hormonal imbalance among females of reproductive age, affecting up to 10–13% of women [167]. Ovulatory dysfunction in women with PCOS is associated with low grade inflammation and an increased cardiometabolic risk [168]. This promotes endothelial dysfunction, independent of obesity, age and other risk factors [169]. Women with PCOS are at substantially increased risk of developing T2DM [124, 170]. The risk for hypertension and dyslipidemia is also moderately increased compared to women without PCOS. Long term data on CVD outcomes are relatively scarce and cardiovascular and metabolic risk profiles are hampered by the heterogeneity of PCOS phenotypes [171–173]. It is controversial that PCOS women with excess androgen production are at high future CVD risk

[174]. Several studies have shown that women with PCOS are at 22% to a twofold increased risk to develop GDM in pregnancy [175, 176]. The Dutch guideline cardiovascular risk management after reproductive and pregnancy-related disorders therefore recommends that women with PCOS should be screened for gestational diabetes (GDM) during pregnancy [177]. When evaluating female patients for their CVD risk it is important to ask about irregular menses and if needed to screen for PCOS by a gynecologist [172]. Women with PCOS should be encouraged to optimize modifiable cardiovascular risk factors such as obesity to reduce their future CVD risk.

Gestational Diabetes (GDM)

Gestational diabetes mellitus (GDM) occurs in 2–10% of pregnancies and confers a 4- to 7-fold higher risk of future type II and the development of the MetS in midlife [178, 179]. Several studies have reported a 66–85% higher risk of CAD, myocardial infarction, and stroke after previous GDM [180]. Women with GDM also have a 1.5 times greater likelihood to develop hypertensive pregnancy disorders (HDP) compared to women without GDM [181]. It is recommended that women with prior GDM receive education about lifestyle modification and regular (yearly) testing for glucose intolerance, since these women are at high risk to develop T2DM [182–184].

Premature Ovarian Insufficiency and Menopause: See Chap. 5

Repeated Miscarriages and Hypertensive Pregnancy Disorders: "stress-test" in Women

In multiple large population-based studies is has been shown that recurrent (≥2) miscarriages convey an increased risk for IHD and other types of CVD [53, 55, 185, 186]. These also occur more often in women having an increased family risk for ASCVD [55]. Spontaneous preterm delivery is also an independent risk factor for the development of IHD, stroke and overall CVD [187]. In high-income countries hypertensive pregnancy disorders (HPD) affect 10% of all pregnancies and account for the majority (16%) of maternal deaths. These are most frequently present in first pregnancies, with a high recurrence rate in subsequent pregnancies. There are several manifestations of HPD, according of the timing and severity of the blood pressure disorders during pregnancy (pregnancy-induced hypertension, early-onset preeclampsia or late-onset preeclampsia) [188]. An uncertain percentage of women has preexisting premature hypertension before conception. Preeclampsia, especially when occurring early in pregnancy, is the severest manifestation of HPD and may degenerate into the Hemolysis Elevated Liver enzymes and Low Platelets (HELLP) syndrome with severe metabolic, vascular and thrombotic complications in the mother [52, 189]. This often results in fetal growth retardation and intrauterine death of the fetus. A low birth weight is an important and reliable indication for the severity of the preeclampsia, which most women are able to recall later in life and thus may be a helpful tool in clinical practice. Worldwide, preeclampsia occurs in 3–5% of pregnancies, defined as de novo blood pressure elevation ≥140/90 mmHg with proteinuria ≥0.3 g/24 h after the 20th week of gestation [190]. In normal pregnancy several components of the metabolic syndrome are temporarily elevated, such as insulin resistance, lipid levels, and coagulation and inflammatory factors. It is hypothesized that normal pregnancy itself stimulates an inflammatory response, which is exaggerated in preeclampsia, and involves dysfunction of the endothelium in the uterine circulation (Fig. 1.3) [191, 192] . The ultimate source of the inflammatory stimulus is presumably the placenta itself. Uteroplacental arterial insufficiency may cause the release of inflammatory stimuli (cytokines) into the maternal circulation, leading to vasoconstriction and activation of the coagulation system. Women after HPD are at increased risk for future CVD, which is strongly related to the timing and severity of the hypertensive disturbances [193–198]. The cardiovascular risk profile after pregnancy importantly reflects the risk of hypertension and CVD later in life [199]. Around 43% of women after early preeclampsia already have hypertension before the age of 40, which is on average 7.7 years earlier than in women with previous uncomplicated pregnancies [54, 184]. In more than 75% of affected women a positive family history for CVD is reported. More arterial stiffness and a higher prevalence of cerebral white matter lesions are also found in women after preeclampsia compared to women after normotensive pregnancies [200–202]. Women after HPD have signs of earlier ovarian ageing as an indication of impaired vascular health [203].

During normal pregnancy, several metabolic factors are temporarily increased such as insulin resistance, lipid levels, as well as coagulation and inflammatory factors [52, 204]. In women who develop HPD or GDM, this physiological response is disturbed, leading to vascular endothelial dysfunction in both the uterine and maternal circulation [192, 205]. Insufficient placentation may be caused by genetic, immunological, vascular and environmental factors and has many pathophysiological mechanisms in common with the initial process of atherosclerosis [204, 206] . Many circulating biomarkers during HPD remain detectable for many years, even decades afterwards [207–209]. These promote early endothelial dysfunction and premature onset of atherosclerosis in the mother [210].

Clinical Symptoms and Treatment Advise in Women After Preeclampsia

Many young women have a variety of symptoms after preeclampsia, that are often not well recognized, but may result in a reduced quality of life [211]. Previously affected women may even state that 'they never have recovered to normal' after their pregnancy (Patient C). Persistent symptoms of fatigue, concentration disturbances and impaired mental well-being may contribute to lower social functioning [212, 213]. In others premature (subclinical) manifestations of CVD may occur within several years after index pregnancy (Patient D). Early preeclampsia is associated with slightly higher levels of depressive symptoms and fatigue on average 14 years after index pregnancy compared to previously unaffected women, but its clinical relevance is not clear yet [214]. It has also been found that during menopause transition women after HPD have an enhanced sympathetic nervous activity which may be associated with more disabling vasomotor symptoms [215]. These preliminary findings will need more attention in future research

Patient C: woman 42 years, persistent symptoms after HELLP

Medical history:

At age 28 years HELLP syndrome, gemelli (1700 and 2200 g, born 33 week by section)

Family risk: hypertension in several first degree relatives

Patient history: In the years following her only, but seriously complicated pregnancy, patient has the feeling that she has "never returned to normal". In stressful sitiations she first had attacks of "near fainting" for several years. She visited a neurologist who could not find anything wrong. After 5 years she returned to het work as a TV producer. Since two years she has symptoms of recurrent headaches, pain between her shoulders, concentration disturbances and a bad condition. She stayed at home for 10 months with a diagnosis of "burn-out".
She is unable to do sports and has chest pain while climbing the stairs.
Recently her blood pressure was 160 mmHg systolic, but this was attributed to stress related to her health problems and a recent divorce.
After her complicated pregnancy in the past she never had regular checks of her blood pressure.
She has never smoked, with a normal weight. Premenopausal state with regular menses. No medication.

Physical exam: length 1.78 m, weight 65 kg, RR 133/80 mmHg, 150/90 mmHg and 145/90 mmHg, auscultation normal.

ECG: sinusrythm 59/min, intermediate axis, normal.

LAB: total cholesterol 5.6 mmol/l, triglyceriden 1.02, HDL 1.63, LDL 3.5 mmol/l.

Discussion: her symptoms can be attributed to premature hypertension, which induces endothelial dysfunction and oxidative stress. She was treated with a combination of a low dose angiotensin-II antagonist in combination with a low dose b-blocker. After a stress-reducing program she is doing well since several years and she enjoys a new relation.

Patient D. Woman 41 years, premature coronary artery disease

Medical history:

migraine since her teens

Hypertension from age 20

3× miscarriage, afterwards 3× hypertensive pregnancies

2015 (last year) : CAC score 237, NOCAD on CTA

Family risk: positive ++. P ACS at 45, M young stroke, hypertension and high family risk.

Patient history:

In the evenings patient often has a nagging pain in her left arm and a feeling of extreme tiredness. This is why she has stopped with regular running.
Symptoms may change from day to day and from week to week.
There is some improvement since medication for her elevated blood pressure was started. With warm weather she often has fluid retention in her ankles.
Menses irregular with IUD. She has smoked between 18 and 26 years.

Physical exam

BMI 20.3 kg/m$_2$, RR 131/85 mmHg, later 160/100 mmHg, auscultation normal.

Lab: T chol 3.7, TG 1.06, HDL 1.7, LDL 1.5 mmol/l (without statin)

ECG: within normal range

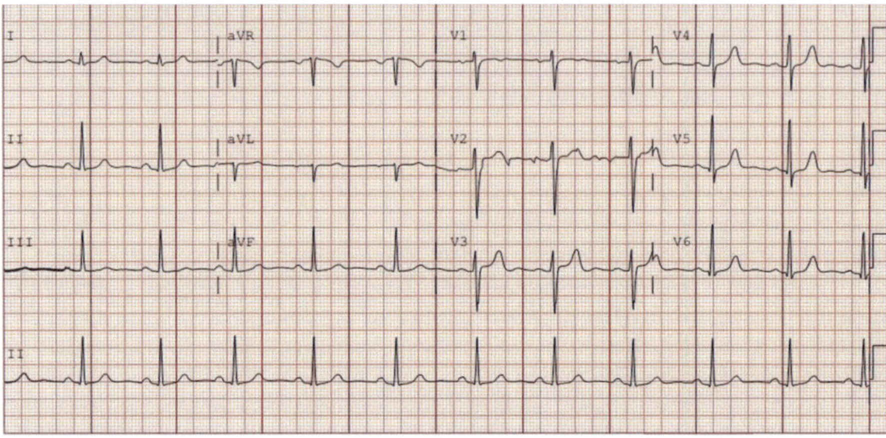

Comments:

Patient at elevated risk for CVD and a high CAC score at young age. No signs of obstructive CAD. There is a typical **'red thread'** (family risk, migraine, miscarriages, hypertensive pregnancies) in her medical history for having premature atherosclerosis. It is therefore crucial to treat her bloodpressure to an optimal level of < 120/80 mmHg at her young age . After initiating an angiotensin-II antagonist her bloodpressure normalized, she regained her energy and was able to restart her running activities.

Thus far, longterm follow-up intervention studies to prevent CVD after high risk pregnancies are lacking. Preeclampsia has now been adopted as a female-specific risk factor in several guidelines, such as the 2011 AHA prevention guideline in women, the 2014 AHA stroke prevention guideline, the 2016 Dutch guideline cardiovascular risk management after reproductive and pregnancy-related disorders, and the 2016 ESC guidelines CVD prevention [40, 42, 182, 187]. First measure after index pregnancy is adherence to a healthy diet- and lifestyle onwards. It remains to be investigated whether early and strict lowering of blood pressure and cholesterol (if appropriate) may prevent the early occurrence of CVD in these potential high risk women [216].

Non-traditional Risk Factors in Women: Co-morbidity with Inflammatory Disorders

An increased CVD mortality risk has been found in patients with rheumatic and endocrine disorders such as rheumatic arthritis (RA), systemic lupus erythematosus (SLE), antiphospholipid syndrome (APS) and thyroid disorders which are more prevalent in women than in men [217–219]. Chronic systemic inflammation itself can be considered as an independent CVD risk factor, but patients with these disorders also have a higher clustering of traditional risk factors which may increase their susceptibility for premature CVD [220]. There are important sex-related differences in immune reactivity, with a relatively increase in women during/after menopause transition [129]. Coronary microvascular dysfunction (CMD) may be the key mechanism involved in accelerated atherosclerosis in chronic inflammatory diseases [221, 222]. Of interest is that women with lichen sclerosis (LS) also have a higher susceptibility for autoimmune disorders such as alopecia areata, vitiligo, thyroid disease and pernicious anemia [223]. Women with CMD regularly report to have concomitant LS, which should be further explored. The main cause of CVD deaths in RA patients is ischemic heart disease (IHD), with a higher ACS related mortality risk compared to the general population [224–227]. The presence of rheumatologic disorders is independently associated with worse outcomes after PCI [228]. It remains to be investigated whether frequently used anti-inflammatory biological agents may also have beneficial anti-atherogenic effects.

Migraine

Until recently, only migraine with aura has been found to be associated with an increased CVD risk in women [229, 230]. In a 20-years follow-up study among participants of the Nurses' Health study however, a consistent increased risk (HR 1.50, CI 1.33–1.69) for cardiac and cerebral manifestations of CVD was found [231]. More than 15% of women had (previous) migraine, which occurs 3–4 times more often in women than in men. Migraine is related to an increased family risk for CVD, premature vascular dysfunction, a higher susceptibility for thrombosis and inflammation (Fig. 1.4) [232, 233]. Several studies have also demonstrated significant associations between migraine and celiac disease, inflammatory bowel disease, and irritable bowel syndrome (IBS) [234]. The case of patient E illustrates the complex co-morbidity of migraine, T1DM, inflammatory diseases and premature CVD.

Patient E. Woman 55 years with T1DM, autoimmune disorders and premature CAD

Medical history:

- at 15 years : Diabetes mellitus Type I
- recurrent migraine in het teens
- at 22 years: colitis ulcerosa.
- reumatic disease with muscle dystrofia both legs
- hypothyroidism
- at 48 years hypertension with LVH
- at 50 years: CABG LIMA-LAD and venous graft AL-MO-PL-RDP.
- afterwards hemolytic anemia, cold agglutines and antigen Diego.
- at 52 years : removal sternum stiches (hypersensitivity)

Discussion:

Over the past years patients has variable periods of severe tiredness with dyspnea and chest pain at exertion. Her symptoms worsen when her chronic bowel disease flares up or when her diabetes is poorly regulated. At other times she feels fairly well and is able to perform light to moderate daily activities. Her wellbeing in general strongly depends on the status of her combined illnesses.

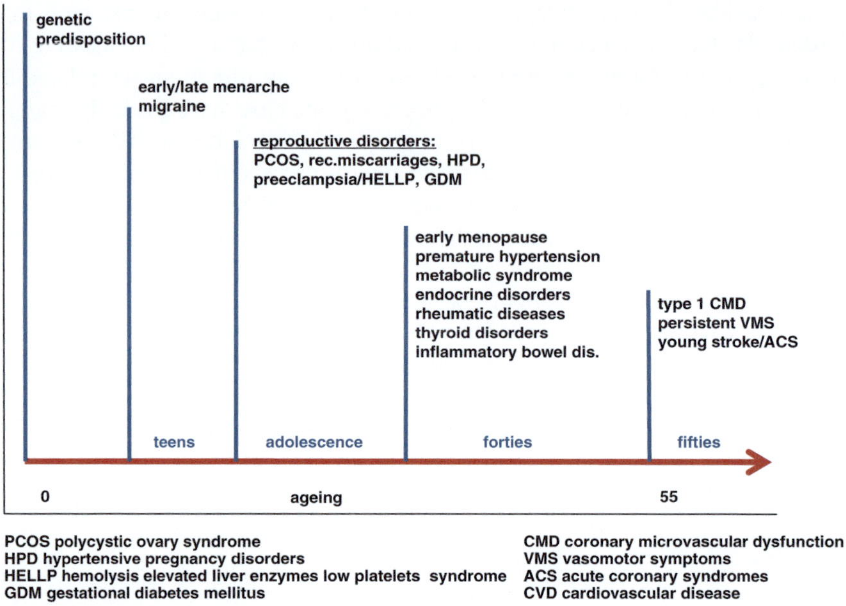

Fig. 1.4 Female-specific and non-traditional risk factors: Risk variables for early endothelial dysfunction/premature CVD. *PCOS* polycystic ovary syndrome, *HPD* hypertensive pregnancy disorders, *HELLP* hemolysis elevated liver enzymes low platelets syndrome, *GDM* gestational diabetes mellitus, *CMD* coronary microvascular dysfunction, *VMS* vasomotor symptoms, *ACS* acute coronary syndromes, *CVD* cardiovascular disease

Know and Manage Your Numbers!

Women with an elevated family risk for CVD should be aware of their CVD risk factors and aim to a healthy lifestyle from early years on. Self-management of blood pressure with modern eHealth applications is less time-consuming than regular office visits and actively involves patients as partners. This may also increase motivation for lifestyle and medication adherence [235]. Recent studies have shown that self monitoring of blood pressure improves treatment outcomes with lower costs compared to office-based therapy [236, 237].

Key Issues

- Clinical manifestations of CVD appear 7–10 years later in women than men
- Smoking and increased family risk are important risk factors in women with premature CVD
- Premenopausal women have a lower CVD risk than similarly aged men

- At old age women have a higher clustering of CVD risk factors than men
- T2DM has a higher relative CVD mortality risk in women than in men
- Female specific risk variables may be helpful to identify women at increased premature ASCVD risk
- HPD and especially preeclampsia/HELLP are important risk factors in women
- Migraine and (autoimmune) inflammatory and rheumatic disorders promote early endothelial dysfunction and are more prevalent in women than in men

References

1. Roth GA, Nguyen G, Forouzanfar MH, Mokdad AH, Naghavi M, Murray CJ. Estimates of global and regional premature cardiovascular mortality in 2025. Circulation. 2015; 132(13):1270–82.
2. Hulsegge G, Picavet HS, Blokstra A, Nooyens AC, Spijkerman AM, van der Schouw YT, et al. Today's adult generations are less healthy than their predecessors: generation shifts in metabolic risk factors: the Doetinchem Cohort Study. Eur J Prev Cardiol. 2014; 21(9):1134–44.
3. Towfighi A, Zheng L, Ovbiagele B. Sex-specific trends in midlife coronary heart disease risk and prevalence. Arch Intern Med. 2009;169(19):1762–6.
4. Puymirat E, Simon T, Steg PG, Schiele F, Gueret P, Blanchard D, et al. Association of changes in clinical characteristics and management with improvement in survival among patients with ST-elevation myocardial infarction. JAMA. 2012;308(10):998–1006.
5. Nichols M, Townsend N, Scarborough P, Rayner M. Cardiovascular disease in Europe: epidemiological update. Eur Heart J. 2013;34(39):3028–34.
6. George J, Rapsomaniki E, Pujades-Rodriguez M, Shah AD, Denaxas S, Herrett E, et al. How Does Cardiovascular Disease First Present in Women and Men? Incidence of 12 Cardiovascular Diseases in a Contemporary Cohort of 1,937,360 People. Circulation. 2015;132(14):1320–8.
7. George J, Rapsomaniki E, Pujades-Rodriguez M, Shah AD, Denaxas S, Herrett E, et al. How does cardiovascular disease first present in women andmen? Incidence of 12 cardiovascular diseases in a contemporary cohort of1,937,360 people, Circulation. 2015;132:1320–8.
8. Leening MJ, Ferket BS, Steyerberg EW, Kavousi M, Deckers JW, Nieboer D, et al. Sex differences in lifetime risk and first manifestation of cardiovascular disease: prospective population based cohort study. BMJ. 2014;349:g5992.
9. Jorstad HT, Colkesen EB, Boekholdt SM, Tijssen JG, Wareham NJ, Khaw KT, et al. Estimated 10-year cardiovascular mortality seriously underestimates overall cardiovascular risk. Heart. 2016;102(1):63–8.
10. Burke AP, Farb A, Malcom G, Virmani R. Effect of menopause on plaque morphologic characteristics in coronary atherosclerosis. Am Heart J. 2001;141(2 Suppl):S58–62.
11. Gierach GL, Johnson BD, Bairey Merz CN, Kelsey SF, Bittner V, Olson MB, et al. Hypertension, menopause, and coronary artery disease risk in the Women's Ischemia Syndrome Evaluation (WISE) Study. J Am Coll Cardiol. 2006;47(3 Suppl):S50–8.
12. Shufelt CL, Johnson BD, Berga SL, Braunstein GD, Reis SE, Bittner V, et al. Timing of hormone therapy, type of menopause, and coronary disease in women: data from the National Heart, Lung, and Blood Institute-sponsored Women's Ischemia Syndrome Evaluation. Menopause. 2011;18(9):943–50.

13. Merz CN. The Yentl syndrome is alive and well. Eur Heart J. 2011;32(11):1313–5.
14. Mosca L, Merz NB, Blumenthal RS, Cziraky MJ, Fabunmi RP, Sarawate C, et al. Opportunity for intervention to achieve American Heart Association guidelines for optimal lipid levels in high-risk women in a managed care setting. Circulation. 2005;111(4):488–93.
15. Kotseva K, Wood D, De Backer G, De Bacquer D, Pyorala K, Keil U, et al. Cardiovascular prevention guidelines in daily practice: a comparison of EUROASPIRE I, II, and III surveys in eight European countries. Lancet. 2009;373(9667):929–40.
16. EugenMed, Cardiovascular Clinical Study G, Regitz-Zagrosek V, Oertelt-Prigione S, Prescott E, Franconi F, et al. Gender in cardiovascular diseases: impact on clinical manifestations, management, and outcomes. Eur Heart J 2016;37(1):24–34.
17. Mosca L, Linfante AH, Benjamin EJ, Berra K, Hayes SN, Walsh BW, et al. National study of physician awareness and adherence to cardiovascular disease prevention guidelines. Circulation. 2005;111(4):499–510.
18. Leifheit-Limson EC, D'Onofrio G, Daneshvar M, Geda M, Bueno H, Spertus JA, et al. Sex differences in cardiac risk factors, perceived risk, and health care provider discussion of risk and risk modification among young patients with acute myocardial infarction: the VIRGO study. J Am Coll Cardiol. 2015;66(18):1949–57.
19. Dallongeville J, De Bacquer D, Heidrich J, De Backer G, Prugger C, Kotseva K, et al. Gender differences in the implementation of cardiovascular prevention measures after an acute coronary event. Heart. 2010;96(21):1744–9.
20. Kotseva K, De Bacquer D, Jennings C, Gyberg V, De Backer G, Ryden L, et al. Time trends in lifestyle, risk factor control, and use of evidence-based medications in patients with Coronary Heart Disease in Europe: results from 3 EUROASPIRE surveys, 1999-2013. Glob Heart. 2016. (PMID: 26994643).
21. Prescott E, Hippe M, Schnohr P, Hein HO, Vestbo J. Smoking and risk of myocardial infarction in women and men: longitudinal population study. BMJ. 1998;316(7137):1043–7.
22. Messner B, Bernhard D. Smoking and cardiovascular disease: mechanisms of endothelial dysfunction and early atherogenesis. Arterioscler Thromb Vasc Biol. 2014;34(3):509–15.
23. Gold EB, Crawford SL, Avis NE, Crandall CJ, Matthews KA, Waetjen LE, et al. Factors related to age at natural menopause: longitudinal analyses from SWAN. Am J Epidemiol. 2013;178(1):70–83.
24. Hayatbakhsh MR, Clavarino A, Williams GM, Sina M, Najman JM. Cigarette smoking and age of menopause: a large prospective study. Maturitas. 2012;72(4):346–52.
25. Lubiszewska B, Kruk M, Broda G, Ksiezycka E, Piotrowski W, Kurjata P, et al. The impact of early menopause on risk of coronary artery disease (PREmature Coronary Artery Disease In Women—PRECADIW case-control study). Eur J Prev Cardiol. 2012;19(1):95–101.
26. Kullo IJ, Rooke TW. Clinical Practice. Peripheral artery disease. N Engl J Med 2016;374(9):861–71.
27. Fowkes FG, Rudan D, Rudan I, Aboyans V, Denenberg JO, McDermott MM, et al. Comparison of global estimates of prevalence and risk factors for peripheral artery disease in 2000 and 2010: a systematic review and analysis. Lancet. 2013;382(9901):1329–40.
28. Putaala J, Yesilot N, Waje-Andreassen U, Pitkaniemi J, Vassilopoulou S, Nardi K, et al. Demographic and geographic vascular risk factor differences in European young adults with ischemic stroke: the 15 cities young stroke study. Stroke. 2012;43(10):2624–30.
29. Jahangir E, Lipworth L, Edwards TL, Kabagambe EK, Mumma MT, Mensah GA, et al. Smoking, sex, risk factors and abdominal aortic aneurysms: a prospective study of 18 782 persons aged above 65 years in the Southern Community Cohort Study. J Epidemiol Community Health. 2015;69(5):481–8.
30. Lederle FA, Larson JC, Margolis KL, Allison MA, Freiberg MS, Cochrane BB, et al. Abdominal aortic aneurysm events in the women's health initiative: cohort study. BMJ. 2008;337:a1724.
31. Iversen B, Jacobsen BK, Lochen ML. Active and passive smoking and the risk of myocardial infarction in 24,968 men and women during 11 year of follow-up: the Tromso Study. Eur J Epidemiol. 2013;28(8):659–67.

32. Twig G, Yaniv G, Levine H, Leiba A, Goldberger N, Derazne E, et al. Body-Mass Index in 2.3 Million Adolescents and Cardiovascular Death in Adulthood. N Engl J Med. 2016;374(25):2430–40.
33. Flegal KM, Carroll MD, Kit BK, Ogden CL. Prevalence of obesity and trends in the distribution of body mass index among US adults, 1999-2010. JAMA. 2012;307(5):491–7.
34. Wilson PW, D'Agostino RB, Sullivan L, Parise H, Kannel WB. Overweight and obesity as determinants of cardiovascular risk: the Framingham experience. Arch Intern Med. 2002;162(16):1867–72.
35. De Smedt D, De Bacquer D, De Sutter J, Dallongeville J, Gevaert S, De Backer G, et al. The gender gap in risk factor control: effects of age and education on the control of cardiovascular risk factors in male and female coronary patients. The EUROASPIRE IV study by the European Society of Cardiology. Int J Cardiol. 2016;209:284–90.
36. Regitz-Zagrosek V, Lehmkuhl E, Mahmoodzadeh S. Gender aspects of the role of the metabolic syndrome as a risk factor for cardiovascular disease. Gender Med. 2007;4 Suppl B:S162–77.
37. Chomistek AK, Manson JE, Stefanick ML, Lu B, Sands-Lincoln M, Going SB, et al. Relationship of sedentary behavior and physical activity to incident cardiovascular disease: results from the Women's Health Initiative. J Am Coll Cardiol. 2013;61(23):2346–54.
38. Oertelt-Prigione S, Seeland U, Kendel F, Rucke M, Floel A, Gaissmaier W, et al. Cardiovascular risk factor distribution and subjective risk estimation in urban women—the BEFRI study: a randomized cross-sectional study. BMC Med. 2015;13:52.
39. Eckel RH, Jakicic JM, Ard JD, de Jesus JM, Houston Miller N, Hubbard VS, et al. 2013 AHA/ACC guideline on lifestyle management to reduce cardiovascular risk: a report of the American College of Cardiology/American Heart Association Task Force on Practice Guidelines. Circulation. 2014;129(25 Suppl 2):S76–99.
40. Bushnell C, McCullough LD, Awad IA, Chireau MV, Fedder WN, Furie KL, et al. Guidelines for the prevention of stroke in women: a statement for healthcare professionals from the American Heart Association/American Stroke Association. Stroke. 2014;45(5):1545–88.
41. Perk J, De Backer G, Gohlke H, Graham I, Reiner Z, Verschuren M, et al. European Guidelines on cardiovascular disease prevention in clinical practice (version 2012). The Fifth Joint Task Force of the European Society of Cardiology and Other Societies on Cardiovascular Disease Prevention in Clinical Practice (constituted by representatives of nine societies and by invited experts). Eur Heart J. 2012;33(13):1635–701.
42. Piepoli MF, Hoes AW, Agewall S, Albus C, Brotons C, Catapano AL, et al. 2016 European Guidelines on cardiovascular disease prevention in clinical practice: The Sixth Joint Task Force of the European Society of Cardiology and Other Societies on Cardiovascular Disease Prevention in Clinical Practice (constituted by representatives of 10 societies and by invited experts): Developed with the special contribution of the European Association for Cardiovascular Prevention & Rehabilitation (EACPR). Eur Heart J. 2016;37(29): 2315–81.
43. Qureshi N, Armstrong S, Dhiman P, Saukko P, Middlemass J, Evans PH, et al. Effect of adding systematic family history enquiry to cardiovascular disease risk assessment in primary care: a matched-pair, cluster randomized trial. Ann Intern Med. 2012;156(4):253–62.
44. Chow CK, Islam S, Bautista L, Rumboldt Z, Yusufali A, Xie C, et al. Parental history and myocardial infarction risk across the world: the INTERHEART Study. J Am Coll Cardiol. 2011;57(5):619–27.
45. Michos ED, Vasamreddy CR, Becker DM, Yanek LR, Moy TF, Fishman EK, et al. Women with a low Framingham risk score and a family history of premature coronary heart disease have a high prevalence of subclinical coronary atherosclerosis. Am Heart J. 2005;150(6):1276–81.
46. Mulders TA, Taraboanta C, Franken LC, van Heel E, Klass G, Forster BB, et al. Coronary artery calcification score as tool for risk assessment among families with premature coronary artery disease. Atherosclerosis. 2016;245:155–60.
47. Patel MJ, de Lemos JA, Philips B, Murphy SA, Vaeth PC, McGuire DK, et al. Implications of family history of myocardial infarction in young women. Am Heart J. 2007;154(3):454–60.

48. Hindieh W, Pilote L, Cheema A, Al-Lawati H, Labos C, Dufresne L, et al. Association between family history, a genetic risk score, and severity of coronary artery disease in patients with premature acute coronary syndromes. Arteriosclerosis Thrombosis and Vasc Biol. 2016;36(6):1286–92.
49. Ranthe MF, Carstensen L, Oyen N, Tfelt-Hansen J, Christiansen M, McKenna WJ, et al. Family history of premature death and risk of early onset cardiovascular disease. J Am Coll Cardiol. 2012;60(9):814–21.
50. Zoller B, Li X, Sundquist J, Sundquist K. Multiplex sibling history of coronary heart disease is a strong risk factor for coronary heart disease. Eur Heart J. 2012;33(22):2849–55.
51. Choi J, Daskalopoulou SS, Thanassoulis G, Karp I, Pelletier R, Behlouli H, et al. Sex- and gender-related risk factor burden in patients with premature acute coronary syndrome. Can J Cardiol. 2014;30(1):109–17.
52. Steegers EA, von Dadelszen P, Duvekot JJ, Pijnenborg R. Pre-eclampsia. Lancet. 2010;376(9741):631–44.
53. Smith GC, Wood AM, Pell JP, Hattie J. Recurrent miscarriage is associated with a family history of ischaemic heart disease: a retrospective cohort study. BJOG. 2011;118(5):557–63.
54. Drost JT, Arpaci G, Ottervanger JP, de Boer MJ, van Eyck J, van der Schouw YT, et al. Cardiovascular risk factors in women 10 years post early preeclampsia: the Preeclampsia Risk EValuation in FEMales study (PREVFEM). Eur J Prev Cardiol. 2012;19(5):1138–44.
55. Ranthe MF, Diaz LJ, Behrens I, Bundgaard H, Simonsen J, Melbye M, et al. Association between pregnancy losses in women and risk of atherosclerotic disease in their relatives: a nationwide cohort studydagger. Eur Heart J. 2016;37(11):900–7.
56. Berger JS, Elliott L, Gallup D, Roe M, Granger CB, Armstrong PW, et al. Sex differences in mortality following acute coronary syndromes. JAMA. 2009;302(8):874–82.
57. Cooney MT, Dudina AL, Graham IM. Value and limitations of existing scores for the assessment of cardiovascular risk: a review for clinicians. J Am Coll Cardiol. 2009;54(14):1209–27.
58. Damen JA, Hooft L, Schuit E, Debray TP, Collins GS, Tzoulaki I, et al. Prediction models for cardiovascular disease risk in the general population: systematic review. BMJ. 2016;353:i2416.
59. Goff Jr DC, Lloyd-Jones DM, Bennett G, Coady S, D'Agostino RB, Gibbons R, et al. 2013 ACC/AHA guideline on the assessment of cardiovascular risk: a report of the American College of Cardiology/American Heart Association Task Force on Practice Guidelines. Circulation. 2014;129(25 Suppl 2):S49 73.
60. Graham I, Atar D, Borch-Johnsen K, Boysen G, Burell G, Cifkova R, et al. European guidelines on cardiovascular disease prevention in clinical practice: full text. Fourth Joint Task Force of the European Society of Cardiology and other societies on cardiovascular disease prevention in clinical practice (constituted by representatives of nine societies and by invited experts). European journal of cardiovascular prevention and rehabilitation: official journal of the European Society of Cardiology, Working Groups on Epidemiology & Prevention and Cardiac Rehabilitation and Exercise Physiology. 2007;14 Suppl 2:S1–113.
61. Vasan RS, Kannel WB. Strategies for cardiovascular risk assessment and prevention over the life course: progress amid imperfections. Circulation. 2009;120(5):360–3.
62. Nasir K, Michos ED, Blumenthal RS, Raggi P. Detection of high-risk young adults and women by coronary calcium and National Cholesterol Education Program Panel III guidelines. J Am Coll Cardiol. 2005;46(10):1931–6.
63. Paixao AR, Ayers CR, El Sabbagh A, Sanghavi M, Berry JD, Rohatgi A, et al. Coronary artery calcium improves risk classification in younger populations. JACC Cardiovasc Imaging. 2015;8(11):1285–93.
64. Bamberg F, Sommer WH, Hoffmann V, Achenbach S, Nikolaou K, Conen D, et al. Meta-analysis and systematic review of the long-term predictive value of assessment of coronary atherosclerosis by contrast-enhanced coronary computed tomography angiography. J Am Coll Cardiol. 2011;57(24):2426–36.

65. Yeboah J, Young R, McClelland RL, Delaney JC, Polonsky TS, Dawood FZ, et al. Utility of nontraditional risk markers in atherosclerotic cardiovascular disease risk assessment. J Am Coll Cardiol. 2016;67(2):139–47.
66. https://www.nice.org.uk/guidance/cg95.
67. Verschuren WM, Boerma GJ, Kromhout D. Total and HDL-cholesterol in The Netherlands: 1987-1992. Levels and changes over time in relation to age, gender and educational level. Int J Epidemiol. 1994;23(5):948–56.
68. Abbey M, Owen A, Suzakawa M, Roach P, Nestel PJ. Effects of menopause and hormone replacement therapy on plasma lipids, lipoproteins and LDL-receptor activity. Maturitas. 1999;33(3):259–69.
69. Reddy Kilim S, Chandala SR. A comparative study of lipid profile and oestradiol in pre- and post-menopausal women. J Clin Diagn Res. 2013;7(8):1596–8.
70. Matthews KA, Meilahn E, Kuller LH, Kelsey SF, Caggiula AW, Wing RR. Menopause and risk factors for coronary heart disease. N Engl J Med. 1989;321(10):641–6.
71. Mora S, Glynn RJ, Hsia J, MacFadyen JG, Genest J, Ridker PM. Statins for the primary prevention of cardiovascular events in women with elevated high-sensitivity C-reactive protein or dyslipidemia: results from the Justification for the Use of Statins in Prevention: An Intervention Trial Evaluating Rosuvastatin (JUPITER) and meta-analysis of women from primary prevention trials. Circulation. 2010;121(9):1069–77.
72. Walsh JM, Pignone M. Drug treatment of hyperlipidemia in women. JAMA. 2004;291(18):2243–52.
73. Kostis WJ, Cheng JQ, Dobrzynski JM, Cabrera J, Kostis JB. Meta-analysis of statin effects in women versus men. J Am Coll Cardiol. 2012;59(6):572–82.
74. Truong QA, Murphy SA, McCabe CH, Armani A, Cannon CP, Group TS. Benefit of intensive statin therapy in women: results from PROVE IT-TIMI 22. Circ Cardiovasc Qual Outcomes. 2011;4(3):328–36.
75. Harrington C, Horne Jr A, Hasan RK, Blumenthal RS. Statin therapy in primary prevention: new insights regarding women and the elderly. Am J Cardiol. 2010;106(9):1357–9.
76. Mizuno K, Nakaya N, Ohashi Y, Tajima N, Kushiro T, Teramoto T, et al. Usefulness of pravastatin in primary prevention of cardiovascular events in women: analysis of the Management of Elevated Cholesterol in the Primary Prevention Group of Adult Japanese (MEGA study). Circulation. 2008;117(4):494–502.
77. Ridker PM, Danielson E, Fonseca FA, Genest J, Gotto Jr AM, Kastelein JJ, et al. Rosuvastatin to prevent vascular events in men and women with elevated C-reactive protein. N Engl J Med. 2008;359(21):2195 207.
78. Cholesterol Treatment Trialists C, Fulcher J, O'Connell R, Voysey M, Emberson J, Blackwell L, et al. Efficacy and safety of LDL-lowering therapy among men and women: meta-analysis of individual data from 174,000 participants in 27 randomised trials. Lancet. 2015;385(9976):1397–405.
79. Stone NJ, Robinson JG, Lichtenstein AH, Bairey Merz CN, Blum CB, Eckel RH, et al. 2013 ACC/AHA guideline on the treatment of blood cholesterol to reduce atherosclerotic cardiovascular risk in adults: a report of the American College of Cardiology/American Heart Association Task Force on Practice Guidelines. Circulation. 2014;129(25 Suppl 2):S1–45.
80. Kavousi M, Leening MJ, Nanchen D, Greenland P, Graham IM, Steyerberg EW, et al. Comparison of application of the ACC/AHA guidelines, adult treatment panel III guidelines, and European Society of Cardiology guidelines for cardiovascular disease prevention in a European cohort. JAMA. 2014;311(14):1416–23.
81. Pavlovic J, Greenland P, Deckers JW, Brugts JJ, Kavousi M, Dhana K, et al. Comparison of ACC/AHA and ESC guideline recommendations following trial evidence for statin use in primary prevention of cardiovascular disease: results from the population-based Rotterdam study. JAMA Cardiol. 2016;1(6):708–13.
82. https://www.nice.org.uk/guidance/cg181.

83. Rosenson RS, Baker SK, Jacobson TA, Kopecky SL, Parker BA. The National Lipid Association's Muscle Safety Expert P. An assessment by the Statin Muscle Safety Task Force: 2014 update. J Clin Lipidol. 2014;8(3 Suppl):S58–71.
84. Sathasivam S. Statin induced myotoxicity. Eur J Intern Med. 2012;23(4):317–24.
85. Thompson PD, Panza G, Zaleski A, Taylor B. Statin-associated side effects. J Am Coll Cardiol. 2016;67(20):2395–410.
86. Ganga HV, Slim HB, Thompson PD. A systematic review of statin-induced muscle problems in clinical trials. Am Heart J. 2014;168(1):6–15.
87. Nissen SE, Stroes E, Dent-Acosta RE, Rosenson RS, Lehman SJ, Sattar N, et al. Efficacy and tolerability of Evolocumab vs Ezetimibe in patients with muscle-related statin intolerance: the GAUSS-3 randomized clinical trial. JAMA. 2016;315(15):1580–90.
88. Hsue PY, Bittner VA, Betteridge J, Fayyad R, Laskey R, Wenger NK, et al. Impact of female sex on lipid lowering, clinical outcomes, and adverse effects in atorvastatin trials. Am J Cardiol. 2015;115(4):447–53.
89. Caspard H, Chan AK, Walker AM. Compliance with a statin treatment in a usual-care setting: retrospective database analysis over 3 years after treatment initiation in health maintenance organization enrollees with dyslipidemia. Clin Ther. 2005;27(10):1639–46.
90. Tomlinson SS, Mangione KK. Potential adverse effects of statins on muscle. Phys Ther. 2005;85(5):459–65.
91. Saxon DR, Eckel RH. Statin intolerance: a literature review and management strategies. Progr Cardiovasc Dis. 2016;59(2):153–64.
92. Taylor BA, Lorson L, White CM, Thompson PD. A randomized trial of coenzyme Q10 in patients with confirmed statin myopathy. Atherosclerosis. 2015;238(2):329–35.
93. Blumel JE, Palacios S, Legorreta D, Vallejo MS, Sarra S. Is fibromyalgia part of the climacteric syndrome? Maturitas. 2012;73(2):87–93.
94. Blumel JE, Cano A, Mezones-Holguin E, Baron G, Bencosme A, Benitez Z, et al. A multinational study of sleep disorders during female mid-life. Maturitas. 2012;72(4):359–66.
95. Rosano GM, Lewis B, Agewall S, Wassmann S, Vitale C, Schmidt H, et al. Gender differences in the effect of cardiovascular drugs: a position document of the Working Group on Pharmacology and Drug Therapy of the ESC. Eur Heart J. 2015;36(40):2677–80.
96. Group SC, Link E, Parish S, Armitage J, Bowman L, Heath S, et al. SLCO1B1 variants and statin-induced myopathy—a genomewide study. N Engl J Med. 2008;359(8):789–99.
97. Voora D, Shah SH, Spasojevic I, Ali S, Reed CR, Salisbury BA, et al. The SLCO1B1*5 genetic variant is associated with statin-induced side effects. J Am Coll Cardiol. 2009;54(17):1609 16.
98. Schirris TJJ, Renkema GH, Ritschel T, Voermans NC, Bilos A, van Engelen BGM, et al. Statin-induced myopathy is associated with mitochondrial complex III inhibition. Cell Metab. 2015;22(3):399–407.
99. Matthews A, Herrett E, Gasparrini A, Van Staa T, Goldacre B, Smeeth L, et al. Impact of statin related media coverage on use of statins: interrupted time series analysis with UK primary care data. BMJ. 2016;353:i3283.
100. Nielsen SF, Nordestgaard BG. Negative statin-related news stories decrease statin persistence and increase myocardial infarction and cardiovascular mortality: a nationwide prospective cohort study. Eur Heart J. 2016;37(11):908–16.
101. Newman CB, Tobert JA. Statin intolerance: reconciling clinical trials and clinical experience. JAMA. 2015;313(10):1011–2.
102. Robinson JG. Lower might be better - It matters how you get there, and in whom. Eur Heart J. 2016;37(17):1380–3.
103. Stroes ES, Thompson PD, Corsini A, Vladutiu GD, Raal FJ, Ray KK, et al. Statin-associated muscle symptoms: impact on statin therapy-European Atherosclerosis Society Consensus Panel Statement on Assessment, Aetiology and Management. Eur Heart J. 2015;36(17):1012–22.
104. Zhang Y, Leach MJ, Hall H, Sundberg T, Ward L, Sibbritt D, et al. Differences between male and female consumers of complementary and alternative medicine in a National US

Population: a secondary analysis of 2012 NIHS Data. Evid Based Complement Alternat Med. 2015;2015:413173.

105. Sabatine MS, Giugliano RP, Wiviott SD, Raal FJ, Blom DJ, Robinson J, et al. Efficacy and safety of evolocumab in reducing lipids and cardiovascular events. N Engl J Med. 2015;372(16):1500–9.
106. Kazi DS, Moran AE, Coxson PG, Penko J, Ollendorf DA, Pearson SD, et al. Cost-effectiveness of PCSK9 inhibitor therapy in patients with heterozygous familial hypercholesterolemia or atherosclerotic cardiovascular disease. JAMA. 2016;316(7):743–53.
107. Cleland JG, Swedberg K, Follath F, Komajda M, Cohen-Solal A, Aguilar JC, et al. The EuroHeart Failure survey programme— a survey on the quality of care among patients with heart failure in Europe. Part 1: patient characteristics and diagnosis. Eur Heart J. 2003;24(5):442–63.
108. Mancusi C, Gerdts E, De Simone G, Abdelhai YM, Lonnebakken MT, Boman K, et al. Impact of isolated systolic hypertension on normalization of left ventricular structure during antihypertensive treatment (the LIFE study). Blood Press. 2014;23(4):206–12.
109. Kingwell BA, Medley TL, Waddell TK, Cole TJ, Dart AM, Jennings GL. Large artery stiffness: structural and genetic aspects. Clin Exp Pharmacol Physiol. 2001;28(12):1040–3.
110. Mao SS, Ahmadi N, Shah B, Beckmann D, Chen A, Ngo L, et al. Normal thoracic aorta diameter on cardiac computed tomography in healthy asymptomatic adults: impact of age and gender. Acad Radiol. 2008;15(7):827–34.
111. Kearney PM, Whelton M, Reynolds K, Muntner P, Whelton PK, He J. Global burden of hypertension: analysis of worldwide data. Lancet. 2005;365(9455):217–23.
112. Lloyd-Sherlock P, Beard J, Minicuci N, Ebrahim S, Chatterji S. Hypertension among older adults in low- and middle-income countries: prevalence, awareness and control. Int J Epidemiol. 2014;43(1):116–28.
113. Lewington S, Clarke R, Qizilbash N, Peto R, Collins R, Prospective SC. Age-specific relevance of usual blood pressure to vascular mortality: a meta-analysis of individual data for one million adults in 61 prospective studies. Lancet. 2002;360(9349):1903–13.
114. Group SR, Wright Jr JT, Williamson JD, Whelton PK, Snyder JK, Sink KM, et al. A randomized trial of intensive versus standard blood-pressure control. N Engl J Med. 2015;373(22):2103–16.
115. Luscher TF, Sudano I. SPRINT: the race for optimal blood pressure control. Eur Heart J. 2016;37(12):937–41.
116. Hendriks SH, van Hateren KJ, Groenier KH, Houweling ST, Maas AH, Kleefstra N, et al. Sex differences in the quality of diabetes care in the Netherlands (ZODIAC-45). PLoS One. 2015;10(12):e0145907.
117. Franzini L, Ardigo D, Cavalot F, Miccoli R, Rivellese AA, Trovati M, et al. Women show worse control of type 2 diabetes and cardiovascular disease risk factors than men: results from the MIND.IT Study Group of the Italian Society of Diabetology. Nutr Metab Cardiovasc Dis. 2013;23(3):235–41.
118. Schroeder EB, Bayliss EA, Daugherty SL, Steiner JF. Gender differences in cardiovascular risk factors in incident diabetes. Womens Health Issues. 2014;24(1):e61–8.
119. Kautzky-Willer A, Handisurya A. Metabolic diseases and associated complications: sex and gender matter! European journal of clinical investigation. 2009;39(8):631–48.
120. Huxley R, Barzi F, Woodward M. Excess risk of fatal coronary heart disease associated with diabetes in men and women: meta-analysis of 37 prospective cohort studies. Bmj. 2006;332(7533):73–8.
121. Anand SS, Islam S, Rosengren A, Franzosi MG, Steyn K, Yusufali AH, et al. Risk factors for myocardial infarction in women and men: insights from the INTERHEART study. European heart journal. 2008;29(7):932–40.
122. Mulnier HE, Seaman HE, Raleigh VS, Soedamah-Muthu SS, Colhoun HM, Lawrenson RA, et al. Risk of myocardial infarction in men and women with type 2 diabetes in the UK: a cohort study using the General Practice Research Database. Diabetologia. 2008;51(9):1639–45.

123. Donahue RP, Rejman K, Rafalson LB, Dmochowski J, Stranges S, Trevisan M. Sex differences in endothelial function markers before conversion to pre-diabetes: does the clock start ticking earlier among women? The Western New York Study. Diabetes Care. 2007;30(2):354–9.
124. Kautzky-Willer A, Harreiter J, Pacini G. Sex and gender differences in risk, pathophysiology and complications of type 2 diabetes mellitus. Endoc Rev. 2016:er20151137.
125. Tamis-Holland JE, Lu J, Korytkowski M, Magee M, Rogers WJ, Lopes N, et al. Sex differences in presentation and outcome among patients with type 2 diabetes and coronary artery disease treated with contemporary medical therapy with or without prompt revascularization: a report from the BARI 2D Trial (Bypass Angioplasty Revascularization Investigation 2 Diabetes). J Am Coll Cardiol. 2013;61(17):1767–76.
126. Novak M, Bjorck L, Welin L, Welin C, Manhem K, Rosengren A. Gender differences in the prevalence of metabolic syndrome in 50-year-old Swedish men and women with hypertension born in 1953. J Hum Hypertens. 2013;27(1):56–61.
127. de Simone G, Devereux RB, Chinali M, Lee ET, Galloway JM, Barac A, et al. Diabetes and incident heart failure in hypertensive and normotensive participants of the Strong Heart Study. J Hypertens. 2010;28(2):353–60.
128. Boonman-de Winter LJ, Rutten FH, Cramer MJ, Landman MJ, Liem AH, Rutten GE, et al. High prevalence of previously unknown heart failure and left ventricular dysfunction in patients with type 2 diabetes. Diabetologia. 2012;55(8):2154–62.
129. Fairweather D. Sex differences in inflammation during atherosclerosis. Clin Med Insights Cardiol. 2014;8(Suppl 3):49–59.
130. Paulus WJ, Tschope C. A novel paradigm for heart failure with preserved ejection fraction: comorbidities drive myocardial dysfunction and remodeling through coronary microvascular endothelial inflammation. J Am Coll Cardiol. 2013;62(4):263–71.
131. Koupenova M, Mick E, Mikhalev E, Benjamin EJ, Tanriverdi K, Freedman JE. Sex differences in platelet toll-like receptors and their association with cardiovascular risk factors. Arterioscler Thromb Vasc Biol. 2015;35(4):1030–7.
132. Major AS, Harrison DG. What fans the fire: insights into mechanisms of inflammation in atherosclerosis and diabetes mellitus. Circulation. 2011;124(25):2809–11.
133. Pasterkamp G. Methods of accelerated atherosclerosis in diabetic patients. Heart. 2013;99(10):743–9.
134. Morling JR, Balkau B, Wild SH. Diabetes in women: a life-course approach. Menopause Int. 2013;19(2):87–95.
135. Monterrosa-Castro A, Blumel JE, Portela-Buelvas K, Mezones-Holguin E, Baron G, Bencosme A, et al. Type II diabetes mellitus and menopause: a multinational study. Climacteric. 2013;16(6):663–72.
136. Authors/Task Force M, Ryden L, Grant PJ, Anker SD, Berne C, Cosentino F, et al. ESC Guidelines on diabetes, pre-diabetes, and cardiovascular diseases developed in collaboration with the EASD: the Task Force on diabetes, pre-diabetes, and cardiovascular diseases of the European Society of Cardiology (ESC) and developed in collaboration with the European Association for the Study of Diabetes (EASD). Eur Heart J 2013;34(39):3035–3087.
137. Carpiuc KT, Wingard DL, Kritz-Silverstein D, Barrett-Connor E. The association of angina pectoris with heart disease mortality among men and women by diabetes status: the Rancho Bernardo Study. J Womens Health. 2010;19(8):1433–9.
138. Barrett-Connor E. The Rancho Bernardo Study: 40 years studying why women have less heart disease than men and how diabetes modifies women's usual cardiac protection. Global Heart. 2013;8(2).
139. Regensteiner JG, Golden S, Huebschmann AG, Barrett-Connor E, Chang AY, Chyun D, et al. Sex differences in the cardiovascular consequences of diabetes mellitus: a scientific statement from the American Heart Association. Circulation. 2015;132(25):2424–47.
140. Esposito K, Chiodini P, Capuano A, Bellastella G, Maiorino MI, Rafaniello C, et al. Metabolic syndrome and postmenopausal breast cancer: systematic review and meta-analysis. Menopause. 2013;20(12):1301–9.

141. Zhou Y, Zhang X, Gu C, Xia J. Influence of diabetes mellitus on mortality in breast cancer patients. ANZ J Surg. 2015;85(12):972–8.
142. Elkeles RS, Godsland IF, Feher MD, Rubens MB, Roughton M, Nugara F, et al. Coronary calcium measurement improves prediction of cardiovascular events in asymptomatic patients with type 2 diabetes: the PREDICT study. Eur Heart J. 2008;29(18):2244–51.
143. Farkouh ME, Dangas G, Leon MB, Smith C, Nesto R, Buse JB, et al. Design of the Future REvascularization Evaluation in patients with Diabetes mellitus: Optimal management of Multivessel disease (FREEDOM) Trial. Am Heart J. 2008;155(2):215–23.
144. Kappetein AP, Head SJ, Morice MC, Banning AP, Serruys PW, Mohr FW, et al. Treatment of complex coronary artery disease in patients with diabetes: 5-year results comparing outcomes of bypass surgery and percutaneous coronary intervention in the SYNTAX trial. Eur J Cardio-Thoracic Surg. 2013;43(5):1006–13.
145. Investigators B. The final 10-year follow-up results from the BARI randomized trial. J Am Coll Cardiol. 2007;49(15):1600–6.
146. Group BDS, Frye RL, August P, Brooks MM, Hardison RM, Kelsey SF, et al. A randomized trial of therapies for type 2 diabetes and coronary artery disease. N Engl J Med. 2009;360(24):2503–15.
147. Hillis LD, Smith PK, Anderson JL, Bittl JA, Bridges CR, Byrne JG, et al. 2011 ACCF/AHA Guideline for Coronary Artery Bypass Graft Surgery. A report of the American College of Cardiology Foundation/American Heart Association Task Force on Practice Guidelines. Developed in collaboration with the American Association for Thoracic Surgery, Society of Cardiovascular Anesthesiologists, and Society of Thoracic Surgeons. J Am Coll Cardiol. 2011;58(24):e123–210.
148. van der Meer MG, van der Graaf Y, Schuit E, Peelen LM, Verschuren WM, Boer JM, et al. Added value of female-specific factors beyond traditional predictors for future cardiovascular disease. J Am Coll Cardiol. 2016;67(17):2084–6.
149. Parikh NI, Jeppson RP, Berger JS, Eaton CB, Kroenke CH, LaBlanc ES, et al. Reproductive Risk Factors and Coronary Heart Disease in the Women's Health Initiative Observational Study. Circulation. 2016;133(22):2149–58.
150. Elias-Smale SE, Gunal A, Maas AH. Gynecardiology: Distinct patterns of ischemic heart disease in middle-aged women. Maturitas. 2015;81(3):348–52.
151. Cirillo PM, Cohn BA. Pregnancy complications and cardiovascular disease death: 50-year follow-up of the Child Health and Development Studies pregnancy cohort. Circulation. 2015;132(13):1234–42.
152. Sorensen MB, Franks S, Robertson C, Pennell DJ, Collins P. Severe endothelial dysfunction in young women with polycystic ovary syndrome is only partially explained by known cardiovascular risk factors. Clin Endocrinol (Oxf). 2006;65(5):655–9.
153. Rao R, Sen S, Han B, Ramadoss S, Chaudhuri G. Gestational diabetes, preeclampsia and cytokine release: similarities and differences in endothelial cell function. Adv Exp Med Biol. 2014;814:69–75.
154. Agatisa PK, Ness RB, Roberts JM, Costantino JP, Kuller LH, McLaughlin MK. Impairment of endothelial function in women with a history of preeclampsia: an indicator of cardiovascular risk. Am J Physiol Heart Circ Physiol. 2004;286(4):H1389–93.
155. Freedman DS, Khan LK, Serdula MK, Dietz WH, Srinivasan SR, Berenson GS, et al. The relation of menarcheal age to obesity in childhood and adulthood: the Bogalusa heart study. BMC Pediatr. 2003;3:3.
156. Kivimaki M, Lawlor DA, Smith GD, Elovainio M, Jokela M, Keltikangas-Jarvinen L, et al. Association of age at menarche with cardiovascular risk factors, vascular structure, and function in adulthood: the Cardiovascular Risk in Young Finns study. Am J Clin Nutr. 2008;87(6):1876–82.
157. Remsberg KE, Demerath EW, Schubert CM, Chumlea WC, Sun SS, Siervogel RM. Early menarche and the development of cardiovascular disease risk factors in adolescent girls: the Fels Longitudinal Study. J Clin Endocrinol Metab. 2005;90(5):2718–24.
158. Colditz GA, Willett WC, Stampfer MJ, Rosner B, Speizer FE, Hennekens CH. A prospective study of age at menarche, parity, age at first birth, and coronary heart disease in women. Am J Epidemiol. 1987;126(5):861–70.

159. Pierce MB, Kuh D, Hardy R. The role of BMI across the life course in the relationship between age at menarche and diabetes, in a British Birth Cohort. Diabet Med. 2012;29(5):600–3.
160. Lakshman R, Forouhi NG, Sharp SJ, Luben R, Bingham SA, Khaw KT, et al. Early age at menarche associated with cardiovascular disease and mortality. J Clin Endocrinol Metab. 2009;94(12):4953–60.
161. Canoy D, Beral V, Balkwill A, Wright FL, Kroll ME, Reeves GK, et al. Age at menarche and risks of coronary heart and other vascular diseases in a large UK cohort. Circulation. 2015;131(3):237–44.
162. Merz CN, Johnson BD, Berga SL, Braunstein GD, Azziz R, Yang Y, et al. Total estrogen time and obstructive coronary disease in women: insights from the NHLBI-sponsored Women's Ischemia Syndrome Evaluation (WISE). J Womens Health. 2009;18(9):1315–22.
163. Carty CL, Spencer KL, Setiawan VW, Fernandez-Rhodes L, Malinowski J, Buyske S, et al. Replication of genetic loci for ages at menarche and menopause in the multi-ethnic Population Architecture using Genomics and Epidemiology (PAGE) study. Hum Reprod. 2013;28(6):1695–706.
164. Morris DH, Jones ME, Schoemaker MJ, Ashworth A, Swerdlow AJ. Familial concordance for age at menarche: analyses from the Breakthrough Generations Study. Paediatr Perinat Epidemiol. 2011;25(3):306–11.
165. He C, Murabito JM. Genome-wide association studies of age at menarche and age at natural menopause. Mol Cell Endocrinol. 2014;382(1):767–79.
166. Rotterdam EA-SPcwg. Revised 2003 consensus on diagnostic criteria and long-term health risks related to polycystic ovary syndrome (PCOS). Hum Reprod 2004;19(1):41–7.
167. Azziz R, Woods KS, Reyna R, Key TJ, Knochenhauer ES, Yildiz BO. The prevalence and features of the polycystic ovary syndrome in an unselected population. J Clin Endocrinol Metab. 2004;89(6):2745–9.
168. Shen SH, Shen SY, Liou TH, Hsu MI, Chang YC, Cheng CY, et al. Obesity and inflammatory biomarkers in women with polycystic ovary syndrome. Eur J Obstet Gynecol Reprod Biol. 2015;192:66–71.
169. Sprung VS, Jones H, Pugh CJ, Aziz NF, Daousi C, Kemp GJ, et al. Endothelial dysfunction in hyperandrogenic polycystic ovary syndrome is not explained by either obesity or ectopic fat deposition. Clin Sci. 2014;126(1):67–74.
170. Moran LJ, Misso ML, Wild RA, Norman RJ. Impaired glucose tolerance, type 2 diabetes and metabolic syndrome in polycystic ovary syndrome: a systematic review and meta-analysis. Hum Reprod Update. 2010;16(4):347–63.
171. Daan NM, Louwers YV, Koster MP, Eijkemans MJ, de Rijke YB, Lentjes EW, et al. Cardiovascular and metabolic profiles amongst different polycystic ovary syndrome phenotypes: who is really at risk? Fertil Steril. 2014;102(5):1444–51. e3
172. Fauser BC, Tarlatzis BC, Rebar RW, Legro RS, Balen AH, Lobo R, et al. Consensus on women's health aspects of polycystic ovary syndrome (PCOS): the Amsterdam ESHRE/ASRM-Sponsored 3rd PCOS Consensus Workshop Group. Fertil Steril. 2012;97(1):28–38. e25
173. Merz CN, Shaw LJ, Azziz R, Stanczyk FZ, Sopko G, Braunstein GD, et al. Cardiovascular disease and 10-year mortality in postmenopausal women with clinical features of polycystic ovary syndrome. J Womens Health. 2016;25(9):875–81.
174. McCartney CR, Marshall JC. Clinical Practice. Polycystic ovary syndrome. N Engl J Med 2016;375(1):54–64.
175. de Wilde MA, Veltman-Verhulst SM, Goverde AJ, Lambalk CB, Laven JS, Franx A, et al. Preconception predictors of gestational diabetes: a multicentre prospective cohort study on the predominant complication of pregnancy in polycystic ovary syndrome. Hum Reprod. 2014;29(6):1327–36.
176. Pan ML, Chen LR, Tsao HM, Chen KH. Relationship between polycystic ovarian syndrome and subsequent gestational diabetes mellitus: a Nationwide Population-Based Study. PLoS One. 2015;10(10):e0140544.
177. Heida KY, Bots ML, de Groot CJ, van Dunne FM, Hammoud NM, Hoek A, et al. Cardiovascular risk management after reproductive and pregnancy-related disorders: a Dutch multidisciplinary evidence-based guideline. Eur J Prev Cardiol. 2016;23(17):1863–79.

178. Noussitou P, Monbaron D, Vial Y, Gaillard RC, Ruiz J. Gestational diabetes mellitus and the risk of metabolic syndrome: a population-based study in Lausanne, Switzerland Diabetes & metabolism 2005;31(4 Pt 1):361–9.
179. Bellamy L, Casas JP, Hingorani AD, Williams D. Type 2 diabetes mellitus after gestational diabetes: a systematic review and meta-analysis. Lancet. 2009;373(9677):1773–9.
180. Gunderson EP, Chiang V, Pletcher MJ, Jacobs DR, Quesenberry CP, Sidney S, et al. History of gestational diabetes mellitus and future risk of atherosclerosis in mid-life: the Coronary Artery Risk Development in Young Adults study. J Am Heart Assoc. 2014;3(2):e000490.
181. Bryson CL, Ioannou GN, Rulyak SJ, Critchlow C. Association between gestational diabetes and pregnancy-induced hypertension. Am J Epidemiol. 2003;158(12):1148–53.
182. Mosca L, Benjamin EJ, Berra K, Bezanson JL, Dolor RJ, Lloyd-Jones DM, et al. Effectiveness-based guidelines for the prevention of cardiovascular disease in women—2011 update: a guideline from the American Heart Association. Circulation. 2011;123(11):1243–62.
183. Landon MB, Gabbe SG. Gestational diabetes mellitus. Obstet Gynecol. 2011; 118(6):1379–93.
184. Heida KY, Franx A, van Rijn BB, Eijkemans MJ, Boer JM, Verschuren MW, et al. Earlier age of onset of chronic hypertension and type 2 diabetes mellitus after a hypertensive disorder of pregnancy or gestational diabetes mellitus. Hypertension. 2015;66(6):1116–22.
185. Kharazmi E, Dossus L, Rohrmann S, Kaaks R. Pregnancy loss and risk of cardiovascular disease: a prospective population-based cohort study (EPIC-Heidelberg). Heart. 2011;97(1):49–54.
186. Wagner MM, Bhattacharya S, Visser J, Hannaford PC, Bloemenkamp KW. Association between miscarriage and cardiovascular disease in a Scottish cohort. Heart. 2015; 101(24):1954–60.
187. Heida KY, Velthuis BK, Oudijk MA, Reitsma JB, Bots ML, Franx A, et al. Cardiovascular disease risk in women with a history of spontaneous preterm delivery: a systematic review and meta-analysis. Eur J Prev Cardiol. 2016;23(3):253–63.
188. Tranquilli AL, Brown MA, Zeeman GG, Dekker G, Sibai BM. The definition of severe and early-onset preeclampsia. Statements from the International Society for the Study of Hypertension in Pregnancy (ISSHP). Pregnancy Hypertension. 2013;3(1):44–7.
189. Cartwright JE, Fraser R, Leslie K, Wallace AE, James JL. Remodelling at the maternal-fetal interface: relevance to human pregnancy disorders. Reproduction. 2010;140(6):803–13.
190. Tranquilli AL, Dekker G, Magee L, Roberts J, Sibai BM, Steyn W, et al. The classification, diagnosis and management of the hypertensive disorders of pregnancy: a revised statement from the ISSHP. Pregnancy Hypertension. 2014;4(2):97–104.
191. Redman CW, Sacks GP, Sargent IL. Preeclampsia: an excessive maternal inflammatory response to pregnancy. Am J Obstet Gynecol. 1999;180(2 Pt 1):499–506.
192. Sattar N, Greer IA. Pregnancy complications and maternal cardiovascular risk: opportunities for intervention and screening? BMJ. 2002;325(7356):157–60.
193. Bellamy L, Casas JP, Hingorani AD, Williams DJ. Pre-eclampsia and risk of cardiovascular disease and cancer in later life: systematic review and meta-analysis. BMJ. 2007;335(7627):974.
194. Ray JG, Vermeulen MJ, Schull MJ, Redelmeier DA. Cardiovascular health after maternal placental syndromes (CHAMPS): population-based retrospective cohort study. Lancet. 2005;366(9499):1797–803.
195. Wikstrom AK, Haglund B, Olovsson M, Lindeberg SN. The risk of maternal ischaemic heart disease after gestational hypertensive disease. BJOG. 2005;112(11):1486–91.
196. McDonald SD, Malinowski A, Zhou Q, Yusuf S, Devereaux PJ. Cardiovascular sequelae of preeclampsia/eclampsia: a systematic review and meta-analyses. Am Heart J. 2008; 156(5):918–30.
197. Wilson BJ, Watson MS, Prescott GJ, Sunderland S, Campbell DM, Hannaford P, et al. Hypertensive diseases of pregnancy and risk of hypertension and stroke in later life: results from cohort study. BMJ. 2003;326(7394):845.
198. Kessous R, Shoham-Vardi I, Pariente G, Sergienko R, Sheiner E. Long-term maternal atherosclerotic morbidity in women with pre-eclampsia. Heart. 2015;101(6):442–6.

199. Veerbeek JH, Hermes W, Breimer AY, van Rijn BB, Koenen SV, Mol BW, et al. Cardiovascular disease risk factors after early-onset preeclampsia, late-onset preeclampsia, and pregnancy-induced hypertension. Hypertension. 2015;65(3):600–6.
200. Hausvater A, Giannone T, Sandoval YH, Doonan RJ, Antonopoulos CN, Matsoukis IL, et al. The association between preeclampsia and arterial stiffness. J Hypertens. 2012; 30(1):17–33.
201. Goel A, Maski MR, Bajracharya S, Wenger JB, Zhang D, Salahuddin S, et al. Epidemiology and mechanisms of de novo and persistent hypertension in the postpartum period. Circulation. 2015;132(18):1726–33.
202. Aukes AM, De Groot JC, Wiegman MJ, Aarnoudse JG, Sanwikarja GS, Zeeman GG. Long-term cerebral imaging after pre-eclampsia. BJOG. 2012;119(9):1117–22.
203. Yarde F, Maas AH, Franx A, Eijkemans MJ, Drost JT, van Rijn BB, et al. Serum AMH levels in women with a history of preeclampsia suggest a role for vascular factors in ovarian aging. J Clin Endocrinol Metab. 2014;99(2):579–86.
204. Visser S, Hermes W, Ket JC, Otten RH, van Pampus MG, Bloemenkamp KW, et al. Systematic review and metaanalysis on nonclassic cardiovascular biomarkers after hypertensive pregnancy disorders. Am J Obstet Gynecol. 2014;211(4):373 e1–9.
205. Roberts JM, Hubel CA. The two stage model of preeclampsia: variations on the theme. Placenta. 2009;30 Suppl A:S32–7.
206. Karumanchi SA, Granger JP. Preeclampsia and pregnancy-related hypertensive disorders. Hypertension. 2016;67(2):238–42.
207. Sattar N, Ramsay J, Crawford L, Cheyne H, Greer IA. Classic and novel risk factor parameters in women with a history of preeclampsia. Hypertension. 2003;42(1):39–42.
208. Drost JT, Maas AH, Holewijn S, Joosten LA, van Eyck J, van der Schouw YT, et al. Novel cardiovascular biomarkers in women with a history of early preeclampsia. Atherosclerosis. 2014;237(1):117–22.
209. Gaugler-Senden IP, Tamsma JT, van der Bent C, Kusters R, Steegers EA, de Groot CJ. Angiogenic factors in women ten years after severe very early onset preeclampsia. PLoS One. 2012;7(8):e43637.
210. Pruthi D, Khankin EV, Blanton RM, Aronovitz M, Burke SD, McCurley A, et al. Exposure to experimental preeclampsia in mice enhances the vascular response to future injury. Hypertension. 2015;65(4):863–70.
211. Roes EM, Raijmakers MT, Schoonenberg M, Wanner N, Peters WH, Steegers EA. Physical well-being in women with a history of severe preeclampsia. J Matern Fetal Neonatal Med. 2005;18(1):39–45.
212. Hoedjes M, Berks D, Vogel I, Franx A, Duvekot JJ, Steegers EA, et al. Poor health-related quality of life after severe preeclampsia. Birth. 2011;38(3):246–55.
213. Brusse IA, Duvekot JJ, Meester I, Jansen G, Rizopoulos D, Steegers EA, et al. Electroencephalography in normotensive and hypertensive pregnancies and subsequent quality of life. PLoS One. 2016;11(5):e0155299.
214. Mommersteeg PM, Drost JT, Ottervanger JP, Maas AH. Long-term follow-up of psychosocial distress after early onset preeclampsia: the Preeclampsia Risk EValuation in FEMales cohort study. J Psychosom Obstet Gynaecol. 2016;37(3):101-9.
215. Drost JT, van der Schouw YT, Herber-Gast GC, Maas AH. More vasomotor symptoms in menopause among women with a history of hypertensive pregnancy diseases compared with women with normotensive pregnancies. Menopause. 2013;20(10):1006–11.
216. Spaan J, Peeters L, Spaanderman M, Brown M. Cardiovascular risk management after a hypertensive disorder of pregnancy. Hypertension. 2012;60(6):1368–73.
217. Amaya-Amaya J, Montoya-Sanchez L, Rojas-Villarraga A. Cardiovascular involvement in autoimmune diseases. Biomed Res Int. 2014;2014:367359.
218. Mason JC, Libby P. Cardiovascular disease in patients with chronic inflammation: mechanisms underlying premature cardiovascular events in rheumatologic conditions. Eur Heart J. 2015;36(8):482-9c.

219. Charakida M, Besler C, Batuca JR, Sangle S, Marques S, Sousa M, et al. Vascular abnormalities, paraoxonase activity, and dysfunctional HDL in primary antiphospholipid syndrome. JAMA. 2009;302(11):1210–7.
220. Agca R, Heslinga SC, van Halm VP, Nurmohamed MT. Atherosclerotic cardiovascular disease in patients with chronic inflammatory joint disorders. Heart. 2016;102(10):790–5.
221. Gianturco L, Bodini BD, Atzeni F, Colombo C, Stella D, Sarzi-Puttini P, et al. Cardiovascular and autoimmune diseases in females: the role of microvasculature and dysfunctional endothelium. Atherosclerosis. 2015;241(1):259–63.
222. Faccini A, Kaski JC, Camici PG. Coronary microvascular dysfunction in chronic inflammatory rheumatoid diseases. Eur Heart J. 2016;37(23):1799–806.
223. Powell J, Wojnarowska F, Winsey S, Marren P, Welsh K. Lichen sclerosus premenarche: autoimmunity and immunogenetics. Br J Dermatol. 2000;142(3):481–4.
224. Shoenfeld Y, Gerli R, Doria A, Matsuura E, Cerinic MM, Ronda N, et al. Accelerated atherosclerosis in autoimmune rheumatic diseases. Circulation. 2005;112(21):3337–47.
225. Sodergren A, Stegmayr B, Lundberg V, Ohman ML, Wallberg-Jonsson S. Increased incidence of and impaired prognosis after acute myocardial infarction among patients with seropositive rheumatoid arthritis. Ann Rheum Dis. 2007;66(2):263–6.
226. Mantel A, Holmqvist M, Jernberg T, Wallberg-Jonsson S, Askling J. Rheumatoid arthritis is associated with a more severe presentation of acute coronary syndrome and worse short-term outcome. Eur Heart J. 2015;36(48):3413–22.
227. Avina-Zubieta JA, Choi HK, Sadatsafavi M, Etminan M, Esdaile JM, Lacaille D. Risk of cardiovascular mortality in patients with rheumatoid arthritis: a meta-analysis of observational studies. Arthritis Rheum. 2008;59(12):1690–7.
228. Nochioka K, Biering-Sorensen T, Hansen KW, Sorensen R, Pedersen S, Jorgensen PG, et al. Long-term outcomes in patients with rheumatologic disorders undergoing percutaneous coronary intervention: a BAsel Stent Kosten-Effektivitats Trial-PROspective Validation Examination (BASKET-PROVE) sub-study. Eur Heart J Acute Cardiovasc Care 2016.
229. Kurth T, Gaziano JM, Cook NR, Logroscino G, Diener HC, Buring JE. Migraine and risk of cardiovascular disease in women. JAMA. 2006;296(3):283–91.
230. Spector JT, Kahn SR, Jones MR, Jayakumar M, Dalal D, Nazarian S. Migraine headache and ischemic stroke risk: an updated meta-analysis. Am J Med. 2010;123(7):612–24.
231. Kurth T, Winter AC, Eliassen AH, Dushkes R, Mukamal KJ, Rimm EB, et al. Migraine and risk of cardiovascular disease in women: prospective cohort study. BMJ. 2016;353:i2610.
232. Napoli R, Guardasole V, Zarra E, Matarazzo M, D'Anna C, Sacca F, et al. Vascular smooth muscle cell dysfunction in patients with migraine. Neurology. 2009;72(24):2111–4.
233. Malik R, Freilinger T, Winsvold BS, Anttila V, Vander Heiden J, Traylor M, et al. Shared genetic basis for migraine and ischemic stroke: a genome-wide analysis of common variants. Neurology. 2015;84(21):2132–45.
234. van Hemert S, Breedveld AC, Rovers JM, Vermeiden JP, Witteman BJ, Smits MG, et al. Migraine associated with gastrointestinal disorders: review of the literature and clinical implications. Front Neurol. 2014;5:241.
235. Richards T, Montori VM, Godlee F, Lapsley P, Paul D. Let the patient revolution begin. BMJ. 2013;346:f2614.
236. McManus RJ, Mant J, Haque MS, Bray EP, Bryan S, Greenfield SM, et al. Effect of self-monitoring and medication self-titration on systolic blood pressure in hypertensive patients at high risk of cardiovascular disease: the TASMIN-SR randomized clinical trial. JAMA. 2014;312(8):799–808.
237. Arrieta A, Woods JR, Qiao N, Jay SJ. Cost-benefit analysis of home blood pressure monitoring in hypertension diagnosis and treatment: an insurer perspective. Hypertension. 2014;64(4):891–6.

Chapter 2
Ischemic Heart Disease in Women

Angela H.E.M. Maas and C. Noel Bairey Merz

Abstract Women have different manifestations of ischemic heart disease (IHD) than men throughout their lifetime. At middle-age they have more often non-obstructive coronary artery disease (NOCAD) and coronary vascular dysfunction rather than obstructive, focal coronary artery disease (CAD). Differences in underlying pathophysiology translate into a different presentation of symptoms among both genders. This needs a more gender-sensitive diagnostic and therapeutic approach as discussed in this chapter.

Keywords Coronary angiography • Coronary artery disease (CAD) • Coronary interventions • Focal coronary artery disease • Fractional flow reserve (FFR) • Functional coronary testing • Gender symptoms • Gender diagnostic testing • Ischemic heart disease (IHD) • Medical treatment • Menopause • Non-obstructive CAD (NOCAD) • Stable angina pectoris

Sex and Gender Differences in Pattern of Ischemic Heart Disease

An important sex difference is the progression of coronary atherosclerosis into more vulnerable plaques which develops later in women than in men [1–3]. The many data that have been obtained from invasive and non-invasive population studies have clearly shown that there is a female- pattern of ischemic heart disease (IHD), as

A.H.E.M. Maas, M.D., Ph.D. (✉)
Department of Cardiology, Women's Cardiac Health Program, Radboud University Medical Center, Nijmegen, The Netherlands
e-mail: angela.maas@radboudumc.nl

C.N. Bairey Merz, M.D.
Director Barbra Streisand Women's Heart Center, Linda Joy Pollin Women's Heart Health Program, Director Preventive Cardiac Center,
Cedars-Sinai, Los Angeles, USA
e-mail: noel.baireymerz@cshs.org

A.H.E.M. Maas, C.N. Bairey Merz (eds.), *Manual of Gynecardiology*,
DOI 10.1007/978-3-319-54960-6_2

summarized in Fig. 2.1 [4–7]. Women have a smaller diameter of the coronary arteries, when corrected for body surface area, compared to men. Plaque morphology shows clinical relevant sex differences with fewer calcifications, less focal obstruction and a more diffuse pattern of atherosclerosis with 'outward remodeling' and 'soft' plaques in women than in men at all ages [8–12]. Combined structural and functional disorders of the coronary circulation are involved in various manifestations of IHD. In the large Swedish coronary angiography and angioplasty register (SCAAR) almost 80% of women under 60 years of age with stable angina symptoms had no visible coronary obstructions at angiography, compared with 40%

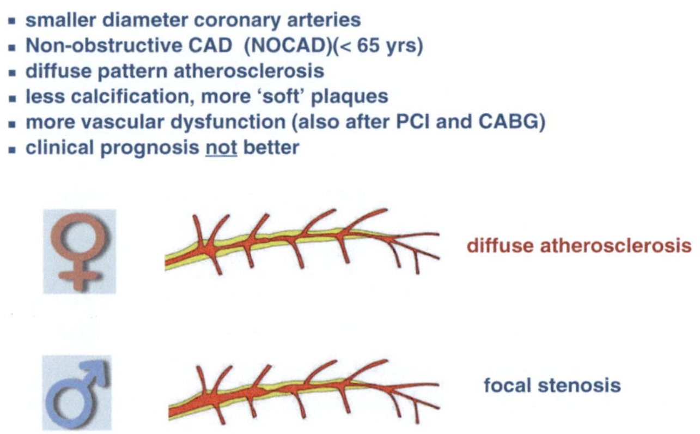

Fig. 2.1 Female pattern of IHD

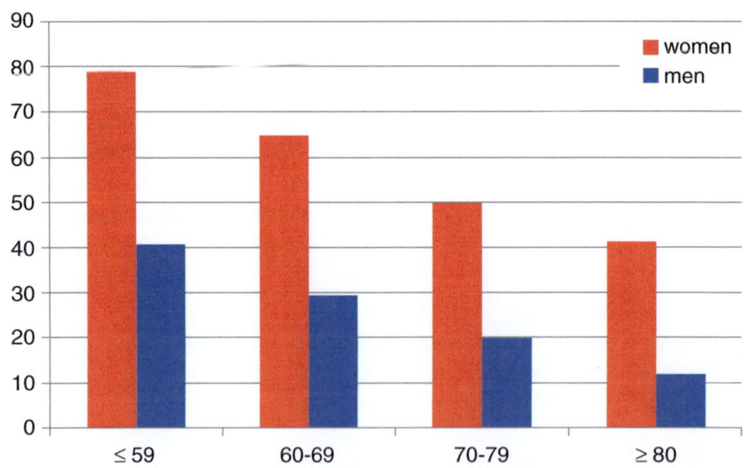

Fig. 2.2 Percentage 'normal' CAG's in patients with stable angina (ref 13)

of men (Fig. 2.2) [13]. Women have twice as often a pattern of non-obstructive coronary artery disease (NOCAD) with coronary vascular dysfunction, which has important consequences for their clinical symptoms, diagnostic strategies, treatment options and outcomes. The prognosis of severe calcified plaques is worse in men than women, while the extent of NOCAD and 'soft' plaques predicts mortality in women but not in men [14, 15]. Women with stable angina and NOCAD are three times more likely to experience a cardiac event within the first year after diagnosis than their male counterparts [16]. In symptomatic women with NOCAD the 5 year IHD event rate is almost 50% higher than in symptomatic women with 'normal' coronary arteries [17, 18]. In the Copenhagen City Heart study the prognosis of NOCAD in women was shown to be comparable to the more obstructive pattern of CAD as it is more frequently present in men [19]. Although atherosclerosis often progresses towards flow-limiting stenoses over time, acute coronary syndromes (ACS) predominantly arise from non-obstructive lesions [20]. The advances in new imaging modalities over the past decades urge clinicians to apply a more sex- and gender-sensitive approach for the detection of IHD and to leave behind coronary angiography as the gold standard [21–23]. This is especially important for female patients, as they are still less well diagnosed and treated than men [24].

Non-obstructive Coronary Artery Disease (NOCAD)

In patients with non-obstructive CAD at coronary angiography, lesions up to 20% can be present, without being noticed [18]. However, with coronary intravascular ultrasound techniques (IVUS) it has been shown that in most patients with suspected IHD without signs of obstructive CAD coronary plaques are already present [25]. Non-obstructive CAD has been found to be associated with a significantly greater 1-year risk of ACS and all-cause mortality, compared with no apparent CAD [26]. Symptoms of IHD are often caused by a combination of atherosclerosis, endothelial dysfunction and spasm in the macro- and microvascular coronary arteries together with activated inflammation and platelet function (Fig. 2.3) [27]. Within all these causative components of IHD important sex differences exist throughout all various stages of life [4]. In clinical practice, an important dilemma is that the agreement between anatomical CAD and functional IHD is rather poor [28, 29]. This is especially disadvantageous for younger women (45–65 years) in whom functional and more diffuse CAD often predominates over focal obstructive CAD (Fig. 2.4). The over-emphasis of obstructive CAD over NOCAD in the current US and ESC guidelines stable CAD is one of the major reasons that symptoms and risk factors in women are still less well treated than in men [30, 31]. Women with recurrent chest pain syndromes and NOCAD need to be diagnosed and treated since they have a twofold increased risk to develop obstructive CAD events in the next 5–8 years and have a four times higher risk for re-hospitalizations and recurrent angiograms than women without these symptoms [32, 33].

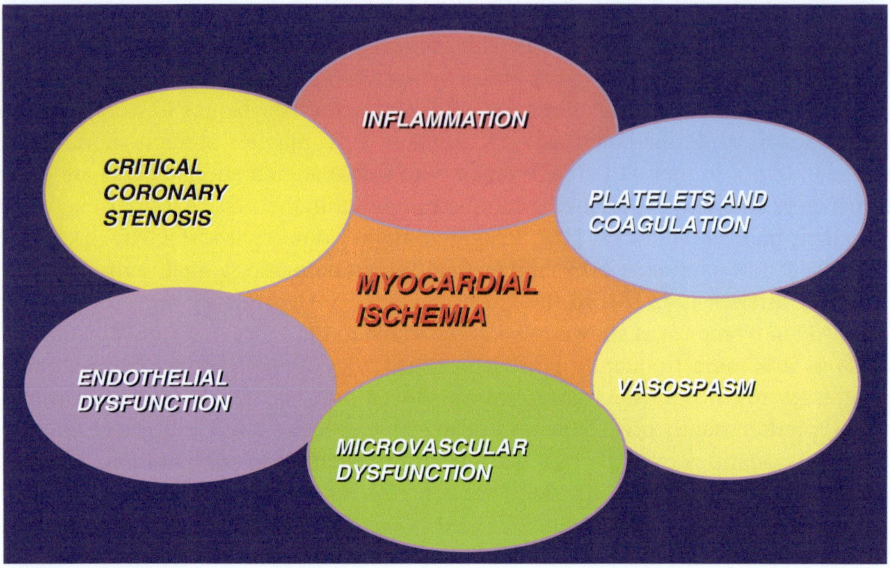

Fig. 2.3 Spectrum of factors involved in ischemic heart disease

Fig. 2.4 Development ischemic heart disease (IHD) in women

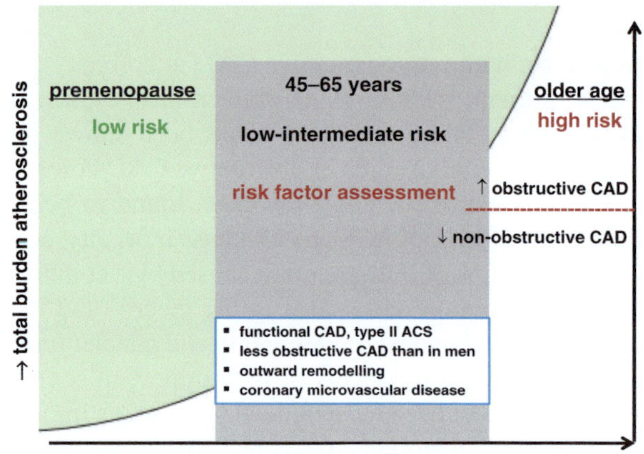

Diagnosis of Ischemic Heart Disease: Need for a More Sex and Gender-appropriate Approach

The clinical evaluation of symptoms of angina pectoris in women is still considered along the male standard. However, the various sex differences in underlying pathophysiological mechanisms involved in IHD often translate into other symptoms than the classical angina pectoris, which is more associated with obstructive CAD (Table 2.1). The combination of NOCAD with endothelial dysfunction

Table 2.1 classification of chest pain[a] with female-specific aspects (–)

Typical angina (definite)	Meets three of the following characteristics: • Oppressive substernal chest discomfort • Provoked by exertion or emotional stress • Relieved by rest and/or nitrates within minutes – **Squeezing, tight, chest discomfort** – **Radiation to chest, jaw(s), left armpit and/or left arm, neck, Shoulders and inter-scapular area** – **May last longer than minutes** – **Crescendo /decrescendo character (spasm)** – **Dyspnea, anxiety, mental stress-related** – **Extreme tiredness, also often after angina**
Atypical angina (probable)	Meets two criteria – **Both typical and atypical symptoms in NOCAD**
Non-anginal chest pain	Lacks or meets only one characteristic criterium – **Beware of cardiac anxiety disorder**

[a]Adapted from Montalescot G et al. 2013 ESC guidelines stable CAD [31]

frequently occurs in young and middle-aged women with a combined typical and atypical symptom presentation, that may be misinterpreted as being of non-cardiac origin [34]. The classification of symptoms in *typical* or *atypical* alone has been shown to be unreliable for the detection of obstructive CAD in women under 55 years of age [35]. Black women have an even more atypical symptom presentation than white women, which may be an extra barrier to appropriate and timely treatment [36]. It is therefore mandatory to simultaneously consider lifestyle behavior and CVD risk factors when evaluating symptoms. In general, women have more symptoms of chest pain than men, leading to recurrent presentations at the emergency department and repeated coronary angiograms (CAG) [4, 32, 37]. The diffuse pattern of CAD can easily be missed at angiography in young high risk women and mistakenly being interpreted as 'small female coronary arteries'. In Patient example A this has mistakenly led to the conclusion that she had a 'false-positive' X-test. After 65 years of age the mode of CAD in women gradually changes into more obstructive stenoses, also depending on the individual CV risk profile. The higher the chance of having focal obstructive CAD, the more classical (male) symptoms of angina pectoris women will have (Patient B). When the underlying degree of obstructive CAD is similar as in men, there is no apparent gender difference any longer in symptom presentation [38]. However, this selection bias in coronary stenoses is not reflecting daily clinical practice. In addition, the increasing prevalence of vascular stiffness and diastolic dysfunction in women at older age leads to additional symptoms of dyspnea, tiredness and loss of condition that can make it more difficult to establish the diagnosis of IHD (Patient C) [39]. At older age (> 70 years) and in diabetic patients symptoms of angina may become more atypical in both women and men. Also, the occurrence of paroxysmal atrial fibrillation (AF) and diastolic heart failure (HFpEF) is a common manifestation of IHD in the elderly and predominates in women over men [40].

Patient A Woman with diffuse CAD at angiography, mistakenly interpreted as 'normal'

46 year old woman has symptoms of chest pain with radiation to the jaws both at rest and during exercise. Her symptoms started 6 months ago and can be provoked by heavy exercise. They also occur at rest and in bed early in the morning. She cannot predict her symptoms very well.
She is premenopausal, non smoking and has several first degree family members with premature CVD and dyslipidemia. She uses no medication.

Physical exam: BMI 23 kg/m², RR 120/80mmHg, no abnormalities at auscultation.

Lab: Total cholesterol 7.3 mmol/l, HDL-C 1.0 mmol/l, LDL-C 5.5 mmol/l , TG 2.8 mmol/l

ECG at rest:

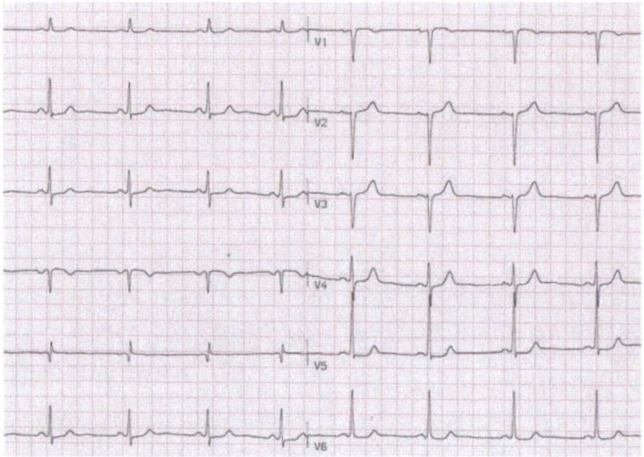

positive ECG at max. exercise (150 W 2 min.)
Chest pain during test.

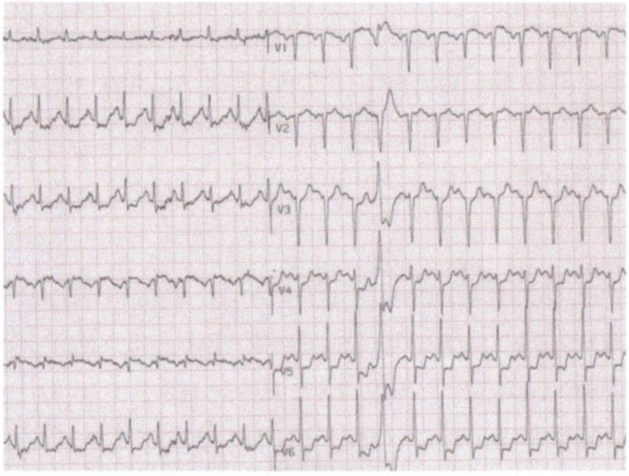

Comments: At CAG the branches of the LCA show very diffuse CAD. (no IVUS done)
Patient was mistakenly sent home with the message of having a false-positive X-test and 'normal coronary arteries'.
Her X-test was real-positive however, due to very diffuse CAD in the LCA, related to her familial dyslipidemia.

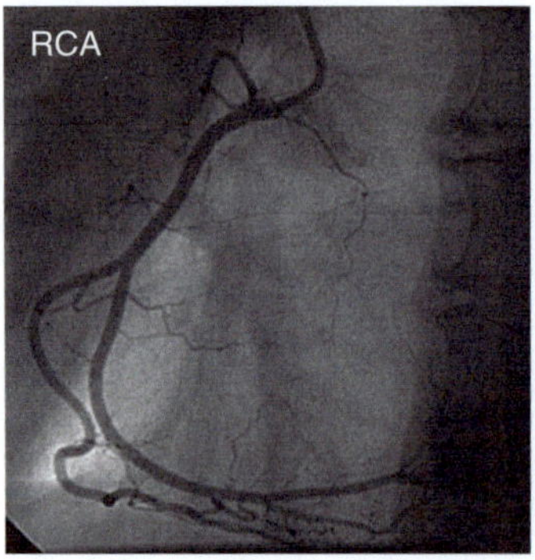

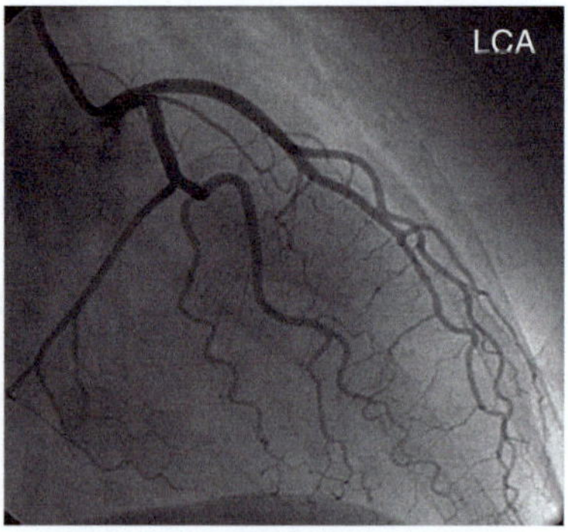

Patient B. Woman 53 years with typical angina

Medical history: at 38 years hysterectomy (ovaria in situ)

Patient history:

Since 10 months patient has gradual increasing symptoms of chest pain during brisk walking, climbing the stairs, cycling and at stress. She has radiation to the jaws and left arm, sometimes between her shoulderblades. Her symptoms are relieved at rest. Gradually she has learned to avoid heavy exercise. She is known with familial hypertension since15 years and has frequent symptoms of hot flushes. She never smoked, had no pregnancies. Her father died (ACS) at 58 years. She has a busy job as an architect. Thus far, her symptoms have been attributed to 'menopause', but she considers heart disease.
Medication use: ARB and b-blocker for her hypertension.

Physical exam: BMI 23 kg/m^2, RR 160/85 mmHg, auscultation normal

Laboratory: Total cholesterol 5.2 mmol/l, HDL 2.2 mmol/l, TG 1.2 mmol/l, LDL 2.5 mmol/l (using simvastatin 10mg)

ECG: sinusrithm 67/min, normal

ECHO: slight hypertrophy proximal septum, LV function normal, no regional wall abnormalities, no signs of LVH or diastolic dysfunction.

X-test: 160Watt , MHR 95% norm (159/min), slight chest pain, non-significant ST-T changes with a blood pressure of 160/85 mmHg before the test, which was Interpreted as a 'doubtful' test.

A SPECT CCTA was performed.

CCTA: CAC50 (80th percentile), with > 70% lesion mid-LAD

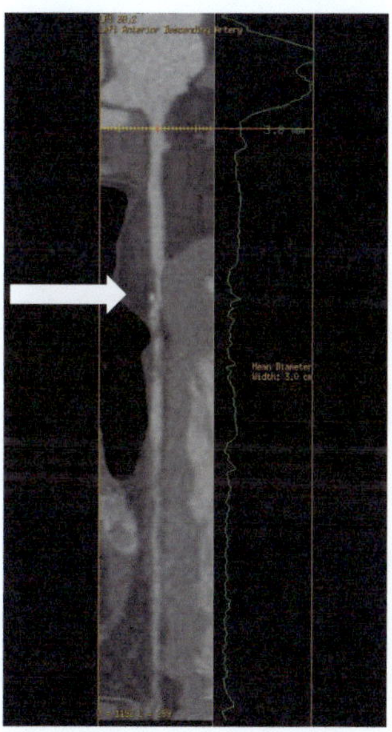

SPECT: reversible ischemia anterior-apical

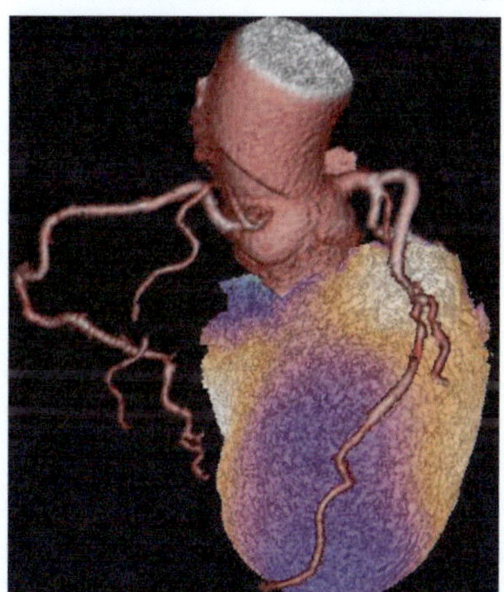

Discussion: At CAG a severe LAD stenosis was found, which was succesfully treated with PCI + stenting with DES. Afterwards she is symptom-free using a statin, antiplatelet therapy and triple medication for her hypertension

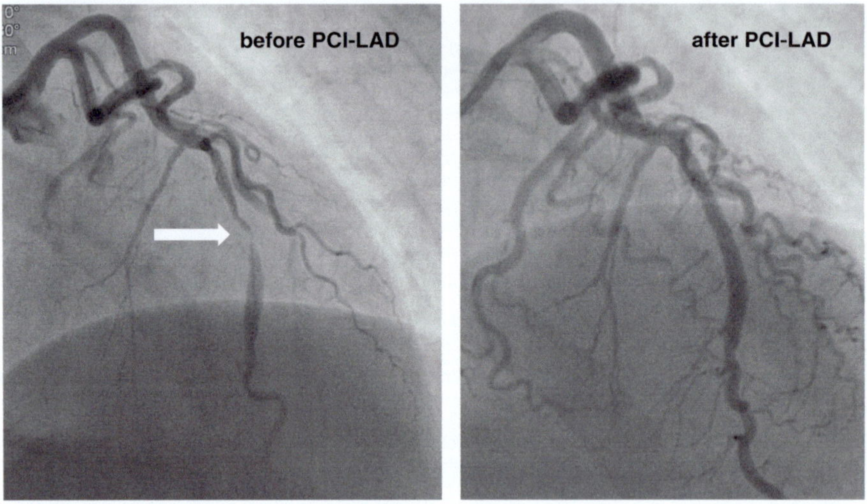

Patient C: **Woman 68 years with multivessel non-obstructive CAD (NOCAD)**

Medical history:
menarche at 18 years; menopause at 40 years
familial hypertension and dyslipidemia
age 58 : PCI-LAD
age 59 : re PCI-LAD
age 64 : PCI-RCX, iatrogenic dissection LM + stent
age 67 : CAG; NOCAD RCA, LAD, < 50% RCX, 95% small D1, conservative.
2× TIA during last 10 years

Patient history:
Since her first PCI 10 years ago, symptoms of chest pain have never disappeard . She often feels a continuous, daily, nagging pain in her back and left arm, which increases at exercise. There is relief with short acting nitrates. Also symptoms of dyspnea, occuring with minor exercise. She has hypertension since many years, just like her parents had. Positive family risk for CVD, one brother has died at 58 years. Sixteen years ago she quitted smoking. Uncomplicated prior pregnancies. Medication: ASA, statin, ACE, B blocker, long-acting nitrates, calcium antagonist, antacids.

Physical examination: BMI 30.4 kg/m^2, RR 143/84 mmHg, at auscultation soft ejection murmur, no wheezingg or peripheral edema.

Lab: normal (with statin)

ECG: SR 66/min, normal axis and repolarization

ECHO: EF 68%, grade 1 diastolic dysfunction

CAG: mid RCA 30%, RCX 30%, stents in LM and LAD good. Prox 70% stenosis small S1.

Comments: this patient has symptoms related to a combination of NOCAD, vascular dysfunction, hypertension and age-related grade1 diastolic dysfunction. This should be treated with healthy lifestyle behaviour and appropriate medication for her blood pressure and anginal symptoms.

Gender differences in communication may hamper the early recognition of angina pectoris in women. Men usually report their symptoms in a direct way, while female patients ask more questions, present more and diverse symptoms and give more detailed histories of their activities [41]. Women's communication is more likely to be emotional, subjective, polite, and self-revealing with more concern and awareness for the feelings of others. This can be misleading to both female patients and their doctors in the correct interpretation of symptoms of IHD.

Non-invasive Testing for IHD: Which Test to Choose for Individual Women

The classic Diamond & Forrester prediction risk model overestimates the chance of having obstructive (≥ 50%) CAD in women and has been updated in 2011 and incorporated in the 2013 ESC guidelines treatment of stable CAD (Fig. 2.5) [31, 42, 43]. Especially in the age-group below 60 years non-invasive imaging techniques should be used more often than invasive angiography. There is still no consensus however for the optimal diagnostic pathway for IHD among the various guidelines in women [31, 44–46]. The 2013 ESC guideline advises stress imaging techniques (SPECT, stress echocardiography) when available as first test of choice, with a preference of non-radiation diagnostics in younger women [31]. The optimal classification criteria of patients into low- intermediate- and high risk categories is also still a matter of debate. The algorithm to classify symptomatic women in IHD risk categories is depicted in Table 2.2 [47–49]. The ESC has recently released the 2016 EU guideline CVD prevention, containing four categories of risk patients (Fig. 2.6) [50].

In 2014 a consensus document for women with suspected IHD was published by the AHA, providing sex- and gender-specific evidence-based guidance to the clinician in the use of diagnostic procedures [51]. In Table 2.3 the most important guidance advice is summarized [52] and in Table 2.4 factors are described that may hamper the sensitivity of non-invasive testing in women. In the large PROMISE trial, performed in predominantly middle-aged patients (m/f) at intermediate IHD

	Typical angina		Atypical angina		Non-anginal pain	
Age	Men	Women	Men	Women	Men	Women
30–39	59	28	29	10	18	5
40–49	69	37	38	14	25	8
50–59	77	47	49	20	34	12
60–69	84	58	59	28	44	17
70–79	89	68	69	37	54	24
>80	93	76	78	47	65	32

Fig. 2.5 Clinical pre-test probabilities in patients with stable chest pain syndromes (ref 43)

Table 2.2 Risk classification of symptomatic women

Low risk when all present: optimal CVD health	• Blood pressure 120/80 mmHg (untreated) • Normal lipid spectrum (untreated) • Normal glucose <6,5 mmol/L • BMI< 25 kg/m^2 • Non-smoking • Healthy diet/regular exercise • Age <45 years /premenopausal
Intermediate risk presence ≥2 RF	– Current smoking – SBP ≥128/80 mmHg, DBP ≥80 mmHg, or medication – Lipid abnormalities; T chol/HDL ratio >4, medication – Obesity, BMI ≥30 kg/m^2 – Unhealthy diet/ sedentary lifestyle – Metabolic syndrome (MetS) – Family: CVD in first degree relatives (<55 M; < 65 F) – Signs subclinical CVD (IMT; CAC etc.) – Systemic disease (SLE; RA, SLE, fibromyalgia) – Previous hypertensive pregnancy; gestational diabetes – Age ≥45 years., postmenopausal
High risk presence ≥1 RF	Documented CAD, previous coronary event Prior stroke Peripheral arterial disease (PAD) Aortic aneurysm Renal dysfunction (GFR < 30) (severe) diabetes mellitus 10-years CVD risk ≥10%

Adapted from Douglas PS, et al., NEJM 1996; Mieres JH, et al., Circulation 2005; Mosca L et al. Circulation 2011; [47–49]

Very high risk	❑ Documented CVD, clinical or unequivocal on imaging. Documented clinical CVD includes previous AMI, ACS, coronary revascularization and other arterial revascularization procedures, stroke, TIA, aortic aneurysm and PAD. ❑ Unequivocally documented CVD on imaging includes plaque on coronary angiography or carotid ultrasound. NOT included: some increase in continuous imaging parameters such as CIMT. ❑ DM with target organ damage such as proteinuria or with a major risk factor such as smoking or marked hypercholesterolemia or hypertension. ❑ Severe CKD (GFR <30 mL/min/1.73 m2). ❑ A calculated SCORE ≥10%.
High risk	❑ Markedly elevated single risk factors, in particular cholesterol >8 mmol/L (>310 mg/dL)(e.g. in familial hypercholesterolemia) or BP ≥180/110 mmHg. ❑ Most other people with DM (with the exception of young people with type 1 DM and without major risk factors that may be at low or moderate risk). ❑ Moderate CKD (GFR 30–59 mL/min/1.73 m2). ❑ A calculated SCORE ≥5% and <10%.
Moderate risk	❑ SCORE is ≥1% and <5% at 10 years. Many middle aged subjects belong to this category.
Low risk	❑ SCORE <1%.

ACS acute coronary syndrome
AMI acute myocardial infarction
BP blood pressure
CKD chronic kidney disease
DM diabetes mellitus
PAD peripheral artery disease
SCORE systematic coronary risk estimation
TIA transient ischemic attack

Fig. 2.6 Risk categories 2016 ESC guidelines CVD prevention (Ref 50)

Table 2.3 Guidance for ischemic heart disease (IHD) testing in women

1. Non-obstructive CAD (NOCAD) is more common in women than in men. The presence of signs of ischemia in NOCAD predisposes to more adverse events
2. Women have more atypical symptoms than men and these are more often provoked by emotional than physical stress
3. Evaluate risk: low-intermediate-high risk. No further testing in *low risk* women
4. **Low risk:** premenopausal, non-smoking and non-diabetic women **Intermediate risk**: presence of several traditional RF **High-risk:** PAD, (poorly controlled) diabetes mellitus, stroke or previous TIA, chronic kidney disease (CKD) and poor exercise capacity (<5 Mets)
5. In *intermediate risk* women initial bicycle (treadmill) exercise (X) testing is first choice of testing
6. In intermediate risk women who are unable to exercise, testing with CCTA, nuclear imaging, MRI or stress echo is preferred (depending on availability and preference)
7. X- test interpretation includes: exercise capacity, chronotropic response, heart rate recovery, blood pressure course and ST- segment changes
8. Post-stress test risk stratification (depending on test) is based on the extent and severity of inducible ischemia as well as detectable CAD, EF reduction and calcium score ≥400

Adapted from Mieres JH et al. [51, 52]

Table 2.4 Factors hampering the sensitivity of noninvasive testing for IHD in women

• Smaller diameter coronary arteries
• More diffuse pattern of CAD
• NOCAD combined with coronary microvascular disease (CMD)
• Hypertension, inducing ECG changes at rest and/or during X testing
• Cardiac co-morbidity (valvular disease/LVH) in the elderly
• Insufficient exercise capacity at older age (& co-morbidity)
• False-positive x-tests in premenopause
Breast tissue artefacts (nuclear imaging)

risk, initial anatomical testing with computed tomographic angiography (CTA) or functional (exercise or pharmacological) testing with electrocardiography, nuclear stress imaging or stress echocardiography, did not show any differences in clinical outcomes over a median follow-up duration of 2 years [53]. However, at a closer sex-specific analysis women had a higher prevalence of traditional CVD risk factors, but were estimated to be at lower risk by their doctors [54]. Women were more often referred for nuclear imaging stress testing than men, but had fewer positive tests. Women seem to derive more prognostic information from a CTA, whereas men tend to derive similar prognostic value from both test types [55]. It is noteworthy that with the use of the current available diagnostic testing the full spectrum of manifestations of IHD is still underestimated in women [56].

In the initial clinical work-up of women at intermediate risk cardiologist should choose for imaging testing that is available and which they are accustomed with. Coronary angiography is indicated in women at intermediate or high risk with functional disability and an abnormal rest-ECG or X-test. New developing non-invasive imaging modalities such as combined fractional flow reserve (FFR)-CT scans are promising for women by the combination of anatomical and functional testing [44, 57]. This also accounts for upcoming combined CTA-PET imaging.

Coronary Angiography, Fractional Flow Reserve and Elective PCI in Women

Invasive coronary angiography has more limited value in women, since they have more outward remodeling, NOCAD and functional IHD that is not well recognized at angiography. However, its diagnostic value increases with age and with a more classical symptom presentation of exercise-induced angina, mimicking the typical 'male' pattern of symptoms. Comparable data from registries show that nearly two thirds of women with stable angina pectoris have (nearly) no abnormalities at angiography [13, 33, 58]. An important limitation of diagnostic angiography is the inability to assess the hemodynamic relevance of a coronary stenosis whereas the functional severity of a lesion can be easily over- or underestimated [28, 29, 59]. As a consequence, an incorrect indication for coronary angiography may also lead to an inappropriate percutaneous coronary intervention (PCI) or even coronary artery bypass graft (CABG). This is especially harmful for women, as they have more residual symptoms after coronary interventions than men [60–62]. The use of fractional flow reserve-guided PCI for stable IHD has improved outcomes in both genders [63, 64]. Fractional flow reserve (FFR) values are found to be higher in women after correction for visually assessed coronary anatomic severity. This may be (partly) caused by the more frequent presence of coronary vascular dysfunction in women [65]. It is currently discussed whether gender-specific guidelines in interpreting fractional flow reserve measurements are indicated [65, 66]. The use of IVUS and or optical coherence tomography (OCT) should be more applied in symptomatic women with NOCAD to characterize coronary plaques as strong arguments for adequate prevention and treatment [25, 46]. Outcomes after coronary stenting have improved in women with the new generations drug eluting stents (DES), which are more safe and effective on the long-term than bare-metal stents (BMS) [67].

Most common peri-procedural complication of coronary angiography or PCI is bleeding at the puncture site. This occurs more frequently in women, but less often with the transradial access [68, 69]. The latter may be more difficult to perform in women, due to spasm-related complications in the radial/brachial artery [70]. Besides the need to adapt dosages of anti-thrombotic agents to body surface are, there are also important sex differences in the thrombotic system that may account for the higher bleeding risk in women [71–73].

Non-invasive and Invasive Testing for Functional Ischemic Heart Disease

The presence of impaired (endothelial) vascular function without occlusive epicardial disease presents as global dysfunction of the macro- and micro vascular coronary circulation. Flow-mediated vasodilatation (FMD) of the brachial artery is perhaps the most known technique to measure endothelial function, and involves measuring response of brachial artery diameter to secondary to hyperemia due to occlusion of the brachial artery [74]. It is associated with coronary artery endothelial function [75]. This test is of limited use however in the clinical setting for IHD detection.

Invasive measurement of vascular dysfunction involves imaging of vasomotor responses of epicardial coronary arteries and functional testing with acetylcholine infusion and measuring coronary flow reserve (CFR) during cardiac catheterization [74]. The main limitation of these techniques however is the invasive nature and potential harmful test in inexperienced hands, making it less applicable for widespread use in cardiology practice. The Coronary Vasomotion Disorders International Study Group (COVADIS) has released a consensus statement as a guidance for coronary vasomotor disorders [76, 77]. The focus of this expert paper was vasospastic angina, which occurs more often in (middle-aged) women than in men. In Tables 2.5 and 2.6 the diagnostic criteria and interpretation of invasive coronary vascular testing are described. In many female patients at intermediate risk, with normal or near normal coronary arteries, having recurrent angina symptoms of presumably vasospastic origin, pragmatic treatment options may be chosen without additional invasive testing, see Patient D.

Patient D:

45 year old woman with recurrent angina symptoms due to hypertension with vascular dysfunction/spasm

Medical history:
Migraine in her teens
Miscarriage first pregnancy
2× preeclampsia and 1 normal pregnancy
Premature hypertension
NSTEMI 5 years ago: normal coronary arteries (type II ACS)

Patient history: Her blood pressure has remained high since her pregnancies with recurrent episodes of migraine. (without aura). Half a year ago she had severe chest pain and pain in both arms during several hours after a stressfull confrontation with her parents. This kind of symptoms occur more often at unexpected and stressful situations. Her blood pressure remains too high, despite combined medication (ACE and calcium antagonist). Family: mother also has hypertension, father migraine. She never smoked.

Physical examination: BMI 23 kg/m^2, RR 145/104 mmHg and 150/95 mmHg, auscultation normal

ECG: normal SR 56/min

ECHO: no structural abnormalities

Comments: young woman with premature hypertension and vascular dysfunction, that has acumulated into a type II ACS 5 years ago. She has residual symptoms related to stress and inappropriately treated hypertension. After better treatment of her blood pressure with triple therapy of ARB, a selective B blocker and diltiazem, she is currently without symptoms.

Table 2.5 Diagnostic criteria for vasospastic angina

1. Nitrate-responsive angina during spontaneous episode, with at least one of the following:	(a) Rest angina—especially between night and early morning (b) Marked diurnal variation in exercise tolerance—reduced in morning (c) Hyperventilation can precipitate an episode (d) Calcium channel blockers (but not b-blockers) suppress episodes
2. Transient ischemic ECG changes—during spontaneous episode in at least two contiguous leads:	(a) ST segment elevation ≥0.1 mV (b) ST segment depression ≥0.1 mV (c) New negative U waves
3. Coronary artery spasm—defined as transient total or subtotal coronary artery occlusion (>90% constriction) with angina and ischemic ECG changes	(a) spontaneously or (b) after provocative stimulus (typically acetylcholine, ergot, or hyperventilation)

Adapted from Beltrame JF et al., Eur Heart J 2015 [76]

Table 2.6 Recommendations for invasive testing of coronary artery spasm

Class I (strong)	History suspicious of VSA without documented episode, especially if: • Nitrate-responsive rest angina, and/or • Marked diurnal variation in symptom onset/exercise tolerance and/or • Rest angina with non-obstructive coronary artery disease (NOCAD) • Unresponsive to empiric therapy ACS presentation in the absence of a culprit lesion Unexplained resuscitated cardiac arrest Unexplained syncope with prior chest pain Recurrent rest angina following successful PCI
Class IIa (good)	Invasive testing for non-invasive diagnosed patients unresponsive to medical therapy Documented spontaneous episode of VSA to determine the 'site and mode' of spasm
Class IIb (controversial)	Invasive testing for non-invasive diagnosed patients responsive to Medical therapy
Class III (contraindications)	Emergent acute coronary syndrome Severe multi-vessel CAD including left main stenosis Severe myocardial dysfunction (Class IIb if symptoms suggestive of vasospasm) Patients without any symptoms suggestive of vasospastic angina

Adapted from Beltrame, JF et al. Eur Heart J 2015. [76]
ACS acute coronary syndrome, *CAD* coronary artery disease, *VSA* vasospastic angina

Medical Treatment of Stable Angina Pectoris in Women: Tailored Approach is the Key

In the 2013 ESC guidelines treatment stable CAD, no gender-specific advice is provided for the treatment of stable symptoms of angina [31]. Despite, from several surveys it is known that women are still undertreated for their symptoms and risk factors [78–80]. This is especially important as the traditional risk factors may serve as triggers for concomitant vascular dysfunction and insufficient treatment of these risk factors worsens future outcomes [17]. Women have more often side-effects of a variety of cardiovascular medications [81]. On the other hand, they tend to use more often (unproven) vitamin and herbal preparations, which is discouraged in the 2011 AHA prevention guidelines in women [49]. When women present with chest pain at the general practitioner or emergency department, they are often directly treated with aspirin, even before the diagnosis IHD has been established. Primary prevention with anti-platelet therapy in low risk women <65 years of age, does not protect against a first cardiac event and has not proven yet to be beneficial in predominantly functional driven IHD [49, 82]. In contrast, inappropriate anti-platelet therapy increases the risk for major bleeding. Most women benefit best from a tailored medical approach for their cardiac symptoms and risk factors that are present. In younger symptomatic women, the threshold for systolic blood pressure should be preferable in the optimal range <120/80 mmHg [50]. With a low blood pressure, there is less oxidative stress as a trigger for (coronary) vascular dysfunction. Caution should be taken in the years after menopause, as total cholesterol and LDL levels rise with 10–15% [83]. The use of calcium antagonists like diltiazem are often very helpful in treatment of persistent angina symptoms in women at middle-age (patient D). It may even be advantageous to combine this with a low-dose selective b-blocker to address autonomic dysfunction that is induced by menopausal hormonal changes [84, 85]. Other women with symptoms of fluid retention due to the enhanced post-menopausal salt sensitivity may profit more from a combination of diltiazem and/or selective b-blocker with an ACE inhibitor or ARB antagonist.

Surgical Treatment for Ischemic Heart Disease

Women have historically a greater short-term mortality with coronary artery bypass grafting (CABG) than men [86–90], however in hospital mortality rates in women are improving over the past decade [60, 91]. In general, women undergoing CABG are older than men with a higher clustering of CVD risk factors. The diffuse character of atherosclerosis may be a reason for the use of fewer anastomoses and arterial grafts in women [90]. There is currently increasing attention for the high prevalence of heart failure with preserved ejection fraction (HFpEF) in elderly women, which is an important and often neglected predictor of short-term and long-term outcomes after CABG [92–94]. It is therefore recommended to pay more attention to heart failure assessment pre- and postoperatively in CABG patients. After CABG women have a poorer health-quality of life than men, with less social support and fewer participation in cardiac rehabilitation programs [86].

Key Issues

- Women have 2x more often non-obstructive CAD (NOCAD) than men
- Angina symptoms in middle-aged women are often a combination of NOCAD and functional CAD
- Women with recurrent chest pain syndromes and NOCAD need to be adequately treated and evaluated for their lifestyle behavior and CVD risk factors
- Women are often estimated at lower risk by their doctors than they actually are
- Women derive more prognostic information from a CTA than men
- Women have more residual symptoms after coronary interventions than men, also related to higher prevalence of vascular dysfunction
- Women have higher rates of bleeding complications after PCI compared to men
- Women have poorer outcomes after CABG due to older age, more clustering of risk factors, fewer arterial grafts and a higher prevalence of HFpEF
- Guidelines indicate a tailored approach to angina management in women

References

1. Burke AP, Farb A, Malcom G, Virmani R. Effect of menopause on plaque morphologic characteristics in coronary atherosclerosis. Am Heart J. 2001;141(2 Suppl):S58–62.
2. Frink RJ. Gender gap, inflammation and acute coronary disease: are women resistant to atheroma growth? Observations at autopsy. J Invasive Cardiol. 2009;21(6):270–7.
3. Han SH, Bae JH, Holmes Jr DR, Lennon RJ, Eeckhout E, Barsness GW, et al. Sex differences in atheroma burden and endothelial function in patients with early coronary atherosclerosis. Eur Heart Journal. 2008;29(11):1359–69.
4. Shaw LJ, Bugiardini R, Merz CN. Women and ischemic heart disease: evolving knowledge. J Am Coll Cardiol. 2009;54(17):1561–75.
5. Maas AH, van der Schouw YT, Regitz-Zagrosek V, Swahn E, Appelman YE, Pasterkamp G, et al. Red alert for women's heart: the urgent need for more research and knowledge on cardiovascular disease in women: proceedings of the workshop held in Brussels on gender differences in cardiovascular disease, 29 September 2010. Eur Heart J. 2011;32(11):1362–8.
6. EugenMed CC. Study G, Regitz-Zagrosek V, Oertelt-Prigione S, Prescott E, Franconi F, et al. Gender in cardiovascular diseases: impact on clinical manifestations, management, and outcomes. Eur Heart J. 2016;37(1):24–34.
7. Vaccarino V, Badimon L, Corti R, de Wit C, Dorobantu M, Hall A, et al. Ischaemic heart disease in women: are there sex differences in pathophysiology and risk factors? Position paper

from the working group on coronary pathophysiology and microcirculation of the European Society of Cardiology. Cardiovasc Res. 2011;90(1):9–17.
8. Erbel R, Mohlenkamp S, Kerkhoff G, Budde T, Schmermund A. Non-invasive screening for coronary artery disease: calcium scoring. Heart. 2007;93(12):1620–9.
9. Nasir K, Gopal A, Blankstein R, Ahmadi N, Pal R, Khosa F, et al. Noninvasive assessment of gender differences in coronary plaque composition with multidetector computed tomographic angiography. Am J Cardiol. 2010;105(4):453–8.
10. Qureshi W, Blaha MJ, Nasir K, Al-Mallah MH. Gender differences in coronary plaque composition and burden detected in symptomatic patients referred for coronary computed tomographic angiography. Int J Cardiovasc Imaging. 2013;29(2):463–9.
11. Smilowitz NR, Sampson BA, Abrecht CR, Siegfried JS, Hochman JS, Reynolds HR. Women have less severe and extensive coronary atherosclerosis in fatal cases of ischemic heart disease: an autopsy study. Am Heart J. 2011;161(4):681–8.
12. Jacobs AK. Coronary intervention in 2009: are women no different than men? Circ Cardiovasc Interv. 2009;2(1):69–78.
13. Johnston N, Schenck-Gustafsson K, Lagerqvist B. Are we using cardiovascular medications and coronary angiography appropriately in men and women with chest pain? Eur Heart J. 2011;32(11):1331–6.
14. Shaw LJ, Min JK, Narula J, Lin F, Bairey-Merz CN, Callister TQ, et al. Sex differences in mortality associated with computed tomographic angiographic measurements of obstructive and nonobstructive coronary artery disease: an exploratory analysis. Circ Cardiovasc Imaging. 2010;3(4):473–81.
15. Raggi P, Gongora MC, Gopal A, Callister TQ, Budoff M, Shaw LJ. Coronary artery calcium to predict all-cause mortality in elderly men and women. J Am Coll Cardiol. 2008;52(1):17–23.
16. Sedlak TL, Lee M, Izadnegahdar M, Merz CN, Gao M, Humphries KH. Sex differences in clinical outcomes in patients with stable angina and no obstructive coronary artery disease. Am Heart J. 2013;166(1):38–44.
17. Gulati M, Cooper-DeHoff RM, McClure C, Johnson BD, Shaw LJ, Handberg EM, et al. Adverse cardiovascular outcomes in women with nonobstructive coronary artery disease: a report from the Women's Ischemia Syndrome Evaluation Study and the St James Women Take Heart Project. Arch Intern Med. 2009;169(9):843–50.
18. Sharaf B, Wood T, Shaw L, Johnson BD, Kelsey S, Anderson RD, et al. Adverse outcomes among women presenting with signs and symptoms of ischemia and no obstructive coronary artery disease: findings from the National Heart, Lung, and Blood Institute-sponsored Women's Ischemia Syndrome Evaluation (WISE) angiographic core laboratory. Am Heart J. 2013;166(1):134–41.
19. Jespersen L, Hvelplund A, Abildstrom SZ, Pedersen F, Galatius S, Madsen JK, et al. Stable angina pectoris with no obstructive coronary artery disease is associated with increased risks of major adverse cardiovascular events. Eur Heart J. 2012;33(6):734–44.
20. Narula J, Strauss HW. The popcorn plaques. Nat Med. 2007;13(5):532–4.
21. Colombo A, Panoulas VF. Diagnostic coronary angiography is getting old! JACC Cardiovasc Imaging. 2015;8(1):11–3.
22. Gaemperli O, Luscher TF, Bax JJ. View point: what should the future design of clinical imaging studies be? Eur Heart J. 2013;34(31):2432–5.
23. Pepine CJ, Ferdinand KC, Shaw LJ, Light-McGroary KA, Shah RU, Gulati M, et al. Emergence of Nonobstructive Coronary Artery Disease: A Woman's Problem and Need for Change in Definition on Angiography. J Am Coll Cardiol. 2015;66(17):1918–33.
24. Garcia M, Mulvagh SL, Bairey Merz CN, Buring JE, Manson JE. Cardiovascular Disease in Women: Clinical Perspectives. Circ Res. 2016;118(8):1273–93.
25. Khuddus MA, Pepine CJ, Handberg EM, Bairey Merz CN, Sopko G, Bavry AA, et al. An intravascular ultrasound analysis in women experiencing chest pain in the absence of obstructive coronary artery disease: a substudy from the National Heart, Lung and Blood Institute-Sponsored Women's Ischemia Syndrome Evaluation (WISE). J Interv Cardiol. 2010;23(6):511–9.

26. Maddox TM, Stanislawski MA, Grunwald GK, Bradley SM, Ho PM, Tsai TT, et al. Nonobstructive coronary artery disease and risk of myocardial infarction. JAMA. 2014;312(17):1754–63.
27. Marzilli M, Merz CN, Boden WE, Bonow RO, Capozza PG, Chilian WM, et al. Obstructive coronary atherosclerosis and ischemic heart disease: an elusive link! J Am Coll Cardiol. 2012;60(11):951–6.
28. Tonino PA, Fearon WF, De Bruyne B, Oldroyd KG, Leesar MA, Ver Lee PN, et al. Angiographic versus functional severity of coronary artery stenoses in the FAME study fractional flow reserve versus angiography in multivessel evaluation. J Am Coll Cardiol. 2010;55(25): 2816–21.
29. Chen SL, Xu B, Chen JB, Xu T, Ye F, Zhang JJ, et al. Diagnostic accuracy of quantitative angiographic and intravascular ultrasound parameters predicting the functional significance of single de novo lesions. Int J Cardiol. 2013;168(2):1364–9.
30. Fihn SD, Gardin JM, Abrams J, Berra K, Blankenship JC, Dallas AP, et al. 2012 ACCF/AHA/ACP/AATS/PCNA/SCAI/STS Guideline for the diagnosis and management of patients with stable ischemic heart disease: a report of the American College of Cardiology Foundation/American Heart Association Task Force on Practice Guidelines, and the American College of Physicians, American Association for Thoracic Surgery, Preventive Cardiovascular Nurses Association, Society for Cardiovascular Angiography and Interventions, and Society of Thoracic Surgeons. J Am Coll Cardiol. 2012;60(24):e44–e164.
31. Task Force Members, Montalescot G, Sechtem U, Achenbach S, Andreotti F, Arden C, et al. 2013 ESC guidelines on the management of stable coronary artery disease: the Task Force on the management of stable coronary artery disease of the European Society of Cardiology. Eur Heart J. 2013;34(38):2949–3003.
32. Robinson JG, Wallace R, Limacher M, Ren H, Cochrane B, Wassertheil-Smoller S, et al. Cardiovascular risk in women with non-specific chest pain (from the Women's Health Initiative Hormone Trials). Am J Cardiol. 2008;102(6):693–9.
33. Jespersen L, Abildstrom SZ, Hvelplund A, Madsen JK, Galatius S, Pedersen F, et al. Burden of hospital admission and repeat angiography in angina pectoris patients with and without coronary artery disease: a registry-based cohort study. PLoS One. 2014;9(4):e93170.
34. Mosca L, Linfante AH, Benjamin EJ, Berra K, Hayes SN, Walsh BW, et al. National study of physician awareness and adherence to cardiovascular disease prevention guidelines. Circulation. 2005;111(4):499–510.
35. Pepine CJ, Balaban RS, Bonow RO, Diamond GA, Johnson BD, Johnson PA, et al. Women's Ischemic Syndrome Evaluation: current status and future research directions: report of the National Heart, Lung and Blood Institute workshop: October 2-4, 2002: Section 1: diagnosis of stable ischemia and ischemic heart disease. Circulation. 2004;109(6):e44–6.
36. Eastwood JA, Johnson BD, Rutledge T, Bittner V, Whittaker KS, Krantz DS, et al. Anginal symptoms, coronary artery disease, and adverse outcomes in Black and White women: the NHLBI-sponsored Women's Ischemia Syndrome Evaluation (WISE) study. J Women's Health. 2013;22(9):724–32.
37. Hemingway H, Langenberg C, Damant J, Frost C, Pyorala K, Barrett-Connor E. Prevalence of angina in women versus men: a systematic review and meta-analysis of international variations across 31 countries. Circulation. 2008;117(12):1526–36.
38. Kreatsoulas C, Shannon HS, Giacomini M, Velianou JL, Anand SS. Reconstructing angina: cardiac symptoms are the same in women and men. JAMA Intern Med. 2013;173(9):829–31.
39. Merz AA, Cheng S. Sex differences in cardiovascular ageing. Heart. 2016;102(11):825–31.
40. Pedrotty DM, Jessup M. "Frailty, thy name is woman": syndrome of women with heart failure with preserved ejection fraction. Circ Cardiovasc Qual Outcomes. 2015;8(2 Suppl 1):S48–51.
41. Elderkin-Thompson V, Waitzkin H. Differences in clinical communication by gender. J Gen Intern Med. 1999;14(2):112–21.
42. Diamond GA, Forrester JS. Analysis of probability as an aid in the clinical diagnosis of coronary-artery disease. N Engl J Med. 1979;300(24):1350–8.

43. Genders TS, Steyerberg EW, Alkadhi H, Leschka S, Desbiolles L, Nieman K, et al. A clinical prediction rule for the diagnosis of coronary artery disease: validation, updating, and extension. Eur Heart J. 2011;32(11):1316–30.
44. Fordyce CB, Douglas PS. Optimal non-invasive imaging test selection for the diagnosis of ischaemic heart disease. Heart. 2016;102(7):555–64.
45. Wolk MJ, Bailey SR, Doherty JU, Douglas PS, Hendel RC, Kramer CM, et al. ACCF/AHA/ASE/ASNC/HFSA/HRS/SCAI/SCCT/SCMR/STS 2013 multimodality appropriate use criteria for the detection and risk assessment of stable ischemic heart disease: a report of the American College of Cardiology Foundation Appropriate Use Criteria Task Force, American Heart Association, American Society of Echocardiography, American Society of Nuclear Cardiology, Heart Failure Society of America, Heart Rhythm Society, Society for Cardiovascular Angiography and Interventions, Society of Cardiovascular Computed Tomography, Society for Cardiovascular Magnetic Resonance, and Society of Thoracic Surgeons. J Am Coll Cardiol. 2014;63(4):380–406.
46. Ng VG, Meller S, Shetty S, Lansky AJ. Diagnosing and characterizing coronary artery disease in women: developments in noninvasive and invasive imaging techniques. J Cardiovasc Transl Res. 2013;6(5):740–51.
47. Douglas PS, Ginsburg GS. The evaluation of chest pain in women. N Engl J Med. 1996;334(20):1311–5.
48. Mieres JH, Shaw LJ, Arai A, Budoff MJ, Flamm SD, Hundley WG, et al. Role of noninvasive testing in the clinical evaluation of women with suspected coronary artery disease: Consensus statement from the Cardiac Imaging Committee, Council on Clinical Cardiology, and the Cardiovascular Imaging and Intervention Committee, Council on Cardiovascular Radiology and Intervention. American Heart Association Circulation. 2005;111(5):682–96.
49. Mosca L, Benjamin EJ, Berra K, Bezanson JL, Dolor RJ, Lloyd-Jones DM, et al. Effectiveness-based guidelines for the prevention of cardiovascular disease in women--2011 update: a guideline from the american heart association. Circulation. 2011;123(11):1243–62.
50. Piepoli MF, Hoes AW, Agewall S, Albus C, Brotons C, Catapano AL, et al. 2016 European Guidelines on cardiovascular disease prevention in clinical practice: The Sixth Joint Task Force of the European Society of Cardiology and Other Societies on Cardiovascular Disease Prevention in Clinical Practice (constituted by representatives of 10 societies and by invited experts): Developed with the special contribution of the European Association for Cardiovascular Prevention & Rehabilitation (EACPR). Eur Heart J. 2016. 37(29): 2315–81.
51. Mieres JH, Gulati M, Bairey Merz N, Berman DS, Gerber TC, Hayes SN, et al. Role of noninvasive testing in the clinical evaluation of women with suspected ischemic heart disease: a consensus statement from the American Heart Association. Circulation. 2014;130(4): 350–79.
52. Mieres JH, Shaw LJ, Wenger NK. Noninvasive testing in women with suspected ischemic heart disease: ten highlights to guide quality clinical care. Clin Cardiol. 2014;37(9):515–6.
53. Douglas PS, Hoffmann U, Patel MR, Mark DB, Al-Khalidi HR, Cavanaugh B, et al. Outcomes of anatomical versus functional testing for coronary artery disease. N Engl J Med. 2015;372(14):1291–300.
54. Hemal K, Pagidipati NJ, Coles A, Dolor RJ, Mark DB, Pellikka PA, et al. Sex Differences in Demographics, Risk Factors, Presentation, and Noninvasive Testing in Stable Outpatients With Suspected Coronary Artery Disease: Insights From the PROMISE Trial. JACC Cardiovasc Imaging. 2016;9(4):337–46.
55. Pagidipati NJ, Hemal K, Coles A, Mark DB, Dolor RJ, Pellikka PA, et al. Sex Differences in Functional and CT Angiography Testing in Patients With Suspected Coronary Artery Disease. J Am Coll Cardiol. 2016;67(22):2607–16.
56. Mieres JH, Bonow RO. Ischemic Heart Disease in Women: A Need for Sex-Specific Diagnostic Algorithms. JACC Cardiovasc Imaging. 2016;9(4):347–9.
57. Min JK, Leipsic J, Pencina MJ, Berman DS, Koo BK, van Mieghem C, et al. Diagnostic accuracy of fractional flow reserve from anatomic CT angiography. JAMA. 2012;308(12): 1237–45.

58. Patel MR, Dai D, Hernandez AF, Douglas PS, Messenger J, Garratt KN, et al. Prevalence and predictors of nonobstructive coronary artery disease identified with coronary angiography in contemporary clinical practice. Am Heart J. 2014;167(6):846–52. e2
59. Tonino PA, De Bruyne B, Pijls NH, Siebert U, Ikeno F. van' t Veer M, et al. Fractional flow reserve versus angiography for guiding percutaneous coronary intervention. N Engl J Med. 2009;360(3):213–24.
60. Tamis-Holland JE, Lu J, Korytkowski M, Magee M, Rogers WJ, Lopes N, et al. Sex differences in presentation and outcome among patients with type 2 diabetes and coronary artery disease treated with contemporary medical therapy with or without prompt revascularization: a report from the BARI 2D Trial (Bypass Angioplasty Revascularization Investigation 2 Diabetes). J Am Coll Cardiol. 2013;61(17):1767–76.
61. Mega JL, Hochman JS, Scirica BM, Murphy SA, Sloan S, McCabe CH, et al. Clinical features and outcomes of women with unstable ischemic heart disease: observations from metabolic efficiency with ranolazine for less ischemia in non-ST-elevation acute coronary syndromes-thrombolysis in myocardial infarction 36 (MERLIN-TIMI 36). Circulation. 2010;121(16): 1809–17.
62. Kok MM, van der Heijden LC, Sen H, Danse PW, Lowik MM, Anthonio RL, et al. Sex Difference in Chest Pain After Implantation of Newer Generation Coronary Drug-Eluting Stents: A Patient-Level Pooled Analysis From the TWENTE and DUTCH PEER Trials. JACC Cardiovasc Interv. 2016;9(6):553–61.
63. De Bruyne B, Fearon WF, Pijls NH, Barbato E, Tonino P, Piroth Z, et al. Fractional flow reserve-guided PCI for stable coronary artery disease. N Engl J Med. 2014;371(13):1208–17.
64. Chandrasekhar J, Mehran R. Sex-Based Differences in Acute Coronary Syndromes: Insights From Invasive and Noninvasive Coronary Technologies. JACC Cardiovasc Imaging. 2016;9(4):451–64.
65. Li J, Rihal CS, Matsuo Y, Elrashidi MY, Flammer AJ, Lee MS, et al. Sex-related differences in fractional flow reserve-guided treatment. Circ Cardiovasc Interv. 2013;6(6):662–70.
66. Kang SJ, Ahn JM, Han S, Lee JY, Kim WJ, Park DW, et al. Sex differences in the visual-functional mismatch between coronary angiography or intravascular ultrasound versus fractional flow reserve. JACC Cardiovasc Interv. 2013;6(6):562–8.
67. Stefanini GG, Baber U, Windecker S, Morice MC, Sartori S, Leon MB, et al. Safety and efficacy of drug-eluting stents in women: a patient-level pooled analysis of randomised trials. Lancet. 2013;382(9908):1879–88.
68. Bertrand OF, Belisle P, Joyal D, Costerousse O, Rao SV, Jolly SS, et al. Comparison of transradial and femoral approaches for percutaneous coronary interventions: a systematic review and hierarchical Bayesian meta-analysis. Am Heart J. 2012;163(4):632–48.
69. Shin JS, Tahk SJ, Yang HM, Yoon MH, Choi SY, Choi BJ, et al. Impact of female gender on bleeding complications after transradial coronary intervention (from the Korean Transradial Coronary Intervention registry). Am J Cardiol. 2014;113(12):2002–6.
70. Abdelaal E, Brousseau-Provencher C, Montminy S, Plourde G, MacHaalany J, Bataille Y, et al. Risk score, causes, and clinical impact of failure of transradial approach for percutaneous coronary interventions. JACC Cardiovasc Interv. 2013;6(11):1129–37.
71. Patti G, De Caterina R, Abbate R, Andreotti F, Biasucci LM, Calabro P, et al. Platelet function and long-term antiplatelet therapy in women: is there a gender-specificity? A 'state-of-the-art' paper. Eur Heart J. 2014;35(33):2213-23b.
72. Mackman N. Triggers, targets and treatments for thrombosis. Nature. 2008;451(7181):914–8.
73. Ahmed B, Dauerman HL. Women, bleeding, and coronary intervention. Circulation. 2013;127(5):641–9.
74. Flammer AJ, Anderson T, Celermajer DS, Creager MA, Deanfield J, Ganz P, et al. The assessment of endothelial function: from research into clinical practice. Circulation. 2012;126(6): 753–67.
75. Anderson TJ, Uehata A, Gerhard MD, Meredith IT, Knab S, Delagrange D, et al. Close relation of endothelial function in the human coronary and peripheral circulations. J Am Coll Cardiol. 1995;26(5):1235–41.

76. Beltrame JF, Crea F, Kaski JC, Ogawa H, Ong P, Sechtem U, et al. International standardization of diagnostic criteria for vasospastic angina. Eur Heart J. 2015. [Epub ahead of print] Review.
77. Beltrame JF, Crea F, Kaski JC, Ogawa H, Ong P, Sechtem U, et al. The Who, What, Why, When, How and Where of Vasospastic Angina. Circ J. 2016;80(2):289–98.
78. Dallongevillle J, De Bacquer D, Heidrich J, De Backer G, Prugger C, Kotseva K, et al. Gender differences in the implementation of cardiovascular prevention measures after an acute coronary event. Heart. 2010;96(21):1744–9.
79. Daly C, Clemens F, Lopez Sendon JL, Tavazzi L, Boersma E, Danchin N, et al. Gender differences in the management and clinical outcome of stable angina. Circulation. 2006;113(4):490–8.
80. Koopman C, Vaartjes I, Heintjes EM, Spiering W, van Dis I, Herings RM, et al. Persisting gender differences and attenuating age differences in cardiovascular drug use for prevention and treatment of coronary heart disease, 1998-2010. Eur Heart J. 2013;34(41):3198–205.
81. Oertelt-Prigione S, Regitz-Zagrosek V. Gender aspects in cardiovascular pharmacology. J Cardiovasc Transl Res. 2009;2(3):258–66.
82. Ridker PM, Cook NR, Lee IM, Gordon D, Gaziano JM, Manson JE, et al. A randomized trial of low-dose aspirin in the primary prevention of cardiovascular disease in women. N Engl J Med. 2005;352(13):1293–304.
83. Abbey M, Owen A, Suzakawa M, Roach P, Nestel PJ. Effects of menopause and hormone replacement therapy on plasma lipids, lipoproteins and LDL-receptor activity. Maturitas. 1999;33(3):259–69.
84. Souza HC, Tezini GC. Autonomic Cardiovascular Damage during Post-menopause: the Role of Physical Training. Aging and Disease. 2013;4(6):320–8.
85. Barnes JN, Hart EC, Curry TB, Nicholson WT, Eisenach JH, Wallin BG, et al. Aging enhances autonomic support of blood pressure in women. Hypertension. 2014;63(2):303–8.
86. Vaccarino V, Lin ZQ, Kasl SV, Mattera JA, Roumanis SA, Abramson JL, et al. Sex differences in health status after coronary artery bypass surgery. Circulation. 2003;108(21):2642–7.
87. Regitz-Zagrosek V, Lehmkuhl E, Hocher B, Goesmann D, Lehmkuhl HB, Hausmann H, et al. Gender as a risk factor in young, not in old, women undergoing coronary artery bypass grafting. J Am Coll Cardiol. 2004;44(12):2413–4.
88. Pollock B, Hamman BL, Sass DM, da Graca B, Grayburn PA, Filardo G. Effect of gender and race on operative mortality after isolated coronary artery bypass grafting. Am J Cardiol. 2015;115(5):614–8.
89. Swaminathan RV, Feldman DN, Pashun RA, Patil RK, Shah T, Geleris JD, et al. Gender differences in in-hospital outcomes after coronary artery bypass grafting. Am J Cardiol. 2016;118(3):362–8.
90. Trienekens MP, Maas AH, Timman ST, Van Swieten HA, Noyez L. Sex differences in patient and procedural characteristics and early outcomes following cardiac surgery. J Cardiovasc Surg. 2015;56(5):817–23.
91. Swaminathan RV, Feldman DN, Pashun RA, Patil RK, Shah T, Geleris JD, et al. Gender Differences in In-Hospital Outcomes After Coronary Artery Bypass Grafting. Am J Cardiol. 2016;118(3):362–8.
92. Ferreira RG, Worthington A, Huang CC, Aranki SF, Muehlschlegel JD. Sex differences in the prevalence of diastolic dysfunction in cardiac surgical patients. J Card Surg. 2015;30(3):238–45.
93. Lehmkuhl E, Kendel F, Gelbrich G, Dunkel A, Oertelt-Prigione S, Babitsch B, et al. Gender-specific predictors of early mortality after coronary artery bypass graft surgery. Clin Res Cardiol. 2012;101(9):745–51.
94. Dalen M, Lund LH, Ivert T, Holzmann MJ, Sartipy U. Survival after coronary artery bypass grafting in patients with preoperative heart failure and preserved vs. reduced ejection fraction. JAMA Cardiol. 2016;1(5):530–8.

Chapter 3
Female Manifestation of Acute Coronary Syndromes

Angela H.E.M. Maas and C. Noel Bairey Merz

Abstract The pathophysiology and clinical manifestation of acute coronary syndromes (ACS) is different among men and women. Women more often have an ACS with 'normal' coronary arteries (MINOCA) than men. Despite, their mortality rates are two times higher. They also have more often variant types of ACS, such as spontaneous coronary artery dissections (SCAD) and a Takotsubo syndrome. Different types of ACS need a different approach in the acute phase and during the lifetime thereafter, which is still insufficiently addressed in the current guidelines.

Keywords Acute coronary syndromes (ACS) • Bleeding risk • Gender mortality • Oral contraceptives • Menopause • Pregnancy • Spontaneous coronary artery dissections (SCAD) • Symptoms ACS • Takotsubo syndrome • Type II ACS • Vaginal bleeding risk

The Role of Age and Gender

Over the past decades there has been a gradual rise in the number of women and men with ischemic heart disease (IHD). Currently, the greatest rise of IHD occurs in Asia and the Eastern European countries, predominantly related to ongoing

A.H.E.M. Maas, M.D., Ph.D. (✉)
Department of Cardiology, Women's Cardiac Health Program,
Radboud University Medical Center, Nijmegen, The Netherlands
e-mail: angela.maas@radboudumc.nl

C.N. Bairey Merz, M.D.
Director Barbra Streisand Women's Heart Center, Linda Joy Pollin Women's Heart Health Program, Director Preventive Cardiac Center, Cedars-Sinai, Los Angeles, CA, USA
e-mail: noel.baireymerz@cshs.org

A.H.E.M. Maas, C.N. Bairey Merz (eds.), *Manual of Gynecardiology*,
DOI 10.1007/978-3-319-54960-6_3

industrialization and a worsening of lifestyle habits [1, 2]. In Western countries, although smoking and elevated cholesterol rates are lower, younger women and men have greater metabolic CVD risk profiles than in prior decades [3], with an increase in acute coronary syndromes (ACS) at middle-age [4–6]. In general, women with an ACS are older than men, with a higher clustering of CVD risk factors [7]. In the younger age-group (<65 years), the risk for an ACS is 3–4 times higher in men compared to women, while after the age of 75 years sex differences in ACS numbers fade with a persistent modest predominance in men [8, 9]. Despite the lower prevalence of ACS in younger women with a less extensive burden of atherosclerosis than in similarly aged men, their ACS mortality rates are almost twice as high [10–15]. This discrepancy is called the 'gender gap' in ACS and is still incompletely understood. Young women with ST-segment–elevation myocardial infarction (STEMI) are less likely to receive reperfusion therapy and more often have reperfusion delays than similarly aged men [16–19]. Gender disparities are found to be more pronounced among patients transferred to percutaneous coronary intervention (PCI) institutions or in those who received fibrinolytic therapy [16].

There are important sex differences in risk factors and underlying pathophysiological mechanisms of ACS, with a more diverse etiology of ACS in women compared to men [20, 21]. Whereas in women <55 years of age current smoking is the leading (>90%) cause for an ACS, in elderly women (>65 years of age) traditional CVD risk factors are most important [8, 22]. In women with premature ACS a genetic inheritance and female-specific risk factors such as an early menopause and/or pregnancy-related complications can often be identified [23–28]. This may also account for co-morbidity with inflammatory diseases, such as rheumatic diseases, inflammatory bowel diseases and thyroid disorders, which frequently occur in women in their forties [29] (see Fig. 1.4, Chap. 1, p18). The clinical relevance of these reproductive and non-traditional risk variables appears to dilute at older age. Depression, marital stress and psychosocial risk factors are relatively more important risk factors related to ACS in especially younger women than men [30–32]. Psychological stress acts more often as a trigger for ACS in women, while vigorous physical activity is more often a provoking trigger in men. Of interest is that the recurrence rate after a premature ACS seems to be related to feminine gender roles and personality traits (anxiety), also when these characteristic are present in younger men [33].

In 2016 the AHA has launched its first scientific statement on ACS in women, summarizing our current knowledge on specific aspects of ACS in female patients [21]. Ischemic heart disease is a complex interaction between anatomical atherosclerosis and functional vascular dysfunction in both the macro- and microvascular coronary vessels, which often overlaps in stable and unstable coronary syndromes [34]. In younger women, coronary vascular dysfunction/spasm predominates over coronary obstruction, leading to distinct clinical and angiographic presentations of ACS and more often a type II ACS, which is predominantly driven by vascular dysfunction/spasm and triggered by traditional and non-traditional risk factors. Fewer women than men present with a STEMI whereas they have more often a non-STEMI (NSTEMI) or unstable angina [35–37]. In Table 3.1 most important gender-specific characteristics of ACS are described.

Table 3.1 Gender-specific characteristics of acute coronary syndromes (ACS).

• Women with ACS are older than men with a higher clustering of traditional RF
• 25–30% all ACS <65 years occur in women
• Smoking women <55 years have a 2× higher relative risk of ACS than men
• Among patients with ACS diabetes is more common in women than men
• Women have more often a type II ACS < 65 years than men
• Women have a longer patient and doctors delay when having an ACS
• Women have more often erosive plaques than plaque ruptures compared to men
• Women more often have an ACS with 'open' coronary arteries than men
• 10–25% ACS in women <65 years are caused by a spontaneous coronary artery dissection (SCAD)
• > 90% of SCAD occur in women
• 10× often Takotsubo ACS in women than in men, especially after 60 years
• Women have fewer STEMI, but relatively more NSTEMI and unstable angina
• Two times higher mortality STEMI and NSTEMI in women over men <60 years

Adapted from: Pagidipati NJ, et al. [14] and Regitz-Zagrosek V et al. [20]

Gender-Differences in the Pathophysiology of Acute Coronary Syndromes

The advances in interventional cardiology over the past decades have literally visualized important sex differences in the extent of coronary atherosclerosis and mechanisms that are involved in ACS. Considering all ages, plaque rupture (type 1 ACS) is the cause of fatal MI in 76% of men and 55% of women [38]. Below 65 years of age women have less obstructive CAD than men and more often an ACS with 'open' coronary arteries with spasm and vascular dysfunction as etiologic factors [38–41]. This has been referred to as a type II ACS in the most recent ESC/AHA 2012 definition of ACS [42]. Despite the associated adverse mortality, there is currently an ongoing discussion whether type II ACS should be more considered as myocardial injury rather than as a distinct infarction. With the introductions of high sensitive (hs) troponin measurements, type II ACS are currently twice as often recognized in women than before [43]. The 'negative' findings at coronary angiography (CAG) during ACS are now called 'myocardial infarction with no obstructive coronary arteries' (MINOCA), which has recently been discussed in an ESC position paper on MINOCA [44–46]. This occurs in 40% of predominantly younger female patients and their coronary arteries are often misinterpreted as being 'clean', while intracoronary non-obstructive plaques are frequently present and can be identified with intravascular ultrasound (IVUS) or optical coherence tomography (OCT) [41, 47–50]. These plaques contain cytokines (vasoactive proteins) that may induce vascular dysfunction and/or spasm in the larger and smaller coronary arteries , presenting in patients as a type II STEMI or NSTEMI [51, 52]. The wrong labeling of these ACS as being 'false positive' may lead to under-treatment of cardiac symptoms and risk factors in women. From pathology studies it is known that younger patients and especially women more often have erosive plaques compared to the classical atherosclerotic plaques that are present in type I ACS [38, 53, 54]. A dysfunctional intima of erosive plaques can induce distal embolization of small thrombi leading to obstruction and necrosis in focal myocardial areas [38]. This can cause elevation of hs-troponins without visible abnormalities at coronary angiography. At older age (>65 years) type I ACS is also the predominant manifestation of ACS in women. Coronary plaque ruptures are more often associated with thrombus formation in women than in men [55]. Age- and sex-related differences in the thrombotic system interfere with the clotting cascade and thrombocyte function within the various manifestations of ACS [56].

Symptom Recognition of Acute Coronary Syndromes in Women

Differences in underlying pathophysiology importantly contribute to another clinical presentation of ACS in women compared to men. When vascular dysfunction/spasm is an important component of ACS, as is often the case in younger women (<65 years), symptoms can vary over time in a crescendo-decrescendo pattern (patient A). This can be very misleading in the interpretation of symptoms by the patient herself and her doctor. This 'atypical' ACS presentation can delay adequate referral to a hospital for several hours or even days [57, 58]. Another barrier for timely referral to the hospital is de lack of awareness in women themselves [59]. The more direct way of symptom expression in men is more accurate and helpful in emergency medical situations. Women tend to 'interpret' their symptoms, while men 'report'. In elderly (>65 years) women with multi-vessel disease, the concomitant presence of diastolic dysfunction or heart failure with preserved ejection fraction (HFpEF), can lead to an ACS presentation with acute decompensated heart failure as the predominant clinical symptom. The most common symptoms when having an ACS in women and men are listed in Table 3.2, with women having more atypical symptoms than men. It is noteworthy to realize that there are often

Table 3.2 Gender differences in symptom presentation during acute coronary syndromes (ACS)

Symptoms	Women	Men
• Acute tight pressing chest pain, squeezing, with radiation to the jaw, left upper arm or both arms	++	+++
• Chest pain, radiation to the throat, left armpit, between shoulder blades, neck, upper abdomen	+++	+
• Crescendo/decrescendo character of symptoms (h/days)	+++	–/+
• Dyspnea, unusual shortness of breath, lightheadedness	+++	+
• 'Flu'-like symptoms, nausea, vomiting, sweating, dry mouth	+++	++
• Anxiety, panic, confusion, scaring distress	+++	+
• Tiredness, unusual fatigue, feeling of exhaustion, weakness, dizziness	+++	+

Adapted from: Mehta LS et al. [21] and Canto JG et al. [61]

overlapping symptoms among both genders and that ACS diagnosis always includes a rapid evaluation of lifestyle and risk factors [60]. Women more often than men report no chest pain at all (37% versus 27%) during ACS, most frequently in patients at older age (>75 years) and in diabetics [61, 62]. This is an important reason why there is still a longer patient-delay in the elderly in seeking medical care after onset of ACS-associated symptoms [63]. Women may experience a period of extreme tiredness, even exhaustion, prior to their ACS [64]. In the ARIC study it was found that silent myocardial infarctions occur in 45% of all ACS, more often in men than women, but with a poorer prognosis in women [65].

Patient A. **Symptom presentation in 44 year old woman with type II ACS**

On her work as a nurse she suddenly experienced symptoms of nausea and a pressing chest pain with radiation to the left jaw. This happened after assisting in a resuscitation of a young patient. In the prior 1-2 weeks she had felt more tired and exhausted than ever before. She was known with (untreated) familial hypertension for several years, no other risk factors. While cycling home after work she still had a continuous pressure on her chest. At home her symptoms almost disappeared, but these returned a few hours later when she went up the stairs to bed. The next day her chest pain came back with a feeling of exhaustion. She doubted whether her symptoms may be heart-related and decided to call the GP, who sent her immediately to the hospital. During the afternoon she has on and off chest pain with ST-T changes on her ECG and elevated hsTroponins.

She went to the cathlab for an emergency CAG**: no abnormalities were found**

The next day she was sent home with the message that 'nothing was wrong', but she was prescribed 5 different medications (2 platelet inhibitors, statin, B blocker and ACS inhibitor). During the weeks thereafter she still had recurrent symptoms of chest pain, tiredness and dyspnea and many side effects of her medication.

It took another 6 months before her symptoms completely disappeared with the use of an ARB, B-blocker and calcium antagonist for treatment of her ***severe hypertension***. During her hospital stay little attention was given to her bloodpressure, which was often around 170/100 mmHg.

Comment: premature hypertension can induce coronary vascular dysfunction and promote te occurrence of a type II ACS in young women.

Management of ACS in Women

Most important determinants for a failure to diagnose ACS at the emergency department (ED) are female gender <55 years, the absence of chest pain, a (near) normal ECG and ethnic diversity [66, 67]. In NSTEMI-ACS it is established that an early invasive strategy results in better survival in men but not in women [68–71]. However, data from different ACS registries such as CRUSADE and the Get With the Guidelines (GWTG) initiatives in the USA and MINAP in the UK suggest that the early mortality in women is not sex-dependent but predominantly related to less frequent use of evidence-based care, such as lower CAG use [72, 73]. In women with NSTEMI, cardiac hs-troponins are less likely to be elevated and the ECG is more often non-diagnostic than in men. These facts may lead to a preferential referral of women with suspected NSTEMI to hospitals without cardiac catheterization facilities, adding further delay to diagnosis and treatment. Recent studies have shown that there is still a less aggressive (invasive) management approach in women with ACS compared to men, also after correction for the severity of underlying CAD [17, 37, 74]. At discharge and by the end of 1 year post ACS fewer women than men receive standard medication, especially when they are young and had MINOCA [75, 76].

Bleeding Risk in Women During and After Coronary Interventions

Women have a more than two times higher bleeding risk after (acute) coronary interventions [77, 78]. This is closely related to their higher in-hospital and one-year mortality. The risk of bleeding following PCI is higher among elderly women, in patients with a low body weight, impaired renal function, and with the administration of multiple antithrombotic drugs [79]. Women also have more bleeding complications after thrombolytic therapy [80]. Using the transradial access for coronary interventions reduces the incidence of peri-procedural bleeding complications and improves clinical outcomes [81]. However, because of the smaller size of the radial/brachial artery with a higher risk of spasm and bleeding, this approach may have more difficulties in women [82, 83].

Vaginal Bleeding Risk in (Premenopausal) Women with Antiplatelet Therapy

With the increase in ACS at middle-age, pre- and perimenopausal women are treated with (dual) platelet therapy (DAPT) including acetylsalicylic acid and clopidogrel (or ticagrelor) for a longer period of time. This can induce excessive uterine bleeding and even anemia, which is especially harmful when the coronary circulation is compromised [84]. Heavy menstrual bleeding is common in women in their forties and may have a variety of underlying causes that require different treatment options. Clinical symptoms of dyspnea and tiredness are often not recognized as being caused by excessive uterine bleeding. Moreover, the majority of cardiologist and other vascular specialists do not ask questions about menstrual status or disorders. See the case of patient B. Importantly, the use of combined oral contraceptives to reduce menstrual bleeding is relatively contraindicated in patients with established CAD (unstable angina, ACS, NSTEMI, STEMI, PCI, CABG) because of the increased risk of myocardial infarction and thrombosis [85, 86]. The use of levonorgestrel releasing intra uterine system (LNG-IUS), endometrial ablation or hysterectomy are alternative options, depending on the gynecology advise. Post ACS antithrombotic therapy may also induce bleeding in postmenopausal women, which is always an indication for consultation of a gynecologist.

Patient B. **Woman 48 yrs with abnormal uterine bleeding after re-PCI**

- **Medical history:** OHCA* at STEMI 1 year ago, treated with PCI-LAD + DES**. EF afterwards < 35%, followed by preventive ICD-implant.
- **Risk factors**: quitted smoking after ACS, hypertension first pregnancy, positive fam. history
- **Patient history:** since ACS 6 months ago she is increasingly tired, with 12 kg weight gain and dyspnea at the slightest exercise, however no chest pain.
- **Medication:** acenocoumarol, clopidogrel 75 mg, long-acting nitrates, furosemide 80 mg, spironolacton 25 mg, metoprolol 100mg, perindopril 4 mg, simvastatin 20mg
- **Physical examination**: BMI 25.9 kg/m2, dyspnea and tachypnea while talking, RR 140/90 mmHg, pulse 92/min regular, at auscultation no murmurs or crepitus, slight ankle edema.
- **Laboratory:** Hb 8.0 mmol/L. Ureum 6.5 mmol/L, creat 77 μmol/L, T chol 4.3 mmol/L, HDL 1.4 mmol/L, LDL 2.2 mmol/L,TG 1.6mmol/L, TSH 2.30
- **ECG:** SR 92/min, intermediate axis, signs of previous anteroseptal myocardial infarction
- Her symptoms were first interpreted as the consequence of her previous ACS. *('you will have to live with it')*

2D ECHO with anteroapical scar and EF 35%

CAG with severe proximal lesion large D1 branch

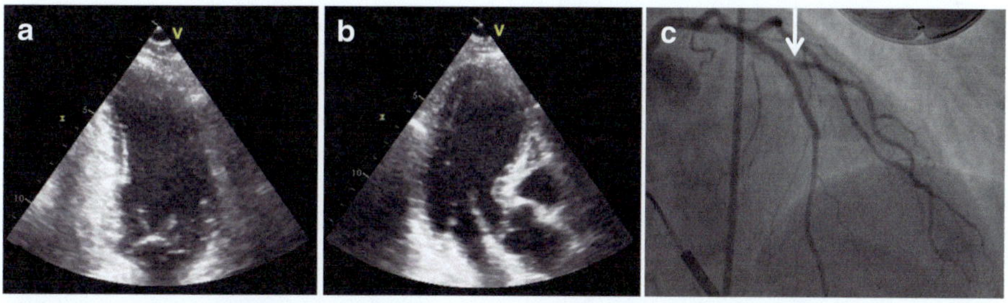

At second opinion her symptoms were interpreted as ongoing ischemia, for which a new CAG was performed. Panel C shows a significant lesion proximal in a large diagonal branch, which was stented with success.

She recovered fast from her symptoms, but 2 weeks later she had a severe vaginal bleeding, due to the combined use of acenocoumarol and clopidogrel. Hb was 5.3 mmol/L. She recovered after blood transfusion and an endometrium ablation by her gynecologist.

Spontaneous Coronary Artery Dissections (SCAD)

Spontaneous coronary artery dissection (SCAD) is a relative rare manifestation of ACS (1.2–2%), of which more than 90% occur in women between 45 and 65 of age [87–89]. In young women its prevalence is estimated at >10% in women <50 years, up to 25% in all women <65 years with ACS (see patient C) [87, 90–92]. A SCAD may also (rarely) occur during pregnancy or in the postpartum period, with a prevalence estimated at 1.8 in 100,000 pregnancies [93–95]. Provoking stressors for a

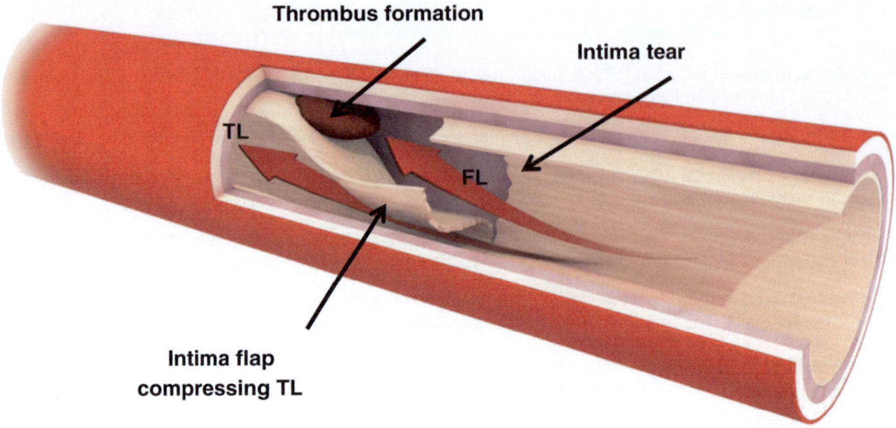

Fig. 3.1 Spontaneous coronary artery dissection (SCAD). *TL* true lumen, *FL* false lumen

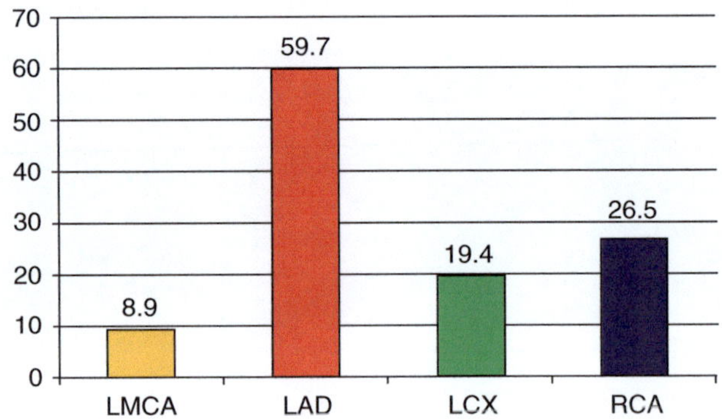

Fig. 3.2 Involved coronary artery in SCAD

SCAD may be emotional, extreme physical exercise, but also coughing, vomiting and heavy lifting. In the majority of SCAD patients a sudden coronary tear is found in the intima of the LAD (60%), followed by the RCA (26%), RCX (19%) and rarely in the LM (9%) (Figs. 3.1 and 3.2) [96]. A SCAD can also be caused by an intramural hematoma in the media of the vessel wall, with or without an intimal flap [94, 97]. Compression of the coronary artery by the false lumen or by a dissecting flap causes obstruction or restriction of flow within the true lumen, resulting in myocardial ischemia or an ACS. The clinical presentation may vary between STEMI, NSTEMI, unstable angina or sudden cardiac death. The diagnosis of SCAD can easily be missed, even in experienced interventional centers, as there are different angiographic features of SCAD that are often interpreted as caused by atherosclerosis [87, 98]. With intracoronary imaging with IVUS or OCT, the true and false lumen can be distinguished from each other, but these manipulations in vulnerable and hemodynamically instable young coronary arteries can be harmful and may lead to secondary iatrogenic dissections.

Patient C. **Female patient 46 yrs with SCAD LAD before (A) and after (B) PCI with DES.**

Elevated family risk CVD, non-smoking, normal weight, no other risk factors.

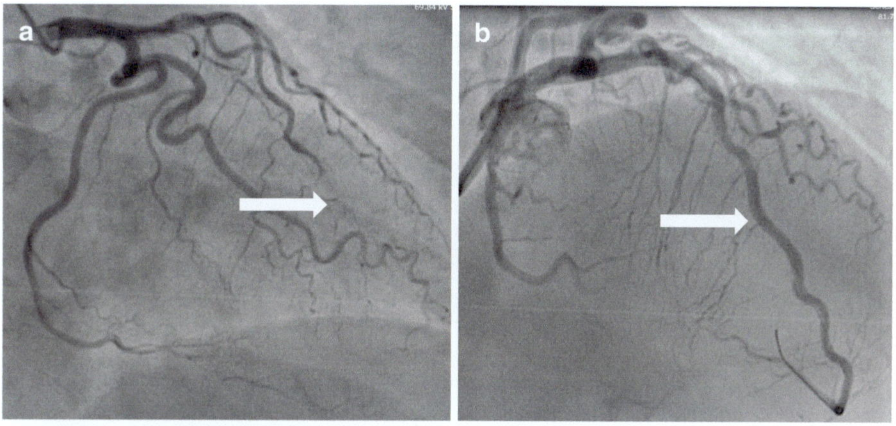

DES drug eluting stent
LAD left anterior descending artery
PCI percutaneous coronary intervention
SCAD spontaneous coronary artery dissection

In several large registries of SCAD patients, an underlying fibromuscular dysplasia (FMD) can be the causative factor, with prevalence estimates in case-series varying from 20 to 72% (Fig. 3.3) [87, 89]. Fibromuscular dysplasia has several angiographic features of coronary artery lesions (smooth stenosis, segmental ectasia and tortuosity) that are often not recognized as such (Fig. 3.4) [99, 100]. In one third of SCAD patients, pre-existent hypertension is present and in 15% signs of atherosclerosis may be involved. In a low percentage of patients (2–8%) mixed connective tissue disorders, such as Ehlers-Danlos and other inflammatory diseases are reported. Only a minority of SCAD patients undergo genetic testing and when performed pathogenic mutations are not frequently found [101]. Given the heterogeneity of this disorder and the relative low prevalence, there are no evidence-based management guidelines yet. When the flow in the dissected artery is higher than TIMI II, a conservative approach is preferred [90]. Coronary stenting may further enlarge the dissection and often leads to more residual symptoms afterwards [102]. It is assumed that most SCAD lesions resolve within 3 months. It is still unclear for how long antithrombotic treatment should be administered and there is no evidence that the use of statins is beneficial in SCAD patients when having normal lipid values. Despite, many young women are sent home with the identical 'big five' medication as a 85 year old man with severe three-vessel disease. This often leads to frustration in younger women who already have a low adherence to long-term medical therapy [76]. The use of beta-blockade reduces arterial shear stress and is (temporarily) advised after SCAD and for prolonged time when hypertension is present [103]. In patients with residual symptoms long-acting diltiazem is often more effective than a beta-blocker.

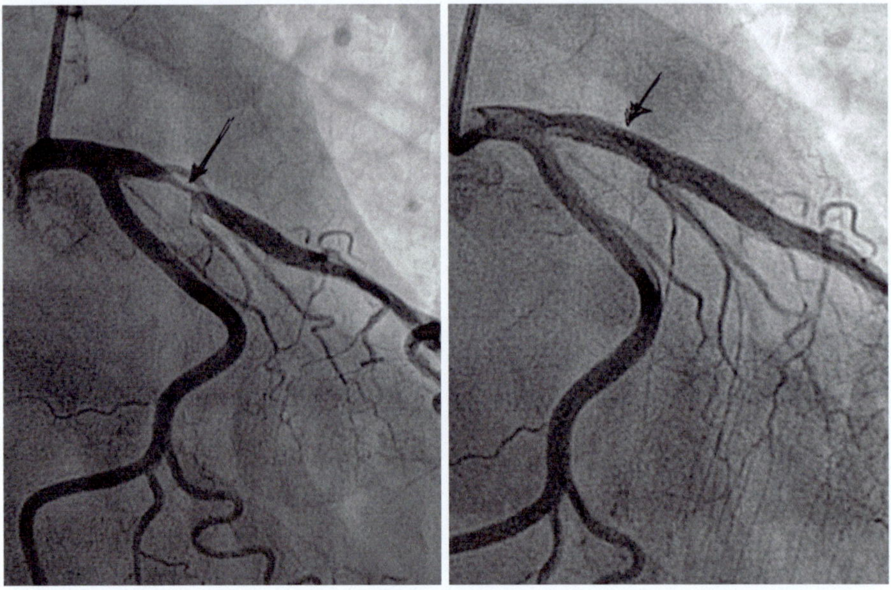

Fig. 3.3 Female patient 48 years with NSTEMI. Fibromuscular dysplasia (FMD), represented as a smooth stenosis with luminal compression proximal in the LAD

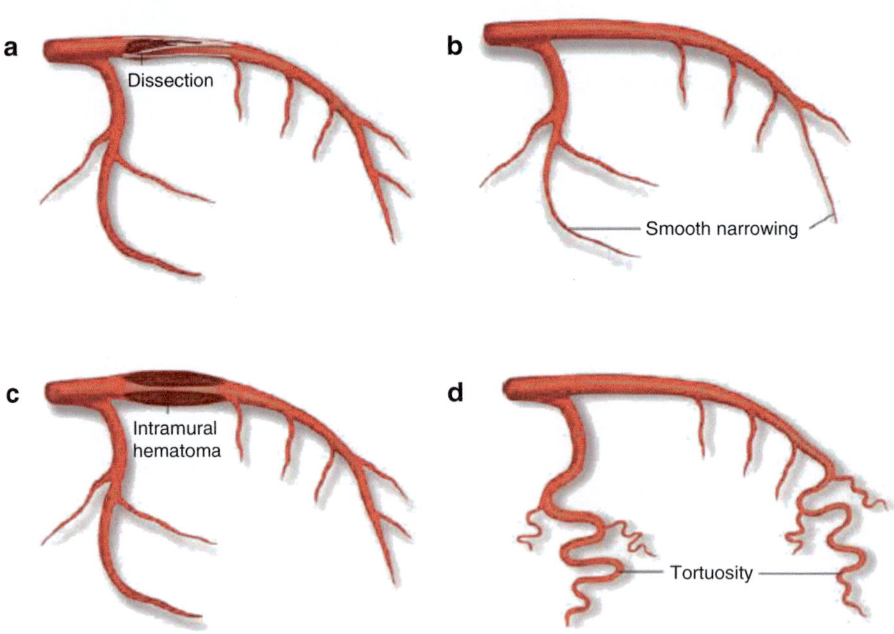

Fig. 3.4 Angiographic manifestations of FMD in coronary arteries. Adapted from: Michelis KC et al. [99]

There is no standardized work-up in patients after SCAD although it is recommended to perform genetic testing for the most common types of mixed connective tissue diseases. Given the relatively high prevalence of FMD in SCAD patients it is advised to perform a CT angiography or MRI of the renal arteries [99, 104]. The recurrence rate of SCAD varies between 10 and 17% [102]. It has been suggested that the degree of tortuosity in the coronary arteries may be a prognostic indicator of SCAD recurrence, but this has not been confirmed by others yet [105].

Takotsubo Cardiomyopathy (Apical Ballooning Syndrome, 'Broken Heart' Syndrome)

Takotsubo cardiomyopathy (TTC), first described in 1990, is a unique predominant female type of ACS characterized by the presence of transient LV wall dysfunction without any significant culprit lesion in the epicardial coronary arteries (Fig. 3.5) [106, 107]. In the majority of cases (>70%) severe emotional-stress acts as a triggering event, resulting is a high-dose catecholamine exposure that induces acute apical LV dysfunction [108, 109]. TTC is nowadays more often recognized than before and occurs in 2–3% of all ACS patients, with a predominance (>90%) in postmenopausal women above 60 years of age [110]. Women have an increased response to adrenergic stress after menopause which may contribute to their increased risk of TTC [111]. Lower estrogen status in postmenopausal women may lead to an impairment in vasodilating and vasoconstrictive reactivity in the microvascular coronary system, resulting in an increased responsiveness to sympathetic activity [112]. In IVUS studies in classical TTC patients no signs of obstructive CAD are seen [113]. In the International Takotsubo

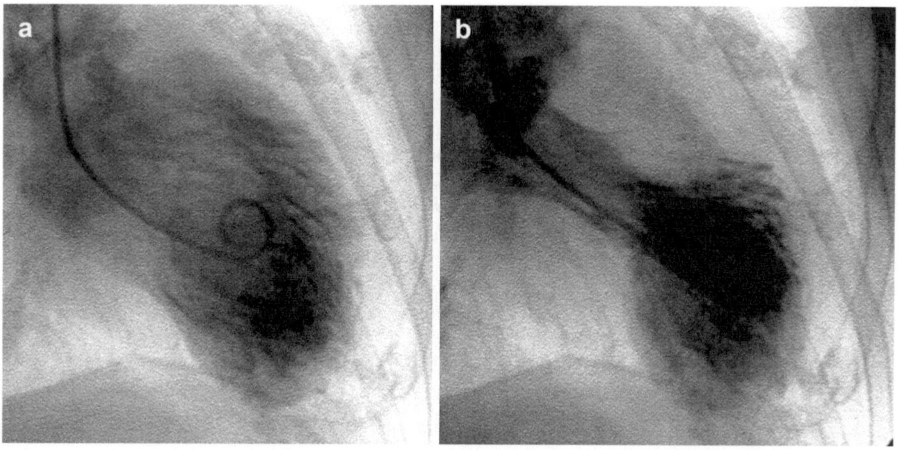

Fig. 3.5 Stress-induced ('tako-tsubo') cardiomyopathy. Adapted from: Teraoka K et al. Circulation. 2005;111:e261–e262

Registry it was found in 1750 patients (90% women) that emotional triggers were not as common as physical triggers (27.7% vs. 36.0%) and that 28.5% of patients had no evident trigger at all prior to their ACS [114]. Rates of neurologic or psychiatric disorders were higher (55.8% vs. 25.7%) compared to patients with standard ACS. In 4% of patients a 'happy' emotional event served as a trigger for TTC-ACS, in these cases named as the 'happy heart syndrome' [115]. In 20% of patients in this cohort more atypical presentations of TTC were noticed, characterized by a younger age of onset, more frequent presence of ST-segment depression, a higher prevalence of neurologic diseases, less pronounced reduction in left ventricular ejection fraction, and lower brain natriuretic peptide values on admission [116]. In general, ECG changes in TTC are comparable with other causes of ACS with a relatively smaller increase in creatinine kinase and hs troponin in proportion to the degree of LV dysfunction. A low serum N-terminal brain natriuretic peptide (NT-proBNP) at admission is a reliable indicator of a favorable prognosis [107]. Cardiac catheterization is still necessary for definitive differentiation between TTC and other causes of ACS and echocardiography or MRI plays a key role in diagnostic and follow-up assessment. A remarkable recovery of systolic LV function is mostly seen within days/weeks after acute onset. In clinical practice it may be difficult to differentiate between a TTC and standard ACS, as is showed in patient D. The use of ACE inhibitors or ARBs after TTC significantly reduces 1-year mortality rates, while this has not been established for the use of beta-blockers [114]. It is unknown yet whether prolonged use of platelet inhibitors and statins may prevent recurrence (0–11.4%) of TTC. Complication rates and mortality in general are comparable between TTC and standard ACS.

Patient D: Woman 72 years withTakotsubo ACS (or type II ACS?)

Medical history:
Known with moderate hypertension, never smoked. Very active for her age.
Negative family history of CVD, T cholesterol 4.6 mol/L, BMI 23.

Patient history: Yesterday evening at 18 hrs acute onset of chest pain, pressing and ongoing crescendo/decrescendo character with symptoms of nausea, vomiting and sweating. Radiation to the left armpit. She had worked all day in the garden and visited her husband in hospital. Two weeks ago she had comparable chest pain symptoms, of short duration, without radiation. These symptoms were not provoked by exercise of emotions. She had a stressful period with a husband having progressive dementia. He was hospitalized 2 days ago.

Medication at admission: Losartan 50 mg; Hydrochloorthiazide 25 mg

Comments: longer duration of stress affects blood pressure negatively and sudden events can induce a Takotsubo ACS. The angiographic features are compatible with a TTC. It may be difficult however to discriminate between a type II ACS.

ECG at admission: STEMI distal anterior leads

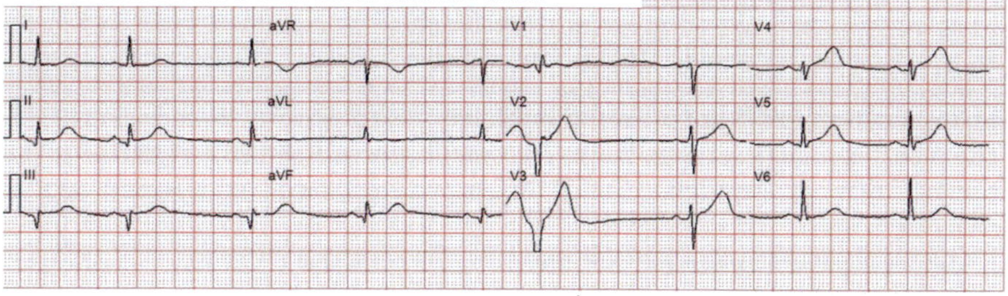

After 12 hrs, with slight residual chest pain

CK	**265**	**445**	**U/L**
hs-Troponin	**360**	**558**	**U/L**

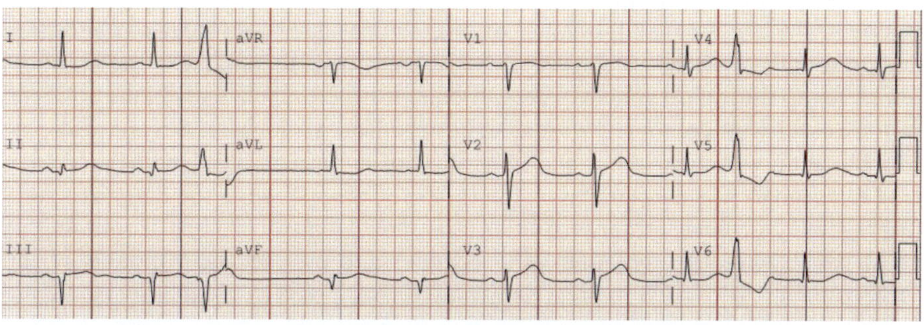

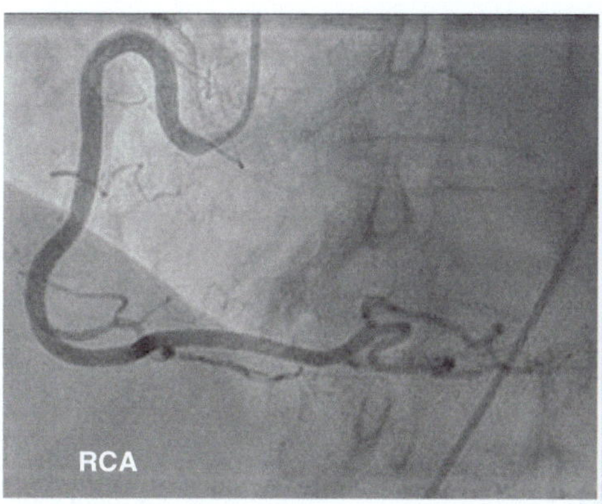

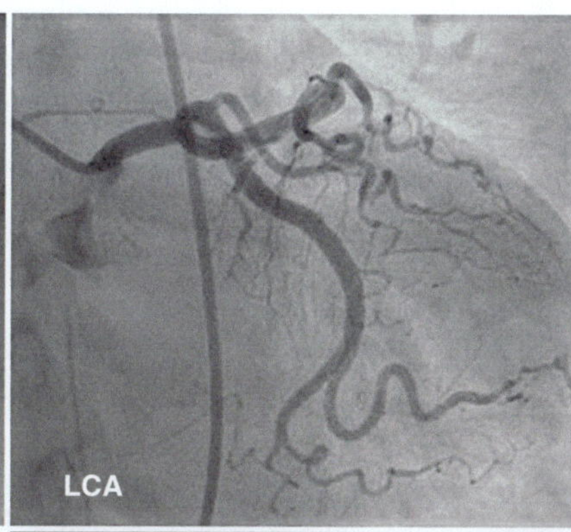

At CAG:

No focal CAD
LV: locally apical dyskinesia

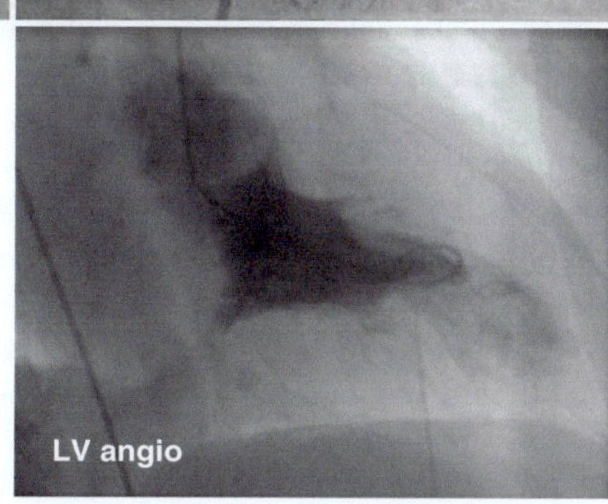

Acute Coronary Syndromes in Pregnancy

As IHD onset occurs at a younger age combined with a rise of maternal pregnancy age, the number of ACS during and immediately after pregnancy is increasing [117]. Estimated maternal death rates due to IHD vary between 5 and 20% [118, 119]. The incidence of pregnancy-related ACS is currently estimated at 1:16,000–32,000 deliveries.

Although patient series are not consistent, traditional CVD risk factors, elevated family risk and smoking account for the majority of atherosclerosis-related ACS during and after pregnancy, whereas spontaneous coronary artery dissection (SCAD) occur relatively more often around delivery and in the early postpartum period [93, 120]. Pregnancy-related ACS can occur during all stages of gestation and present most often as a STEMI. A SCAD may be associated with high progesterone levels during pregnancy with subsequent structural changes in the collagen of the vessel wall combined with a higher prothrombotic state. Severe post-partum bleeding with or without administration of ergonovine-like medication may lead to coronary vasospasm and a type II ACS. Cornerstone of the diagnosis ACS in pregnancy or puerperium is similar as in non-pregnant women, consisting of chest pain symptoms, dynamic ECG changes and elevated hs-troponins [121]. Timely diagnosis of ACS in pregnancy may be hampered by frequently occurring symptoms during pregnancy itself, such as dyspnea and extreme tiredness. Main differential diagnoses of acute ischemic chest pain are preeclampsia, acute pulmonary embolism and aortic dissection. In STEMI it is advised to do a CAG at a skilled lab with PCI facilities to perform an intervention when indicated. The radial access site is preferred for lower radiation and bleeding risk and the type of PCI is not different from non-pregnant women and depends on the findings at angiography.

Pregnancy in Women at Increased Cardiovascular Risk

In women with preexisting IHD, the risk of a subsequent pregnancy depends on higher maternal age, residual ischemia, LV function <40% and medication use [122, 123]. It is therefore strongly advised to apply preconception counseling in women at increased risk and to advise them according to the 2011 ESC guidelines during pregnancy [121]. Pregnancy should be strongly discouraged in women with severe left ventricular dysfunction (LVEF < 30%, NYHA III–IV) and in women with symptoms and signs of ischemia. In women after a previous IHD event, the use of acetylsalicylic acid and beta -blockers is safe during pregnancy, but the use of almost all other preventive cardiac medications should be (temporarily) interrupted. This should be well discussed before gestation.

Key Issues

- Women with ACS are in general older than men, with a relatively higher clustering of CVD risk factors
- 25–30% of all ACS concern women <65 years
- ACS in younger women (<65 years) has a lower burden of atherosclerosis than in men, with relatively more often a type II ACS, and more 'open' coronary arteries (MINOCA)
- ACS symptom presentation is more atypical in women with a longer patient delay and a twofold higher mortality than in men
- Women have a more than twice the rate of bleeding risk after acute coronary interventions as men
- Combined oral contraceptives to reduce menstrual bleeding are relatively contraindicated in patients with ACS and other established CAD
- Levonorgestrel releasing intra-uterine system (LNG-IUS), endometrial ablation or hysterectomy are alternative options
- 10–25% of ACS in women <65 years is a spontaneous coronary artery dissection (SCAD)
- Takotsubo ACS occurs 9–10 times more often in women (>60 years) than in men
- Women receive less often evidence-based therapy post-ACS than men
- Pre-pregnancy counseling is needed after SCAD and in women after a previous CVD event

References

1. Shepard D, VanderZanden A, Moran A, Naghavi M, Murray C, Roth G. Ischemic heart disease worldwide, 1990 to 2013: estimates from the global burden of disease study 2013. Circ Cardiovasc Qual Outcomes. 2015;8(4):455–6.
2. Hartley A, Marshall DC, Salciccioli JD, Sikkel MB, Maruthappu M, Shalhoub J. Trends in mortality from ischaemic heart disease and cerebrovascular disease in Europe: 1980–2009. Circulation. 2016;133(20):1916–26.
3. Hulsegge G, Picavet HS, Blokstra A, Nooyens AC, Spijkerman AM, van der Schouw YT, et al. Today's adult generations are less healthy than their predecessors: generation shifts in metabolic risk factors: the Doetinchem Cohort Study. Eur J Prev Cardiol. 2014;21(9): 1134–44.
4. Puymirat E, Simon T, Steg PG, Schiele F, Gueret P, Blanchard D, et al. Association of changes in clinical characteristics and management with improvement in survival among patients with ST-elevation myocardial infarction. JAMA. 2012;308(10):998–1006.
5. Ford ES, Capewell S. Coronary heart disease mortality among young adults in the U.S. from 1980 through 2002: concealed leveling of mortality rates. J Am Coll Cardiol. 2007;50(22): 2128–32.
6. Vedanthan R, Seligman B, Fuster V. Global perspective on acute coronary syndrome: a burden on the young and poor. Circ Res. 2014;114(12):1959–75.

7. Kragholm K, Halim SA, Yang Q, Schulte PJ, Hochman JS, Melloni C, et al. Sex-stratified trends in enrollment, patient characteristics, treatment, and outcomes among non-ST-segment elevation acute coronary syndrome patients: insights from clinical trials over 17 years. Circ Cardiovasc Qual Outcomes. 2015;8(4):357–67.
8. Berger JS, Elliott L, Gallup D, Roe M, Granger CB, Armstrong PW, et al. Sex differences in mortality following acute coronary syndromes. JAMA. 2009;302(8):874–82.
9. Albrektsen G, Heuch I, Lochen ML, Thelle DS, Wilsgaard T, Njolstad I, et al. Lifelong gender gap in risk of incident myocardial infarction: the Tromso Study. JAMA Intern Med. 2016;176(11):1673–9.
10. Champney KP, Frederick PD, Bueno H, Parashar S, Foody J, Merz CN, et al. The joint contribution of sex, age and type of myocardial infarction on hospital mortality following acute myocardial infarction. Heart. 2009;95(11):895–9.
11. Otten AM, Maas AH, Ottervanger JP, Kloosterman A, van't Hof AW, Dambrink JH, et al. Is the difference in outcome between men and women treated by primary percutaneous coronary intervention age dependent? Gender difference in STEMI stratified on age. Eur Heart J Acute Cardiovasc Care. 2013;2(4):334–41.
12. Gupta A, Wang Y, Spertus JA, Geda M, Lorenze N, Nkonde-Price C, et al. Trends in acute myocardial infarction in young patients and differences by sex and race, 2001 to 2010. J Am Coll Cardiol. 2014;64(4):337–45.
13. Chandrasekhar J, Baber U, Sartori S, Faggioni M, Aquino M, Kini A, et al. Sex-related differences in outcomes among men and women under 55 years of age with acute coronary syndrome undergoing percutaneous coronary intervention: results from the PROMETHEUS Study. Catheter Cardiovasc Interv. 2016;89(4):629–37.
14. Pagidipati NJ, Peterson ED. Acute coronary syndromes in women and men. Nat Rev Cardiol. 2016;13(8):471–80.
15. Dreyer RP, Wang Y, Strait KM, Lorenze NP, D'Onofrio G, Bueno H, et al. Gender differences in the trajectory of recovery in health status among young patients with acute myocardial infarction: results from the variation in recovery: role of gender on outcomes of young AMI patients (VIRGO) study. Circulation. 2015;131(22):1971–80.
16. D'Onofrio G, Safdar B, Lichtman JH, Strait KM, Dreyer RP, Geda M, et al. Sex differences in reperfusion in young patients with ST-segment-elevation myocardial infarction: results from the VIRGO study. Circulation. 2015;131(15):1324–32.
17. Donataccio MP, Puymirat E, Parapid B, Steg PG, Eltchaninoff H, Weber S, et al. In-hospital outcomes and long-term mortality according to sex and management strategy in acute myocardial infarction. Insights from the French ST-elevation and non-ST-elevation Myocardial Infarction (FAST-MI) 2005 Registry. Int J Cardiol. 2015;201:265–70.
18. Khera S, Kolte D, Gupta T, Subramanian KS, Khanna N, Aronow WS, et al. Temporal trends and sex differences in revascularization and outcomes of ST-segment elevation myocardial infarction in younger adults in the United States. J Am Coll Cardiol. 2015;66(18):1961–72.
19. Milcent C, Dormont B, Durand-Zaleski I, Steg PG. Gender differences in hospital mortality and use of percutaneous coronary intervention in acute myocardial infarction: microsimulation analysis of the 1999 nationwide French hospitals database. Circulation. 2007;115(7):833–9.
20. EUGenMed; Cardiovascular Clinical Study Group, Regitz-Zagrosek V, Oertelt-Prigione S, Prescott E, Franconi F, Gerdts E, Foryst-Ludwig A, Maas AH, Kautzky-Willer A, Knappe-Wegner D, Kintscher U, Ladwig KH, Schenck-Gustafsson K, Stangl V. Gender in cardiovascular diseases: impact on clinical manifestations management, and outcomes. Eur Heart J. 2016;37(1):24–34.
21. Mehta LS, Beckie TM, DeVon HA, Grines CL, Krumholz HM, Johnson MN, et al. Acute myocardial infarction in women: a scientific statement from the American Heart Association. Circulation. 2016;133(9):916–47.
22. Prescott E, Hippe M, Schnohr P, Hein HO, Vestbo J. Smoking and risk of myocardial infarction in women and men: longitudinal population study. BMJ. 1998;316(7137):1043–7.
23. Ranthe MF, Carstensen L, Oyen N, Tfelt-Hansen J, Christiansen M, McKenna WJ, et al. Family history of premature death and risk of early onset cardiovascular disease. J Am Coll Cardiol. 2012;60(9):814–21.

24. Choi J, Daskalopoulou SS, Thanassoulis G, Karp I, Pelletier R, Behlouli H, et al. Sex- and gender-related risk factor burden in patients with premature acute coronary syndrome. Can J Cardiol. 2014;30(1):109–17.
25. Hahmann HW, Schatzer-Klotz D, Bunte T, Becker D, Schieffer HJ. The significance of high levels of lipoprotein (a) compared with established risk factors in premature coronary artery disease: differences between men and women. Atherosclerosis. 1999;144(1):221–8.
26. Elias-Smale SE, Gunal A, Maas AH. Gynecardiology: distinct patterns of ischemic heart disease in middle-aged women. Maturitas. 2015;81(3):348–52.
27. Mu F, Rich-Edwards J, Rimm EB, Spiegelman D, Missmer SA. Endometriosis and risk of coronary heart disease. Circ Cardiovasc Qual Outcomes. 2016;9(3):257–64.
28. Ossewaarde ME, Bots ML, Verbeek AL, Peeters PH, van der Graaf Y, Grobbee DE, et al. Age at menopause, cause-specific mortality and total life expectancy. Epidemiology. 2005;16(4):556–62.
29. Mason JC, Libby P. Cardiovascular disease in patients with chronic inflammation: mechanisms underlying premature cardiovascular events in rheumatologic conditions. Eur Heart J. 2015;36(8):482–9c.
30. Low CA, Thurston RC, Matthews KA. Psychosocial factors in the development of heart disease in women: current research and future directions. Psychosom Med. 2010; 72(9):842–54.
31. Parashar S, Rumsfeld JS, Reid KJ, Buchanan D, Dawood N, Khizer S, et al. Impact of depression on sex differences in outcome after myocardial infarction. Circ Cardiovasc Qual Outcomes. 2009;2(1):33–40.
32. Bucholz EM, Strait KM, Dreyer RP, Lindau ST, D'Onofrio G, Geda M, et al. Sex differences in young patients with acute myocardial infarction: a VIRGO study analysis. Eur Heart J Acute Cardiovasc Care. 2016. pii: 2048872616661847. [Epub ahead of print].
33. Pelletier R, Khan NA, Cox J, Daskalopoulou SS, Eisenberg MJ, Bacon SL, et al. Sex versus gender-related characteristics: which predicts outcome after acute coronary syndrome in the young? J Am Coll Cardiol. 2016;67(2):127–35.
34. Crea F, Camici PG, Bairey Merz CN. Coronary microvascular dysfunction: an update. Eur Heart J. 2014;35(17):1101–11.
35. Hochman JS, Tamis JE, Thompson TD, Weaver WD, White HD, Van de Werf F, et al. Sex, clinical presentation, and outcome in patients with acute coronary syndromes. Global use of strategies to open occluded coronary arteries in acute coronary syndromes IIb investigators. N Engl J Med. 1999;341(4):226–32.
36. Jneid H, Fonarow GC, Cannon CP, Hernandez AF, Palacios IF, Maree AO, et al. Sex differences in medical care and early death after acute myocardial infarction. Circulation. 2008;118(25):2803–10.
37. Lichtman JH, Wang Y, Jones SB, Leifheit-Limson EC, Shaw LJ, Vaccarino V, et al. Age and sex differences in inhospital complication rates and mortality after percutaneous coronary intervention procedures: evidence from the NCDR®. Am Heart J. 2014;167(3):376–83.
38. Yahagi K, Davis HR, Arbustini E, Virmani R. Sex differences in coronary artery disease: pathological observations. Atherosclerosis. 2015;239(1):260–7.
39. Shaw LJ, Bugiardini R, Merz CN. Women and ischemic heart disease: evolving knowledge. J Am Coll Cardiol. 2009;54(17):1561–75.
40. Smilowitz NR, Sampson BA, Abrecht CR, Siegfried JS, Hochman JS, Reynolds HR. Women have less severe and extensive coronary atherosclerosis in fatal cases of ischemic heart disease: an autopsy study. Am Heart J. 2011;161(4):681–8.
41. Chandrasekhar J, Mehran R. Sex-based differences in acute coronary syndromes: insights from invasive and noninvasive coronary technologies. JACC Cardiovasc Imaging. 2016;9(4):451–64.
42. Thygesen K, Alpert JS, Jaffe AS, Simoons ML, Chaitman BR, White HD, et al. Third universal definition of myocardial infarction. Circulation. 2012;126(16):2020–35.
43. Shah AS, Griffiths M, Lee KK, McAllister DA, Hunter AL, Ferry AV, et al. High sensitivity cardiac troponin and the under-diagnosis of myocardial infarction in women: prospective cohort study. BMJ. 2015;350:g7873.

44. Beltrame JF. Assessing patients with myocardial infarction and nonobstructed coronary arteries (MINOCA). J Intern Med. 2013;273(2):182–5.
45. Pasupathy S, Tavella R, Beltrame JF. The what, when, who, why, how and where of myocardial infarction with non-obstructive coronary arteries (MINOCA). Circ J. 2015;80(1):11–6.
46. Agewall S, Beltrame JF, Reynolds HR, Niessner A, Rosano G, Caforio AL, et al. ESC working group position paper on myocardial infarction with non-obstructive coronary arteries. Eur Heart J. 2017;38(3):143–53.
47. Kovacic JC, Fuster V. Smoking gun theory: angiographically normal or mild coronary plaque as a cause of myocardial infarction. Circulation. 2012;126(25):2918–20.
48. Pasupathy S, Air T, Dreyer RP, Tavella R, Beltrame JF. Systematic review of patients presenting with suspected myocardial infarction and nonobstructive coronary arteries. Circulation. 2015;131(10):861–70.
49. Prati F, Uemura S, Souteyrand G, Virmani R, Motreff P, Di Vito L, et al. OCT-based diagnosis and management of STEMI associated with intact fibrous cap. JACC Cardiovasc Imaging. 2013;6(3):283–7.
50. Reynolds HR, Srichai MB, Iqbal SN, Slater JN, Mancini GB, Feit F, et al. Mechanisms of myocardial infarction in women without angiographically obstructive coronary artery disease. Circulation. 2011;124(13):1414–25.
51. Ong P, Athanasiadis A, Hill S, Vogelsberg H, Voehringer M, Sechtem U. Coronary artery spasm as a frequent cause of acute coronary syndrome: The CASPAR (Coronary Artery Spasm in Patients With Acute Coronary Syndrome) Study. J Am Coll Cardiol. 2008;52(7):523–7.
52. Tousoulis D, Oikonomou E, Economou EK, Crea F, Kaski JC. Inflammatory cytokines in atherosclerosis: current therapeutic approaches. Eur Heart J. 2016;37(22):1723–32.
53. Burke AP, Farb A, Malcom GT, Liang Y, Smialek J, Virmani R. Effect of risk factors on the mechanism of acute thrombosis and sudden coronary death in women. Circulation. 1998;97(21):2110–6.
54. Farb A, Burke AP, Tang AL, Liang TY, Mannan P, Smialek J, et al. Coronary plaque erosion without rupture into a lipid core. A frequent cause of coronary thrombosis in sudden coronary death. Circulation. 1996;93(7):1354–63.
55. Ruiz-Garcia J, Lerman A, Weisz G, Maehara A, Mintz GS, Fahy M, et al. Age- and gender-related changes in plaque composition in patients with acute coronary syndrome: the PROSPECT study. EuroIntervention. 2012;8(8):929–38.
56. Mackman N. Triggers, targets and treatments for thrombosis. Nature. 2008;451(7181):914–8.
57. Diercks DB, Owen KP, Kontos MC, Blomkalns A, Chen AY, Miller C, et al. Gender differences in time to presentation for myocardial infarction before and after a national women's cardiovascular awareness campaign: a temporal analysis from the Can Rapid Risk Stratification of Unstable Angina Patients Suppress ADverse Outcomes with Early Implementation (CRUSADE) and the National Cardiovascular Data Registry Acute Coronary Treatment and Intervention Outcomes Network-Get with the Guidelines (NCDR ACTION Registry-GWTG). Am Heart J. 2010;160(1):80–7.
58. Kaul P, Armstrong PW, Sookram S, Leung BK, Brass N, Welsh RC. Temporal trends in patient and treatment delay among men and women presenting with ST-elevation myocardial infarction. Am Heart J. 2011;161(1):91–7.
59. Lichtman JH, Leifheit-Limson EC, Watanabe E, Allen NB, Garavalia B, Garavalia LS, et al. Symptom recognition and healthcare experiences of young women with acute myocardial infarction. Circ Cardiovasc Qual Outcomes. 2015;8(2 Suppl. 1):S31–8.
60. Kreatsoulas C, Crea-Arsenio M, Shannon HS, Velianou JL, Giacomini M. Interpreting angina: symptoms along a gender continuum. Open Heart. 2016;3(1):e000376.
61. Canto JG, Goldberg RJ, Hand MM, Bonow RO, Sopko G, Pepine CJ, et al. Symptom presentation of women with acute coronary syndromes: myth vs reality. Arch Intern Med. 2007;167(22):2405–13.
62. Coventry LL, Finn J, Bremner AP. Sex differences in symptom presentation in acute myocardial infarction: a systematic review and meta-analysis. Heart Lung. 2011;40(6):477–91.

63. Makam RP, Erskine N, Yarzebski J, Lessard D, Lau J, Allison J, et al. Decade long trends (2001–2011) in duration of pre-hospital delay among elderly patients hospitalized for an acute myocardial infarction. J Am Heart Assoc. 2016;5(4):e002664.
64. McSweeney JC, Cody M, O'Sullivan P, Elberson K, Moser DK, Garvin BJ. Women's early warning symptoms of acute myocardial infarction. Circulation. 2003;108(21):2619–23.
65. Zhang ZM, Rautaharju PM, Prineas RJ, Rodriguez CJ, Loehr L, Rosamond WD, et al. Race and sex differences in the incidence and prognostic significance of silent myocardial infarction in the Atherosclerosis Risk in Communities (ARIC) Study. Circulation. 2016;133(22):2141–8.
66. Lee TH, Rouan GW, Weisberg MC, Brand DA, Acampora D, Stasiulewicz C, et al. Clinical characteristics and natural history of patients with acute myocardial infarction sent home from the emergency room. Am J Cardiol. 1987;60(4):219–24.
67. Pope JH, Aufderheide TP, Ruthazer R, Woolard RH, Feldman JA, Beshansky JR, et al. Missed diagnoses of acute cardiac ischemia in the emergency department. N Engl J Med. 2000;342(16):1163–70.
68. Lagerqvist B, Husted S, Kontny F, Stahle E, Swahn E, Wallentin L, et al. 5-year outcomes in the FRISC-II randomised trial of an invasive versus a non-invasive strategy in non-ST-elevation acute coronary syndrome: a follow-up study. Lancet. 2006;368(9540):998–1004.
69. Fox KA, Poole-Wilson PA, Henderson RA, Clayton TC, Chamberlain DA, Shaw TR, et al. Interventional versus conservative treatment for patients with unstable angina or non-ST-elevation myocardial infarction: the British Heart Foundation RITA 3 randomised trial. Randomized Intervention Trial of unstable Angina. Lancet. 2002;360(9335):743–51.
70. Swahn E, Alfredsson J, Afzal R, Budaj A, Chrolavicius S, Fox K, et al. Early invasive compared with a selective invasive strategy in women with non-ST-elevation acute coronary syndromes: a substudy of the OASIS 5 trial and a meta-analysis of previous randomized trials. Eur Heart J. 2012;33(1):51–60.
71. Roffi M, Patrono C, Collet JP, Mueller C, Valgimigli M, Andreotti F, et al. 2015 ESC guidelines for the management of acute coronary syndromes in patients presenting without persistent ST-segment elevation: task force for the management of acute coronary syndromes in patients presenting without persistent ST-segment elevation of the European Society of Cardiology (ESC). Eur Heart J. 2016;37(3):267–315.
72. Blomkalns AL, Chen AY, Hochman JS, Peterson ED, Trynosky K, Diercks DB, et al. Gender disparities in the diagnosis and treatment of non-ST-segment elevation acute coronary syndromes: large-scale observations from the CRUSADE (Can Rapid Risk Stratification of Unstable Angina Patients Suppress Adverse Outcomes With Early Implementation of the American College of Cardiology/American Heart Association Guidelines) National Quality Improvement Initiative. J Am Coll Cardiol. 2005;45(6):832–7.
73. Gale CP, Cattle BA, Woolston A, Baxter PD, West TH, Simms AD, et al. Resolving inequalities in care? Reduced mortality in the elderly after acute coronary syndromes. The Myocardial Ischaemia National Audit Project 2003-2010. Eur Heart J. 2012;33(5):630–9.
74. Nante N, Messina G, Cecchini M, Bertetto O, Moirano F, McKee M. Sex differences in use of interventional cardiology persist after risk adjustment. J Epidemiol Community Health. 2009;63(3):203–8.
75. Ramanath VS, Armstrong DF, Grzybowski M, Rahnama-Mohagdam S, Tamhane UU, Gordon K, et al. Receipt of cardiac medications upon discharge among men and women with acute coronary syndrome and nonobstructive coronary artery disease. Clin Cardiol. 2010;33(1):36–41.
76. Smolina K, Ball L, Humphries KH, Khan N, Morgan SG. Sex disparities in post-acute myocardial infarction pharmacologic treatment initiation and adherence: problem for young women. Circ Cardiovasc Qual Outcomes. 2015;8(6):586–92.
77. Ahmed B, Dauerman HL. Women, bleeding, and coronary intervention. Circulation. 2013;127(5):641–9.
78. Ndrepepa G, Schulz S, Neumann FJ, Byrne RA, Hoppmann P, Cassese S, et al. Bleeding after percutaneous coronary intervention in women and men matched for age, body mass index, and type of antithrombotic therapy. Am Heart J. 2013;166(3):534–40.

79. Feit F, Voeltz MD, Attubato MJ, Lincoff AM, Chew DP, Bittl JA, et al. Predictors and impact of major hemorrhage on mortality following percutaneous coronary intervention from the REPLACE-2 trial. Am J Cardiol. 2007;100(9):1364–9.
80. Mehta RH, Stebbins AS, Lopes RD, Califf RM, Pieper KS, Armstrong PW, et al. Comparison of incidence of bleeding and mortality of men versus women with ST-elevation myocardial infarction treated with fibrinolysis. Am J Cardiol. 2012;109(3):320–6.
81. Bertrand OF, Belisle P, Joyal D, Costerousse O, Rao SV, Jolly SS, et al. Comparison of transradial and femoral approaches for percutaneous coronary interventions: a systematic review and hierarchical Bayesian meta-analysis. Am Heart J. 2012;163(4):632–48.
82. Abdelaal E, Brousseau-Provencher C, Montminy S, Plourde G, MacHaalany J, Bataille Y, et al. Risk score, causes, and clinical impact of failure of transradial approach for percutaneous coronary interventions. JACC Cardiovasc Interv. 2013;6(11):1129–37.
83. Shin JS, Tahk SJ, Yang HM, Yoon MH, Choi SY, Choi BJ, et al. Impact of female gender on bleeding complications after transradial coronary intervention (from the Korean Transradial Coronary Intervention registry). Am J Cardiol. 2014;113(12):2002–6.
84. Maas AH, Euler M, Bongers MY, Rolden HJ, Grutters JP, Ulrich L, et al. Practice points in gynecardiology: abnormal uterine bleeding in premenopausal women taking oral anticoagulant or antiplatelet therapy. Maturitas. 2015;82(4):355–9.
85. Shufelt CL, Bairey Merz CN. Contraceptive hormone use and cardiovascular disease. J Am Coll Cardiol. 2009;53(3):221–31.
86. Roos-Hesselink JW, Cornette J, Sliwa K, Pieper PG, Veldtman GR, Johnson MR. Contraception and cardiovascular disease. Eur Heart J. 2015;36(27):1728–34, 34a–34b.
87. Saw J, Aymong E, Sedlak T, Buller CE, Starovoytov A, Ricci D, et al. Spontaneous coronary artery dissection: association with predisposing arteriopathies and precipitating stressors and cardiovascular outcomes. Circ Cardiovasc Interv. 2014;7(5):645–55.
88. Vrints CJ. Spontaneous coronary artery dissection. Heart. 2010;96(10):801–8.
89. Tweet MS, Gulati R, Hayes SN. What clinicians should know about spontaneous coronary artery dissection. Mayo Clin Proc. 2015;90(8):1125–30.
90. Otten AM, Ottervanger JP, Kloosterman A, van't Hof AW, Marcel Gosselink AT, Dambrink JH, et al. Treatment assignment in young women with spontaneous coronary artery dissection. Int J Cardiol. 2014;176(3):1223–4.
91. Vanzetto G, Berger-Coz E, Barone-Rochette G, Chavanon O, Bouvaist H, Hacini R, et al. Prevalence, therapeutic management and medium-term prognosis of spontaneous coronary artery dissection: results from a database of 11,605 patients. Eur J Cardiothorac Surg. 2009;35(2):250–4.
92. Nakashima T, Noguchi T, Haruta S, Yamamoto Y, Oshima S, Nakao K, et al. Prognostic impact of spontaneous coronary artery dissection in young female patients with acute myocardial infarction: A report from the Angina Pectoris-Myocardial Infarction Multicenter Investigators in Japan. Int J Cardiol. 2016;207:341–8.
93. Roth A, Elkayam U. Acute myocardial infarction associated with pregnancy. J Am Coll Cardiol. 2008;52(3):171–80.
94. Vijayaraghavan R, Verma S, Gupta N, Saw J. Pregnancy-related spontaneous coronary artery dissection. Circulation. 2014;130(21):1915–20.
95. Faden MS, Bottega N, Benjamin A, Brown RN. A nationwide evaluation of spontaneous coronary artery dissection in pregnancy and the puerperium. Heart. 2016;102(24):1974–79.
96. Giacoppo D, Capodanno D, Dangas G, Tamburino C. Spontaneous coronary artery dissection. Int J Cardiol. 2014;175(1):8–20.
97. Alfonso F, Bastante T, Cuesta J, Rodriguez D, Benedicto A, Rivero F. Spontaneous coronary artery dissection: novel insights on diagnosis and management. Cardiovasc Diagn Ther. 2015;5(2):133–40.
98. Hill SF, Sheppard MN. Non-atherosclerotic coronary artery disease associated with sudden cardiac death. Heart. 2010;96(14):1119–25.
99. Michelis KC, Olin JW, Kadian-Dodov D, d'Escamard V, Kovacic JC. Coronary artery manifestations of fibromuscular dysplasia. J Am Coll Cardiol. 2014;64(10):1033–46.

100. Saw J, Bezerra H, Gornik HL, Machan L, Mancini GB. Angiographic and intracoronary manifestations of coronary fibromuscular dysplasia. Circulation. 2016;133(16):1548–59.
101. Henkin S, Negrotto SM, Tweet MS, Kirmani S, Deyle DR, Gulati R, et al. Spontaneous coronary artery dissection and its association with heritable connective tissue disorders. Heart. 2016;102(11):876–81.
102. Tweet MS, Hayes SN, Pitta SR, Simari RD, Lerman A, Lennon RJ, et al. Clinical features, management, and prognosis of spontaneous coronary artery dissection. Circulation. 2012;126(5):579–88.
103. Saw J, Mancini GB, Humphries KH. Contemporary review on spontaneous coronary artery dissection. J Am Coll Cardiol. 2016;68(3):297–312.
104. Persu A, Giavarini A, Touze E, Januszewicz A, Sapoval M, Azizi M, et al. European consensus on the diagnosis and management of fibromuscular dysplasia. J Hypertens. 2014;32(7):1367–78.
105. Eleid MF, Guddeti RR, Tweet MS, Lerman A, Singh M, Best PJ, et al. Coronary artery tortuosity in spontaneous coronary artery dissection: angiographic characteristics and clinical implications. Circ Cardiovasc Interv. 2014;7(5):656–62.
106. Prasad A, Lerman A, Rihal CS. Apical ballooning syndrome (Tako-Tsubo or stress cardiomyopathy): a mimic of acute myocardial infarction. Am Heart J. 2008;155(3):408–17.
107. Bossone E, Lyon A, Citro R, Athanasiadis A, Meimoun P, Parodi G, et al. Takotsubo cardiomyopathy: an integrated multi-imaging approach. Eur Heart J Cardiovasc Imaging. 2014;15(4):366–77.
108. Paur H, Wright PT, Sikkel MB, Tranter MH, Mansfield C, O'Gara P, et al. High levels of circulating epinephrine trigger apical cardiodepression in a beta2-adrenergic receptor/Gi-dependent manner: a new model of Takotsubo cardiomyopathy. Circulation. 2012;126(6):697–706.
109. Lyon AR, Rees PS, Prasad S, Poole-Wilson PA, Harding SE. Stress (Takotsubo) cardiomyopathy—a novel pathophysiological hypothesis to explain catecholamine-induced acute myocardial stunning. Nat Clin Pract Cardiovasc Med. 2008;5(1):22–9.
110. Otten AM, Ottervanger JP, Symersky T, Suryapranata H, de Boer MJ, Maas AH. Diagnosis of takotsubo cardiomyopathy is increasing over time in patients presenting as ST-elevation myocardial infarction. Neth Heart J. 2016;24(9):520–9.
111. Martin EA, Tan SL, MacBride LR, Lavi S, Lerman LO, Lerman A. Sex differences in vascular and endothelial responses to acute mental stress. Clin Auton Res. 2008;18(6):339–45.
112. Otten AM, Ottervanger JP, Symersky T, Suryapranata H, de Boer MJ, Maas AH. Tako-tsubo cardiomyopathy is age-dependent in men, but not in women. Int J Cardiol. 2015;188:65–6.
113. Haghi D, Roehm S, Hamm K, Harder N, Suselbeck T, Borggrefe M, et al. Takotsubo cardiomyopathy is not due to plaque rupture: an intravascular ultrasound study. Clin Cardiol. 2010;33(5):307–10.
114. Templin C, Ghadri JR, Diekmann J, Napp LC, Bataiosu DR, Jaguszewski M, et al. Clinical features and outcomes of takotsubo (stress) cardiomyopathy. N Engl J Med. 2015; 373(10):929–38.
115. Ghadri JR, Sarcon A, Diekmann J, Bataiosu DR, Cammann VL, Jurisic S, et al. Happy heart syndrome: role of positive emotional stress in takotsubo syndrome. Eur Heart J. 2016;37(37):2823–29.
116. Ghadri JR, Cammann VL, Napp LC, Jurisic S, Diekmann J, Bataiosu DR, et al. Differences in the clinical profile and outcomes of typical and atypical takotsubo syndrome: data from the International Takotsubo Registry. JAMA Cardiol. 2016;1(3):335–40.
117. Callaghan WM, Creanga AA, Kuklina EV. Severe maternal morbidity among delivery and postpartum hospitalizations in the United States. Obstet Gynecol. 2012;120(5):1029–36.
118. Cantwell R, Clutton-Brock T, Cooper G, Dawson A, Drife J, Garrod D, et al. Saving mothers' lives: reviewing maternal deaths to make motherhood safer: 2006–2008. The eighth report of the confidential enquiries into maternal deaths in the United Kingdom. BJOG. 2011;118(Suppl. 1):1–203.
119. James AH, Jamison MG, Biswas MS, Brancazio LR, Swamy GK, Myers ER. Acute myocardial infarction in pregnancy: a United States population-based study. Circulation. 2006;113(12):1564–71.

120. Elkayam U, Jalnapurkar S, Barakkat MN, Khatri N, Kealey AJ, Mehra A, et al. Pregnancy-associated acute myocardial infarction: a review of contemporary experience in 150 cases between 2006 and 2011. Circulation. 2014;129(16):1695–702.
121. European Society of G, Association for European Paediatric C, German Society for Gender M, Regitz-Zagrosek V, Blomstrom Lundqvist C, Borghi C, et al. ESC guidelines on the management of cardiovascular diseases during pregnancy: the task force on the management of cardiovascular diseases during pregnancy of the European Society of Cardiology (ESC). Eur Heart J. 2011;32(24):3147–97.
122. Roos-Hesselink JW, Ruys TP, Stein JI, Thilen U, Webb GD, Niwa K, et al. Outcome of pregnancy in patients with structural or ischaemic heart disease: results of a registry of the European Society of Cardiology. Eur Heart J. 2013;34(9):657–65.
123. Burchill LJ, Lameijer H, Roos-Hesselink JW, Grewal J, Ruys TP, Kulikowski JD, et al. Pregnancy risks in women with pre-existing coronary artery disease, or following acute coronary syndrome. Heart. 2015;101(7):525–9.

Chapter 4
Stable Ischemic Heart Disease Beyond Stenoses: Coronary Microvascular Dysfunction

Suzette Elias-Smale

Abstract At least half of (predominant) female patients with recurrent angina, without signs of obstructive CAD, have underlying coronary microvascular dysfunction (CMD). Especially when signs of ischemia are present, this syndrome has an adverse prognosis. Patients with CMD have a characteristic symptom presentation, with a variety of traditional and non-traditional risk factors. Diagnostic testing and treatment are still a challenge, with much room for improvement.

Keywords Cardiac syndrome X • Classification CMD • Coronary flow reserve (CFR) • Coronary microvascular disease (CMD) • Coronary reactivity testing (CRT) • Intravascular ultrasound (IVUS) • Microvascular angina • Non-obstructive CAD (NOCAD) • Transthoracic Doppler echocardiography (TTDE) • Vasospasm

Background Stable Angina Without Obstructive Coronary Artery Disease

Evolving knowledge regarding sex differences in ischemic heart disease (IHD) has emerged over the last decades. Prevalence, symptom manifestation, and pathophysiology for IHD vary between women and men. Paradoxical sex differences are observed where women have more often non-obstructive coronary artery disease (NOCAD) and yet greater rates of myocardial ischemia and mortality than men [1, 2]. These differences are associated with women's smaller coronary arteries, higher coronary blood flow, and higher endothelial shear stress, which have major effects on endothelial function and the distribution of coronary atherosclerosis [3].

Approximately 60–70% of women versus 30% of men undergoing a clinically indicated coronary angiography for suspected stable IHD do not have obstructive

S. Elias-Smale, M.D., Ph.D.
Department of Cardiology, Radboud University Medical Center, Nijmegen, The Netherlands
e-mail: Suzette.Elias-Smale@radboudumc.nl

A.H.E.M. Maas, C.N. Bairey Merz (eds.), *Manual of Gynecardiology*,
DOI 10.1007/978-3-319-54960-6_4

CAD [4]. These rates are especially high in women below 60 years of age, in which up to 80% of women have (near) normal coronary arteries [5]. In these patients, endothelial and/or microvascular dysfunction, and many other processes (e.g. coronary spasm or myocardial bridging), may contribute to myocardial ischemia [6, 7]. In 80–100% of such patients, atherosclerosis was observed in the coronary arteries using intravascular ultrasound (IVUS) [8, 9]. This suggests that atherosclerosis might be linked to these other mechanisms, especially to endothelial and coronary microvascular dysfunction (CMD). This broadens our traditional concepts of coronary atherosclerosis to be not only involved in obstructive CAD, but also in dysfunction of the coronary epicardial vessels and microcirculation (See Fig. 2.3, Chap. 2).

It is estimated that at least half of patients with IHD without obstructive CAD have underlying CMD [10]. However, particularly in women, complex interactions of diffuse epicardial coronary narrowing and CMD often make a definitive underlying diagnosis difficult. The previously used term 'cardiac syndrome X', revealing the puzzle this condition has been given many physicians over the last decades, is now obsolete.

In contrast to what was previously thought, large prospective studies indicate that patients with NOCAD, especially when ischemia is present, do not have benign cardiovascular outcomes, but an increased risk of myocardial infarction, heart failure, stroke and cardiovascular and overall mortality [4, 11–15].

Coronary Microvascular Dysfunction

The primary task of the coronary microcirculation, which comprises 90% of the coronary circulation, is to match coronary blood flow supply and myocardial demand by processes involving endothelial and non-endothelial dependent vasoreactivity of the small (pre) arterioles [16]. Dysfunction of the microvasculature can lead to ischemia by limited microvascular vasodilator capacity or inappropriate vasoconstriction [17].

In 2007, Camici and Crea proposed original clinical and pathogenic classifications of CMD [18]. Accordingly, CMD was classified into four main types on the basis of the clinical setting in which it occurs: (1) CMD in the absence of myocardial diseases and obstructive CAD, (2) CMD in myocardial diseases, (3) CMD in obstructive CAD, and (4) iatrogenic CMD. Furthermore, they proposed that several pathogenic mechanisms can contribute to CMD and their importance varies in different clinical settings, although many of them may coexist in the same condition (Table 4.1).

In this chapter, we will focus on type I CMD while it typically occurs in women and is the most challenging condition regarding proper diagnosis and treatment.

Symptom Evaluation in Coronary Microvascular Dysfunction

In patients with microvascular angina, chest pain is frequently provoked by exercise, resembling 'classical' stable angina caused by severe epicardial vessel narrowing. However, the presence of CMD is more likely if there is a variable threshold of physical activity that provokes angina, if the chest pain persists for several minutes

Table 4.1 Types of CMD, adapted from Camici and Crea NEJM 2007 [18]

Type of MCD	Description
Primary MCD: MCD in the absence of obstructive CAD and myocardial disease	This type is related to traditional cardiovascular risk factors. Both endothelial dependent and non-endothelial dependent vasoreactivity plays a role
MCD in myocardial disease	This type is sustained by adverse remodeling of intramural coronary arterioles and found in primary and secondary cardiomyopathies
MCD in obstructive CAD	This type accompanies stable CAD or ACS
Iatrogenic MCD	This type occurs after PCI and seems to be caused by distal embolization and or vasoconstriction

Table 4.2 Symptoms of CMD

Exertional angina ('typical' angina)
Angina provoked by a variable threshold of physical activity
Angina persisting for minutes to hours after exertion is interrupted
Angina at rest and or at night/early morning
Angina triggered by palpitations or mental arousal
Poor/slow response to nitroglycerin
Dyspnea at exertion
Tiredness/loss of energy (can also be reported on the day after a busy day)

after effort is interrupted and/or whether there is slow or poor response to nitroglycerin [19, 20]. In addition to exercise induced angina, (prolonged) chest pain at rest and or at night/early morning is often reported, which may be provoked by vasospasm [21, 22]. Also, low heart rate activities such as mental arousal, or palpitation are more common triggers of angina than in patients with obstructive atherosclerosis [23]. In many patients, dyspnea at exertion is also reported an equivalent of a disturbed oxygen demand, with a general feeling of tiredness and loss of energy (see patient example) (Table 4.2). Microvascular angina has now been incorporated in the 2013 European Society of Cardiology (ESC) guidelines on management of stable CAD [20].

Risk Factors for Coronary Microvascular Dysfunction Type 1

Common cardiovascular risk factors such as hypertension, dyslipidemia, diabetes mellitus, and smoking are also known to be involved in CMD [18]. Most CMD type 1 patients have multiple ACSVD risk factors, despite data suggesting that a poor relation exists between these risk factors and CMD severity [24]. Female-specific cardiovascular risk factors (e.g. gestational diabetes and hypertension, pre-eclampsia, HELLP syndrome) and non-traditional risk factors, such as migraine and chronic inflammatory rheumatoid diseases are more commonly seen in women than in men. It is assumed that CMD may be the key mechanism involved in accelerated atherosclerosis in chronic inflammatory diseases [25, 26].

Diagnostic Testing of Coronary Microvascular Dysfunction

The diagnosis of CMD requires the exclusion of obstructive CAD by coronary computed tomography angiography (CTA) or coronary angiography (CAG). Since women often express a more diffuse pattern of atherosclerosis instead of stenotic disease, It is important to not merely focus on significant anatomical stenoses (commonly defined as >50% luminal narrowing) [1]. Excluding the hemodynamic relevance of evident coronary plaque—yet without the appearance of stenosis—by fractional reserve measurement (FFR) may be helpful in selected patients before making a diagnosis of microvascular disease as the most probable cause of the patient's symptoms [27].

Apart from exclusion of hemodynamic relevant epicardial CAD, attempts should be made to obtain objective evidence of CMD. The diagnosis can be established if a symptomatic patient has normal or non-obstructed coronary arteries by arteriography (coronary CTA or CAG), but with objective signs of cardiac ischemia (e.g. ST segment depression on exercise ECG, ischemic changes by myocardial perfusion imaging). It is of note that in CMD patients wall motion abnormalities usually cannot be induced during dobutamine stress echocardiography [28].

Since ischemia cannot always be detected by commonly used methods in cardiology practice, diagnostic tests for CMD are focused on the evaluation of coronary vascular function. Invasive coronary reactivity testing (CRT) using vaso-active agents to evaluate macrovascular and microvascular responses is still considered the reference standard for a definitive diagnosis of CMD [29]. During invasive coronary angiography non-endothelial mediated vasoreactivity is tested by measurement of coronary flow reserve (CFR). This is defined as the ratio of hyperemic myocardial blood flow, as induced by administration of adenosine or dipirydamole, divided by resting flow. A CFR ≤ 2.5 is indicative of coronary microvascular dysfunction. In both symptomatic men and women, a CFR < 2.0 has been shown to be an important predictor of adverse outcomes [13]. Endothelial dependent microvascular function is tested by injection of acetylcholine. A reduction of coronary blood flow >50% in response to high dose acetylcholine is regarded as abnormal endothelial microvascular function. In extent, acetylcholine, in different dosages, is used to assess macrovascular endothelial function and micro- and macrovascular vasospasm. Furthermore, non-endothelial macrovascular function is tested using nitroglycerin [29]. Invasive coronary reactivity testing is a very complete and thorough study of macro- and microvascular coronary (dys)function, and an invasive established diagnosis of CMD has been associated with a worse outcome [13, 30, 31]. Despite, this test is not routinely performed for a variety of reasons, including a lack of standardized protocols and concerns over catheterization laboratory time and safety. Several studies, however, have shown this method to have acceptably low complication rates and recently guidelines have been published for vasoreactivity testing [29, 32, 33].

In recent years, technological advances have led to the development of several non-invasive imaging techniques that allow sufficiently reliable measures of CMD. Using transthoracic Doppler echocardiography (TTDE), CFR can be assessed by measuring diastolic coronary blood flow in the left anterior descending (LAD) coronary at peak vasodilatation and at rest. Although this technique needs practice, reproducibility studies have shown acceptable intra-observer and inter-observer variability of TTDE–CFR performed by skilled operators [34]. Validation studies have shown that TTDE is feasible in the majority of patients and show a high agreement with CFR obtained with invasive coronary reactivity testing [35]. Positron emission tomography (PET) can also measure CFR and detect coronary vasomotor abnormalities caused by microvascular disease. PET has been shown to be a reliable tool to quantify myocardial blood flow (MBF) and CFR. Unfortunately, availability of PET scanning for diagnosis of CMD is limited. The nuclear tracers that can measure MBF and CFR most reliably are oxygen-15 labeled water and nitrogen-13 labeled ammonia [36]. However, an on-site cyclotron is mandatory for usage of these tracers. There is no consensus yet on whether contrast stress echocardiography or cardiac magnetic resonance (CMR) can reliably quantify perfusion abnormalities caused by CMD [35].

Therapeutic Options for Coronary Microvascular Dysfunction

First of all, it is of note that therapy studies for CMD are limited and often suffer from small sample sizes and a heterogeneous patient selection. Current ESC guidelines recommend that in all patients with microvascular angina optimal coronary risk factor control should be achieved and all patients should receive secondary cardiovascular prevention medications including aspirin and statins [20]. However, the benefits of long-term aspirin use in CMD patients is uncertain. Risk factor control should also include non-pharmacological therapy including weight loss, healthy diet and exercise [37]. For some patients, stress reduction therapy, like mindfulness based cognitive therapy, can be beneficial in reducing symptoms [SE, unpublished data].

Anti-anginal treatment is empirical while underlying mechanisms of CMD are often diverse and overlapping with macrovascular coronary disease. Treatment approaches should be tailored to the underlying mechanism whenever possible. In patients with exercise induced angina beta-blockers are first choice. Research has shown more favorable results from nebivolol compared to metoprolol [38]. Calcium antagonists and long-acting nitrates have shown variable results in clinical trials and are more helpful when used in addition to beta-blockers in the case of insufficient control of symptoms. However, in patients with predominant angina at rest, indicating an underlying vasospastic component, calcium antagonists are recommended as first line of therapy [37]. Short acting nitrates are recommended to relieve spontaneous attacks of angina. However, patients often report a limited effect of this treatment. In patients with angina refractory to various combinations of traditional anti-anginal medication, non-traditional forms of anti-anginal treatment can be added. Options include xanthine derivatives (aminophylline, bamiphylline), ivabradine, ranolazine, and nicorandil [20]. In patients in who enhanced pain

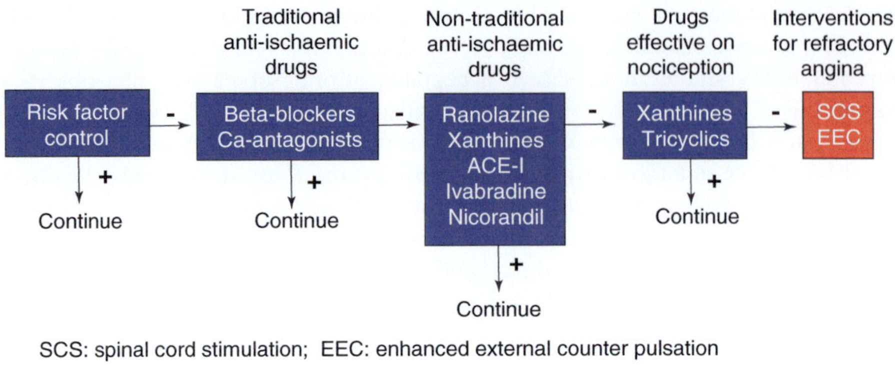

Fig. 4.1 Therapeutic options for CMD (ESC guidelines on management of stable angina [20]). *SCS* spinal cord stimulation, *EEC* enhanced external counter pulsation

perception is suspected drugs which modulate pain perception, like tricyclic antidepressants, are indicated [23]. Unfortunately, in patients with microvascular angina, the susceptibility of symptoms to medical treatment is extremely variable. Trialing of different drug combinations is often needed before establishing satisfactory symptom control and about 30% patients have refractory angina despite optimization of pharmacotherapy [39]. In those patients, additional interventions for pain relief like spinal cord stimulation or enhanced external counterpulsation may be discussed [see Fig. 4.1. Schematic overview therapy ESC guideline].

While most cardiologists still focus on obstructive CAD, the diagnosis CMD is often overlooked leading to preventable visits to the emergency room, repeat coronary angiograms, high treatment costs, diminished quality of life and even a worse cardiovascular prognosis [5].

The following patient story illustrates this.

Netty, 56 years, CMD type 1 patient: "I was not taken seriously with my complaints".

"Six years ago I started to have oppressive chest pain, shortness of breath on exertion and fatigue. The chest pain often came up after physical exertion, and could keep on for hours. Symptoms were also triggered by emotional stress. If I could not resolve the pain with relaxation methods, I took sublingual nitroglycerin, on which the pain usually subsided.

I was rushed to the hospital several times. On each occasion a coronary angiogram was made to see if there was an obstruction in my coronary arteries, but time and again the cardiologists told me that there was nothing wrong with my heart.

My symptoms, however, persisted, and I went from one doctor/cardiologist to another, but nobody could help me. The whole time I felt like I was not taken seriously with my complaints, while I strongly felt that there had to be some kind of underlying disease. After 2 years I came in contact with a cardiologist specialized in coronary microvascular disease, by whom my disease was finally diagnosed. Now I am treated with various medications. And although my symptoms have not completely subsided, I am doing a lot better. Also the fact that finally a diagnosis was made, helped me and my family a lot."

References

1. Shaw LJ, et al. Insights from the NHLBI-Sponsored Women's Ischemia Syndrome Evaluation (WISE) Study: part I: gender differences in traditional and novel risk factors, symptom evaluation, and gender-optimized diagnostic strategies. J Am Coll Cardiol. 2006;47(3 Suppl): S4–S20.
2. Bairey Merz CN, et al. Insights from the NHLBI-Sponsored Women's Ischemia Syndrome Evaluation (WISE) Study: part II: gender differences in presentation, diagnosis, and outcome with regard to gender-based pathophysiology of atherosclerosis and macrovascular and microvascular coronary disease. J Am Coll Cardiol. 2006;47(3 Suppl):S21–9.
3. Patel MB, et al. Imaging microvascular dysfunction and mechanisms for female-male differences in CAD. JACC Cardiovasc Imaging. 2016;9(4):465–82.
4. Jespersen L, et al. Stable angina pectoris with no obstructive coronary artery disease is associated with increased risks of major adverse cardiovascular events. Eur Heart J. 2012;33(6):734–44.
5. Johnston N, Schenck-Gustafsson K, Lagerqvist B. Are we using cardiovascular medications and coronary angiography appropriately in men and women with chest pain? Eur Heart J. 2011;32(11):1331–6.
6. Pepine CJ. Multiple causes for ischemia without obstructive coronary artery disease: not a short list. Circulation. 2015;131(12):1044–6.
7. Pepine CJ, et al. Emergence of nonobstructive coronary artery disease: a woman's problem and need for change in definition on angiography. J Am Coll Cardiol. 2015;66(17):1918–33.
8. Khuddus MA, et al. An intravascular ultrasound analysis in women experiencing chest pain in the absence of obstructive coronary artery disease: a substudy from the National Heart, Lung and Blood Institute-Sponsored Women's Ischemia Syndrome Evaluation (WISE). J Interv Cardiol. 2010;23(6):511–9.
9. Lee BK, et al. Invasive evaluation of patients with angina in the absence of obstructive coronary artery disease. Circulation. 2015;131(12):1054–60.
10. Marinescu MA, et al. Coronary microvascular dysfunction, microvascular angina, and treatment strategies. JACC Cardiovasc Imaging. 2015;8(2):210–20.
11. Lin FY, et al. Mortality risk in symptomatic patients with nonobstructive coronary artery disease: a prospective 2-center study of 2,583 patients undergoing 64-detector row coronary computed tomographic angiography. J Am Coll Cardiol. 2011;58(5):510–9.
12. Maddox TM, et al. Nonobstructive coronary artery disease and risk of myocardial infarction. JAMA. 2014;312(17):1754–63.
13. Murthy VL, et al. Effects of sex on coronary microvascular dysfunction and cardiac outcomes. Circulation. 2014;129(24):2518–27.
14. Johnson BD, et al. Persistent chest pain predicts cardiovascular events in women without obstructive coronary artery disease: results from the NIH-NHLBI-sponsored Women's Ischaemia Syndrome Evaluation (WISE) study. Eur Heart J. 2006;27(12):1408–15.

15. Gulati M, et al. Adverse cardiovascular outcomes in women with nonobstructive coronary artery disease: a report from the Women's Ischemia Syndrome Evaluation Study and the St James Women Take Heart Project. Arch Intern Med. 2009;169(9):843–50.
16. Herrmann J, Kaski JC, Lerman A. Coronary microvascular dysfunction in the clinical setting: from mystery to reality. Eur Heart J. 2012;33(22):2771–2782b.
17. Camici PG, d'Amati G, Rimoldi O. Coronary microvascular dysfunction: mechanisms and functional assessment. Nat Rev Cardiol. 2015;12(1):48–62.
18. Camici PG, Crea F. Coronary microvascular dysfunction. N Engl J Med. 2007;356(8): 830–40.
19. Lanza GA, Crea F. Primary coronary microvascular dysfunction: clinical presentation, pathophysiology, and management. Circulation. 2010;121(21):2317–25.
20. Task Force M, et al. 2013 ESC guidelines on the management of stable coronary artery disease: the Task Force on the management of stable coronary artery disease of the European Society of Cardiology. Eur Heart J. 2013;34(38):2949–3003.
21. Ong P, et al. Increased coronary vasoconstrictor response to acetylcholine in women with chest pain and normal coronary arteriograms (cardiac syndrome X). Clin Res Cardiol. 2012;101(8):673–81.
22. Cosin-Sales J, et al. C-reactive protein, clinical presentation, and ischemic activity in patients with chest pain and normal coronary angiograms. J Am Coll Cardiol. 2003;41(9):1468–74.
23. Crea F, Camici PG, Bairey Merz CN. Coronary microvascular dysfunction: an update. Eur Heart J. 2014;35(17):1101–11.
24. Wessel TR, et al. Coronary microvascular reactivity is only partially predicted by atherosclerosis risk factors or coronary artery disease in women evaluated for suspected ischemia: results from the NHLBI Women's Ischemia Syndrome Evaluation (WISE). Clin Cardiol. 2007;30(2):69–74.
25. Gianturco L, et al. Cardiovascular and autoimmune diseases in females: the role of microvasculature and dysfunctional endothelium. Atherosclerosis. 2015;241(1):259–63.
26. Faccini A, Kaski JC, Camici PG. Coronary microvascular dysfunction in chronic inflammatory rheumatoid diseases. Eur Heart J. 2016;37(23):1799–806.
27. Rodes-Cabau J, et al. Importance of diffuse atherosclerosis in the functional evaluation of coronary stenosis in the proximal-mid segment of a coronary artery by myocardial fractional flow reserve measurements. Am J Cardiol. 2011;108(4):483–90.
28. Panza JA, et al. Investigation of the mechanism of chest pain in patients with angiographically normal coronary arteries using transesophageal dobutamine stress echocardiography. J Am Coll Cardiol. 1997;29(2):293–301.
29. Wei J, et al. Safety of coronary reactivity testing in women with no obstructive coronary artery disease: results from the NHLBI-sponsored WISE (Women's Ischemia Syndrome Evaluation) study. JACC Cardiovasc Interv. 2012;5(6):646–53.
30. von Mering GO, et al. Abnormal coronary vasomotion as a prognostic indicator of cardiovascular events in women: results from the National Heart, Lung, and Blood Institute-Sponsored Women's Ischemia Syndrome Evaluation (WISE). Circulation. 2004;109(6):722–5.
31. Pepine CJ, et al. Coronary microvascular reactivity to adenosine predicts adverse outcome in women evaluated for suspected ischemia results from the National Heart, Lung and Blood Institute WISE (Women's Ischemia Syndrome Evaluation) study. J Am Coll Cardiol. 2010;55(25):2825–32.
32. Ong P, et al. Clinical usefulness, angiographic characteristics, and safety evaluation of intracoronary acetylcholine provocation testing among 921 consecutive white patients with unobstructed coronary arteries. Circulation. 2014;129(17):1723–30.
33. Beltrame JF, Crea F, Kaski JC, Ogawa H, Ong P, Sechtem U, Shimokawa H, Bairey Merz CN; Coronary Vasomotion Disorders International Study Group (COVADIS).International standardization of diagnostic criteria for vasospastic angina. Eur Heart J. 2015;4. pii:ehv351. [Epub ahead of print] Review.
34. Meimoun P, Tribouilloy C. Non-invasive assessment of coronary flow and coronary flow reserve by transthoracic Doppler echocardiography: a magic tool for the real world. Eur J Echocardiogr. 2008;9(4):449–57.

35. Lanza GA, et al. Methods to investigate coronary microvascular function in clinical practice. J Cardiovasc Med (Hagerstown). 2013;14(1):1–18.
36. Schindler TH, et al. Cardiac PET imaging for the detection and monitoring of coronary artery disease and microvascular health. JACC Cardiovasc Imaging. 2010;3(6):623–40.
37. Ong P, Athanasiadis A, Sechtem U. Treatment of angina pectoris associated with coronary microvascular dysfunction. Cardiovasc Drugs Ther. 2016;30(4):351–6.
38. Sen N, et al. Nebivolol therapy improves endothelial function and increases exercise tolerance in patients with cardiac syndrome X. Anadolu Kardiyol Derg. 2009;9(5):371–9.
39. Lamendola P, et al. Long-term prognosis of patients with cardiac syndrome X. Int J Cardiol. 2010;140(2):197–9.

Chapter 5
Menopause and Cardiovascular Risk

Angela H.E.M. Maas and C. Noel Bairey Merz

Abstract Men are at higher comparative CVD risk than women throughout their lifespan. During menopause transition the traditional CVD risk factors change into a more adverse direction in women with an up-regulation of hormonal systems such as the renin-angiotensin system (RAS) and the sympathetic nervous system. Primary ovarian insufficiency (POI) and persistent vasomotor symptoms are considered to be modest additive risk factors in women. Hypertension is a key-risk factor and may cause a variety of symptoms in middle-aged women that are often not well recognized. This chapter may be an eye-opener for many clinical cardiologists.

Keywords Arterial stiffness • Blood pressure • BRCA 1/2 mutation carriers • Endometriosis • Endothelial dysfunction • Estrogen • Hormone therapy (HT) • Hypertension • Hysterectomy • Menopause • Oral contraceptives • Primary ovarian insufficiency (POI) • Sex-hormones • Symptoms hypertension • Vasomotor symptoms (VMS) • Vaginal bleeding • Venous thrombo-embolism (VTE)

Menopause Transition

During menopause transition many women report bothersome symptoms, which may persist for a number of years and are often associated with a reduced health-related quality of life. The mean age at onset of menopause is 51 years, which is rather constant over time and populations worldwide, but there is substantial

---

A.H.E.M. Maas, M.D., Ph.D. (✉)
Department of Cardiology, Women's Cardiac Health Program,
Radboud University Medical Center, Nijmegen, The Netherlands
e-mail: angela.maas@radboudumc.nl

C.N. Bairey Merz, M.D.
Director Barbra Streisand Women's Heart Center, Linda Joy Pollin
Women's Heart Health Program, Director Preventive Cardiac Center,
Cedars-Sinai, Los Angeles, CA, USA
e-mail: noel.baireymerz@cshs.org

A.H.E.M. Maas, C.N. Bairey Merz (eds.), *Manual of Gynecardiology*,
DOI 10.1007/978-3-319-54960-6_5

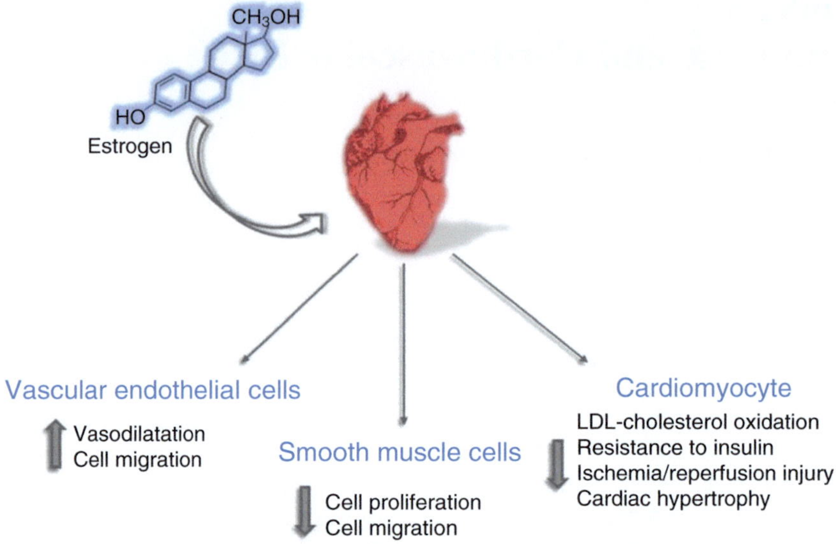

Fig. 5.1 Estrogen and the heart. In healthy premenopausal women estrogen may promote vasodilatation, reduces smooth muscle cell proliferation and prevents cardiac hypertrophy. Adapted from Menazza S et al. Circ Res, 2016 [3]

inter-individual variation, varying roughly between 40 and 60 years [1]. If natural menopause occurs before the age of 40, it is considered as primary ovarian insufficiency (POI). To establish age at menopause may be difficult in women using oral contraceptives, in those with a levonorgestrel releasing intra uterine system (LNG-IUS) or in women after previous hysterectomy without ovariectomy. Estrogen in experimental investigation appears to have important effects on cardiovascular function including vascular reactivity, blood pressure, endothelial relaxation, and cardiac remodeling [2–5]. These effects are mediated by both (acute) direct and (later) genomic effects of the estrogen receptors (ERα and ERβ) that are present in the vascular wall and in cardiomyocytes. Circulating estrogens also have regulating effects on several metabolic factors that are pro- and anti-atherosclerotic, such as lipids, inflammatory markers and the coagulation system [6–9]. During the fertile years of life the estrogen status is often ascribed to the later onset and differences in manifestation of ischemic heart disease (IHD) and myocardial remodelling in women compared to men (Fig. 5.1), however specific studies to address this are lacking. While healthy endothelium is sensitive to the vasodilator properties of estrogens, this may reverse when vascular stiffness and signs of atherosclerotic disease gradually develop over time [10–12]. While risk factor prevalence and CVD risk increases with the menopause, this could be distinguished from aging [13]. Nevertheless, men are at higher comparative risk than women throughout their lifespan. Lower estrogen levels after menopause appear to be related to altered vascular function, inflammation and upregulation of other hormonal systems such as the renin-angiotensin system (RAS) and the sympathetic nervous system [14–19].

Vasomotor Symptoms and Cardiovascular Disease Risk

Besides a diversity of gynecological symptoms, 50–70% of Caucasian women experience vasomotor symptoms (VMS) during menopause transition, consisting of hot flushes, night sweats, palpitations, sleeping disturbances, concentration problems, headaches etc. These symptoms may also be related to oxidative stress and an adverse CVD risk profile [20], although the literature is mixed regarding relations between hot flashes and CVD. Severe VMS in women have been associated with hypertension, elevated total cholesterol levels and increased CVD events [21–23]. Several studies have suggested that subclinical atherosclerosis is more prevalent in women with VMS compared to women without these symptoms [24, 25]. Menopausal vasomotor symptoms are associated with increased sympathetic and decreased parasympathetic function that may enhance the risk of cardiovascular events [17, 26–28]. Vasomotor symptoms are also exacerbated by an increase in insulin resistance and inflammatory factors derived from visceral adipose tissue, which has an increased activity after menopause [29]. In the Women's Health Initiative Observational Study (WHI-OS) it was found that early VMS (before/around cessation of menstruation) are associated with a lower CVD risk (HR 0.89, 95% CI 0.81–0.97), while VMS in late menopause indicate an elevated CVD risk profile (HR 1.23, 95% CI 1.00–1.52) [30]. The mechanisms of VMS may therefore be different within separate stages of menopause transition and may vary over time. It is assumed that early VMS are associated with estrogen-dependent lowering of the thermo-neutral zone in the brain, whereas late VMS (age 55+) are more related to a higher sympathetic nervous system activity after menopause [19, 31]. Women at increased CVD risk, such as after previous hypertensive pregnancy disorders (HPD), have a higher sympathetic nerve activity and more disabling VMS compared to women after normotensive pregnancies [32, 33].

Premature Natural Menopause

Primary ovarian insufficiency (POI), formerly known as premature ovarian failure (POF), is characterized by secondary amenorrhea for at least 4 months accompanied by an elevated FSH above 40 IU/L, occurring prior to age of 40 years [34, 35]. The incidence of POI is reported to be 1–2%. Earlier menopausal age than normal is associated with an increased incidence of CVD [36–38]. In a systematic review of 32 studies, including more than 310.000 women, it was found that women who experienced a menopause younger than 45 years have a relative risk of 1.19 (CI 1.08–1.31) for CVD mortality [39]. Other epidemiological data have led to a calculated 2% decrease of CVD mortality risk for each year that menopause is delayed [40]. Women who have recently been diagnosed with POI have a slightly unfavorable serum lipid profile compared to healthy controls with a normal ovarian function [41]. Early menopause is also a predictor of recurrent angina symptoms after myocardial infarction [42]. In a case-control study of 83 respectively 266 women >45 years, women with POI exhibited an unfavorable cardiovascular risk profile, including higher abdominal fat, elevated chronic inflammatory factors, and a trend towards increased blood pressure, and an impaired kidney function compared to controls, but no difference in subclinical signs of atherosclerosis was found [43]. Despite the association of premature cessation of ovarian function and short term health problems such as decreased fertility and climacteric symptoms, current available data indicate that POI is only a modest risk factor for IHD and overall CVD risk but not for stroke [44]. Age at onset of menopause is (partly) heritable with a link to DNA repair and immune mediator pathways [45].

Cardiovascular Risk in BRCA1/2 Mutation Carriers

BRCA1/2 mutation carriers are at high risk of breast and ovarian cancer. To reduce the risk of ovarian cancer a risk-reducing salpingo-oophorectomy (RRSO) is advised to all *BRCA1/2* mutation carriers at age 35–40 years (*BRCA1*) and at age 40–45 years (*BRCA2*) [46]. In women without previous breast cancer, hormone therapy may be considered until natural age at menopause after premature surgical menopause [47]. As BRCA genes play an important role in DNA damage repair, they may also interfere with the pathophysiology of atherosclerosis. This hypothesis is supported by finding that BRCA1/2 deficient cells are more sensitive to oxidative stress [48, 49]. The potential increased intrinsic and extrinsic susceptibility of BRCA1/2 mutation carriers to CVD needs further research.

Hysterectomy, Endometriosis and Cardiovascular Risk

In the Nurses' Health Study it was found that that a bilateral ovariectomy after hysterectomy is associated with a two times higher risk for CVD, especially when performed before 50 years of age [50]. In the Women's Health Initiative (WHI) Observational Study this disadvantage was found to be importantly associated with a lower socio-economic status (SES) and a more adverse CVD risk profile in women undergoing a hysterectomy [51]. Large population-based data from Sweden however confirmed a positive association between hysterectomy with/without oophorectomy and CVD in women <50 years, but not at older age [52].

In many cases the indication for a hysterectomy is related to endometriosis, which promotes inflammation, oxidative stress and an adverse lipid profile [53]. It is therefore warranted that gynecologists and cardiovascular specialists seek collaboration to optimize CVD prevention in these patients.

Endothelial Dysfunction in Menopause-Transition

Postmenopausal women have over a threefold greater risk of atherosclerosis when compared to premenopausal women, however after adjustment for age and other potential confounders it is controversial whether menopause is associated with increased risk independent of aging [13]. The decline in endothelial function appears to start in early menopause before signs of subclinical atherosclerosis are present [54, 55]. This could provoke undetermined symptoms of chest pain and dyspnea which is often labeled as "stress" or complaints secondary to menopause. However, women who are diagnosed with 'undetermined' chest pain syndromes have a two-fold increased risk to develop a IHD event in the next 5–7 years and improvement of lifestyle factors and risk factor modification is therefore crucial [56, 57].

Smoking induces premature endothelial dysfunction in premenopausal women by downregulation of the estrogen receptors in the vascular wall, activation of inflammation and the thrombotic system and promoting LDL cholesterol oxidation [58].

The ability to detect endothelial dysfunction, as a first sign of vascular ageing, may be important in assessing cardiovascular risk in women more accurately, although the variability of response limits the application in clinical practice [59]. This can be done non-invasively by peripheral techniques such as ultrasound of the brachial artery (FMD: flow mediated dilatation) or digital arterial tonometry (endoPAT) [60]. With measurements of pulse wave velocity (PWV) the degree of arterial stiffness can be established, functioning as a predictor of future CVD events [61, 62]. The gold standard of assessing coronary endothelial function invasively involves the responses of both the epicardial arteries and the microcirculation to an endothelium dependent vasodilator such as acetylcholine [63]. Measurements of peripheral endothelial function correlates modestly with coronary artery endothelial function and predicts future cardiovascular events in population studies [64]. A potential disadvantage is that functional tests are time-consuming, have day-to-day variability similar to blood pressure that requires repeated testing and are importantly dependent on the expertise of the vascular laboratory [65]. An advantage of these techniques is that functional vascular abnormalities can be noticed before any signs of subclinical atherosclerosis are seen, as is the case with carotid intima media thickness measurements (CIMT) or a coronary artery calcium score with CT angiography (CCTA).

Hypertension As a Key Risk Factor in Menopause

Hypertension is a critically important risk factor that affects women in the early postmenopausal years and elevated blood pressure is often poorly treated [66, 67]. There is anecdotal concern that when a man has an elevated blood pressure we call it 'hypertension', but when it affects a woman we call it 'stress'. This may be one reason why women with elevated blood pressure are treated differently than men in primary care [68]. About 30–50% of women develop hypertension (RR >140/90 mmHg) before the age of 60 and the onset of hypertension can cause a variety of symptoms that are often attributed to menopause [69, 70]. Detection and control of elevated blood pressure in the perimenopause is crucial for the prevention of future hypertension [71]. There are more missed opportunities for treating hypertension adequately in women at middle-age than in similarly aged men [72]. Also, in normotensive women, higher normal blood pressures are associated with greater cardiovascular risk compared to lower blood pressures even when in the normal range [73]. The socalled "white-coat" hypertension at the doctor's office occurs more often in women and may progress over time to sustained hypertension [74, 75]. Systolic blood pressure is the best predictor of CV risk and increases more with the white coat response than does diastolic blood pressure. As blood pressure is characterized by a considerable variability over time additional ambulatory monitoring is recommended in these patients. Self-monitoring with modern eHealth applications is getting more popular and may improve quality of blood pressure monitoring and adherence to medical therapy [76, 77]. In the 2014 AHA guidelines hypertension in adults treatment goals are stricter for patients <60 years than in elderly [78]. However, this was before publication of the Systolic Blood Pressure Intervention Trial (SPRINT) trial that found evidence of cardiovascular benefit with more intensive lowering of systolic blood pressure (goal <120 mmHg) compared with the currently recommended goal (<140 mmHg) in older patients (>75 years) with cardiovascular risk but without diabetes or stroke [79]. This has led to an ongoing debate to which extent blood pressure should be lowered in men/women, within various age-categories and different levels of CVD risk [80, 81]. Publication already suggests lowering the threshold for normal systolic blood pressure to 130 mmHg in upcoming guidelines with a particular emphasis on women [80, 82].

The rise in systolic blood pressure with ageing is caused by an increase in vascular stiffness of the great arteries in combination with atherosclerotic changes in the vessel wall. Systolic blood pressure is considered to be the most important arbiter of risk with ageing, and rises more steeply in women compared to men [83–85]. This is also related to the additional effects of hormonal changes during menopause [69, 86–88]. Several other sex-hormone related factors and weight gain have an additive effect on the rise in blood pressure during menopausal transition (Table 5.1) [89–92]. Also, sodium sensitivity increases during menopausal transition, frequently leading to intermittent fluid retention (edema legs, hands, lower eyelids) [93–96]. Physicians should intensify the detection of hypertension in middle-aged women after previous hypertensive pregnancy disorders and preeclampsia [97, 98]. Women develop more vascular and myocardial stiffness than men with ageing [99–101]. This is closely associated with their higher prevalence of diabetes, obesity and hypertension, resulting in more strokes, left ventricular hypertrophy and heart failure with preserved ejection fraction (HFpEF) [102–104].

Table 5.1 Associations between menopause-related estrogen decline and blood pressure

• Relative increase in androgen levels
• Activation RAS, higher renin levels
• Increase plasma-endothelin levels
• Higher salt sensitivity
• Increase in insulin resistance
• Higher sympathetic activity
• Increase in weight

RAS renin angiotensin system

Elevated Blood Pressure Is Often Symptomatic

Whereas hypertension may be asymptomatic in elderly patients with stiffened and atherosclerotic arteries, it can induce many diverse symptoms in younger patients [105]. Higher blood pressure causes shear stress on the arterial wall promoting endothelial dysfunction that may translate into symptoms of chest pain [106, 107]. This often responds well to short acting nitrates causing vasodilatation and lowering blood pressure. In the WISE study hypertension was prevalent in 55% of females, mean age 58 years, who were referred for coronary angiography for chest pain syndromes [13, 108]. Many frequently occurring complaints at middle-age can be related to a higher blood pressure, such as an oppressive chest pain or continuous band sensation at rest, with or without radiation to the shoulder blades, jaws and left (or both) arm(s). Many hypertensive women report that they prefer "to take off their bra" when being at home (patient A). Other symptoms such as sleep disturbances, palpitations, paroxysmal atrial fibrillation (AF), headaches, dizzyness, fluid retention, dyspnea, extreme tiredness and lack of energy are also frequently mentioned. Symptoms may vary over time (days/weeks/months) and increase during stressful situations and exercise. Many women experience symptoms of dyspnea while climbing the stairs or running to a bus and interchange their bike into an electric bike to catch up with their husbands. In Table 5.2 frequently reported symptoms related to elevated blood pressure in middle-aged women are described. In women having severe VMS mean 24-h blood pressure is 10 mmHg higher than in asymptomatic women, while treatment of hypertension reduces these symptoms [109, 110]. Drospirenone, a progestin with anti-mineralocorticoid properties, combined with 17-beta estradiol at various doses, lowers blood pressure in hypertensive subjects with moderate hypertension, whilst effectively alleviating VMS [111]. Patient A and B are common examples of middle-aged women with symptomatic hypertension. These kind of patients often visit outpatient clinics where a traditional cardiac work-up is done to rule out obstructive CAD, ending up without a diagnosis, treatment and plausible explanation for their symptoms. The choice for the most appropriate type of anti-hypertensive medication should be importantly based on the predominant symptoms that patients have, their resting heart rate and tolerance of various medications.

Table 5.2 Reported symptoms in middle-aged women with elevated blood pressure

• Tight, nagging and often continuous chest pain at rest
• Radiating pain to the jaws, left arm, shoulder blades
• Stress-related chest pain, with or without radiation
• Dyspnea at physical exercise (stairs, climbing, hurrying)
• Lack of physical condition, tiredness, lack of energy, exhaustion
• Hot flushes, severe sweating (day and night)
• Headaches, concentration disturbances, dizziness
• Palpitations at rest, paroxysmal supraventricular tachycardia/atrial fibrillation
• Intermittent fluid retention (ankles, hands, eyes)
• Sleeping disorders, inability to lie/sleep on left side
• 'bra feels too tight'

Patient A: Woman 56 years-second opinion for undetermined symptoms of chest pain

Medical history:
Hypertension last trimester first pregnancy
Curettage (abnormal menstrual bleeding)
Meniscus operation

Patient history: She recently had a coronary angiography elsewhere showing no abnormalities. Since several years, she has an intermittent feeling of chest pain, as if her bra is too tight. These symptoms occur several times a week, mostly unexpected and at rest. Duration of symptoms varies between half an hour up to several hours . She often awakes at night with sweating, palpitations and a feeling of shortness of breath. She is postmenopausal since 2 years. Other symptoms are swollen ankles from time to time and sudden feelings of extreme tiredness. Her physical condition is worse than it used to be. She never smoked. Family history is positive for hypertension. She recently started with 50 mg metoprolol daily, which slightly relieved her symptoms.

Physical exam: BMI 26, RR 150-160/90 mmHg both arms, soft systolic ejection murmur, normal pulmonary sounds.

ECG: SR 67/min, normal axis, slight repolarization abnormalities, but overall normal.

ECHO: borderline septal hypertrophy, normal ejectionfraction. No diastolic dysfunction.

Lab: normal, including lipids and TSH

Comments: patient has persistent and variable symptoms of chest pain, tiredness and loss of condition, caused by a developing familial hypertension. In her first pregnancy she already showed that she is predisposed to develop hypertension at a later age. After the addition of an ARB to her medication , her blood pressure lowered to 130/ 85 mmHg with a concomitant reduction of her symptoms. Within a few weeks time her chest pain has gradually disappeared and she feels as if she has "renewed" her energy level.

Patient B: 43 year old woman with chest pain and unexplained tiredness

Medical history: 1x miscarriage and 1x preeclampsia
early menopause 42 years

Patient history: She has recurrent chest pain since a year both at rest and during exercise, such as cycling. Radiation to the left arm. She feels tired and has shortness of breath during exercise. She stopped with sports because of these symptoms. She needs to urinate 2-3x at night. She stopped taking oral contraceptives a year ago, and her her periods did not resume. She quit her job last year with feelings of "burn-out". She never smoked. Family history positive for premature CVD on mother's side. Her diastolic BP is often 100 mmHg. After an inconclusive X-test, a CAG was done a year ago, showing normal coronary arteries. Total cholesterol 5.5 mmol/L.

Physical examination: BMI 26 , RR 167/100 mmHg and 160/100 mmHg, normal auscultation.

ECG: SR 103/min, intermed axis, normal repolarization

Comments: patient with pos. family history and premature menopause with symptoms secondary to hypertension. She was given the combination of metoprolol 50 mg and irbesartan150 mg, later 300 mg, whereafter her symptoms gradually disappeared and her BP normalized.

Elevated blood pressure may induce extrasystoles, paroxysmal supraventricular tachycardia or AF with variable strain-related ST-T changes on the resting ECG. The latter may be caused by shear stress on the myocardium, often in combination with endothelial dysfunction and/or subendocardial ischemia in the smaller coronary arteries. In the Women's Health initiative study it was found that non-specific repolarisation abnormalities are associated with an increased long-term cardiovascular risk [112]. Dynamic ECG changes are frequently present during high peak systolic blood pressures at the emergency department and dissolve well with nitrates. In younger women at low chance of having obstructive CAD this often lead to unnecessary and repeated coronary angiograms.

Use of Oral Contraceptives, VTE/CVD Risk and Abnormal Uterine Bleeding

Thus far, the currently used newer generations of oral contraceptives (OC) have not been associated with an increased risk for hypertension or IHD, but with a persistent increased risk of venous thrombo-embolism (VTE) [113–116]. In the MEGA-study, women who were current smokers and used OC had an 8.8-fold higher risk (OR 8.79, CI 95 5.73–13.49) for VTE than nonsmoking women who did not use oral contraceptives [117]. The higher risk of ACS in young women on OC has been predominantly attributed to the combined deleterious effects of smoking [118]. Smoking acts synergistically with OC use and counteracts the protective vasodilating effects of endogenous estrogens in women before menopause. Prolonged OC use for many years lowers the risk of ovarian, endometrium and colon cancer [119]. Long-term OC use has not been found to be associated with a higher coronary atherosclerosis burden as measured by quantitative coronary angiography [120]. Recent data derived from almost five million French women indicate that that levonorgestrel-containing pills should be the first choice when prescribing a combined OC [121]. However, these are still contraindicated in women after an ischemic cardiac or neurologic event and in women after VTE/pulmonary embolism [116, 122]. Also, in women >35 years with multiple CVD risk factors OC are not recommended [123]. In women receiving therapeutic anticoagulation with vitamin K antagonists or novel oral anticoagulants (NOACs) the risk for a recurrent VTE is not increased [124]. The elevated risk for abnormal uterine bleeding (AUB) in high risk premenopausal women, induced by the use of (dual) platelet therapy, NOACs or vitamin K antagonists, may demand specific individual gynaecological advise such as for the levonorgestrel releasing intra uterine system (LNG-IUS) or endometrial ablation [125]. Concomitant long-term use of a NOAC with acetylsalicylicacid or other antiplatelet drugs (clopidogrel, ticagrelor, prasugrel) should be avoided, because combination therapy increases the risk of AUB and does not improve efficacy for stroke or VTE prevention [126, 127].

Postmenopausal Hormone Therapy: When Is It Safe for the Heart and Brain?

The apparent vasoprotective effects of estrogens during the fertile years of life have been the basis for the assumption that hormone therapy (HT) may protect against CVD [128]. This "estrogen-hypothesis" was initially supported by large observational studies, such as the Nurses' Health Study, in which it was found that the prevalence of CVD was lower in HRT users that in non-users [129]. Despite, in the large randomized HT trials, such as the Women's Health Initiative (WHI) studies, a CVD protective effect of HT could not be demonstrated and in contrast even more harm was seen in elderly (>60 years) women at elevated CVD risk [130]. In a meta-analysis of randomized-controlled trials a significantly lower risk of IHD and death from any cause (HR 0.72, CI 0.62–0.82) was found in HT users younger than 60 years who were less than 10 years since menopause [131]. The Danish Osteoporosis Prevention Study (DOPS), included women on average 50 years and 7 months past menopause, to HT with estradiol alone or in combination with a progesterone and showed a significantly lower risk of IHD at 10 and 16 years of follow-up among HT users compared to non-users [132]. The effects of HT on CVD are therefore importantly dependent on the timing of therapy initiation relative to menopause [12, 133]. Moreover, the type of HT, the dose and the route of administration should be also considered. In the Kronos Early Estrogen Prevention Study (KEEPS), low-dose treatment with oral conjugated estrogens or combined estradiol patch with oral progesterone among young women (42–58 years) at low risk for CVD showed no significant effect on CIMT progression compared to placebo after 2 years of treatment [134]. Conversely, in the Early versus Late Intervention Trial with Estradiol (ELITE) HT was associated with less progression of subclinical atherosclerosis (measured as CIMT) compared to placebo when therapy was initiated within 6 years after menopause but not when it was started after 10 or more years after menopause [135]. The risk of VTE risk is higher in users of systemic combined estrogen–progestogen treatment than in users of estrogen only [136]. Several studies have shown that transdermal estrogen and vaginal estrogen do not appear to increase the risk of VTE [136, 137]. Hormone therapy improvement in cognitive function has not been supported [138], and longer term trials demonstrate increased dementia and mild cognitive impairment with HT compared to placebo [139, 140].

For women with premature menopause it is advised that HT should be administered at least until the median age of natural menopause which is 51 years [141, 142]. Longer duration of treatment can be considered when severe menopausal VMS are present. After the publications of the WHI results there had been a 80% decline in the prescription of HT, leaving many patients and doctors in confusion [143]. This has led to an overuse of untested potentially harmful alternative treatments. Although HT is not recommended for the primary or secondary prevention of IHD in postmenopausal women, its (temporary) use can be relatively safe in the hands of well-trained physicians, weighing risks and benefits with the patient. Women with known IHD or with many coronary risk factors seeking HT because of

Table 5.3 Cardiovascular risk estimation when considering hormone therapy (HT)

Risk category		HT advise
High risk ≥1 RF	Clinically manifest vascular disease (IHD, cerebrovascular disease, PAD, aortic disease, CKD)	–
	Diabetes mellitus	
	10-y predicted CVD risk ≥10%	
	Age >60 years	
	Previous VTE	
Intermediate risk ≥1 major RF	Cigarette smoking	+/–
	SBP ≥120, DBP ≥80 mmHg, or treated hypertension	
	Total cholesterol ≥5.5 mmol/L, or treated for dyslipidemia	
	Obesity, poor diet, insufficient physical activity	
	Family history of premature CVD	
	Metabolic syndrome	
	Evidence of subclinical atherosclerosis (e.g., coronary calcification, carotid plaque, or thickened IMT)	
	Systemic autoimmune disease (e.g. rheumatoid arthritis)	
	History of preeclampsia, gestational diabetes, or pregnancy induced hypertension	
Low CVD risk	Total cholesterol <200 mg/dL (untreated)	+
	BP <120/<80 (untreated)	
	Fasting blood glucose <100 mg/dL (untreated)	
	Body mass index <25 kg/m^2	
	Non-smoking, adequate physical activity	
	Healthy diet	

Adapted from Mosca L, et al. Effectiveness-based guidelines for the prevention of cardiovascular disease in women—2011 update: a guideline from the American Heart Association. Circulation. 2011;123(11):1243–62

CKD chronic kidney disease, *CVD* cardiovascular disease, *IHD* ischemic heart disease, *IMT* intima media thickness, *PAD* peripheral arterial disease, *VTE* venous thromboembolic event

troublesome climacteric symptoms should be properly counselled for their individual baseline risk of developing breast cancer, VTE and CVD (recurrence) (see Table 5.3).

Appropriate counselling and treatment of VMS and CVD risk factors is essential for women during midlife, also because the impact of menopausal symptoms on work ability is high [144, 145]. In 2015 the European menopause and andropause society (EMAS) has released a clinical guide for postmenopausal health, emphasizing the need for an individual patient approach with appropriate choice of HT and route of administration [146]. This is also the starting point of the NICE guidelines on menopause management that were released in November 2015 (https://www.nice.org.uk/guidance/NG23) and the revised global consensus statement on menopausal hormone therapy [147]. For the possibilities of non-hormonal management of VMS the EMAS has recently provided a separate position statement [148].

Key Issues

- Traditional RF profile worsens in postmenopausal women predominantly due to aging
- Persistent VMS in women aged >55 years may be related to an adverse CVD risk profile
- Premature ovarian insufficiency (POI) is a modest risk factor for overall CVD risk
- Women who undergo hysterectomy/ovariectomy <50 years should be screened for CVD risk factors
- Endothelial dysfunction occurs earlier in women at elevated risk and may contribute to symptoms
- Hypertension is highly prevalent at middle-age and can contribute to symptoms
- Postmenopausal hormone therapy for VMS is relatively safe in low risk for CVD women <6–10 years after onset menopause
- Postmenopausal hormone therapy is not indicated for CVD prevention

References

1. Morabia A, Costanza MC. International variability in ages at menarche, first livebirth, and menopause. World Health Organization Collaborative Study of Neoplasia and Steroid Contraceptives. Am J Epidemiol. 1998;148(12):1195–205.
2. Miller VM, Duckles SP. Vascular actions of estrogens: functional implications. Pharmacol Rev. 2008;60(2):210–41.
3. Menazza S, Murphy E. The expanding complexity of estrogen receptor signaling in the cardiovascular system. Circ Res. 2016;118(6):994–1007.
4. Salerni S, Di Francescomarino S, Cadeddu C, Acquistapace F, Maffei S, Gallina S. The different role of sex hormones on female cardiovascular physiology and function: not only oestrogens. Eur J Clin Investig. 2015;45(6):634–45.
5. Turgeon JL, Carr MC, Maki PM, Mendelsohn ME, Wise PM. Complex actions of sex steroids in adipose tissue, the cardiovascular system, and brain: insights from basic science and clinical studies. Endocr Rev. 2006;27(6):575–605.
6. Cushman M, Legault C, Barrett-Connor E, Stefanick ML, Kessler C, Judd HL, et al. Effect of postmenopausal hormones on inflammation-sensitive proteins: the Postmenopausal Estrogen/Progestin Interventions (PEPI) Study. Circulation. 1999;100(7):717–22.
7. Hulley S, Grady D, Bush T, Furberg C, Herrington D, Riggs B, et al. Randomized trial of estrogen plus progestin for secondary prevention of coronary heart disease in postmenopausal women. Heart and Estrogen/Progestin Replacement Study (HERS) Research Group. JAMA. 1998;280(7):605–13.
8. Koh KK. Effects of estrogen on the vascular wall: vasomotor function and inflammation. Cardiovasc Res. 2002;55(4):714–26.
9. Pradhan AD, Manson JE, Rossouw JE, Siscovick DS, Mouton CP, Rifai N, et al. Inflammatory biomarkers, hormone replacement therapy, and incident coronary heart disease: prospective analysis from the Women's Health Initiative Observational Study. JAMA. 2002;288(8):980–7.
10. Rossouw JE, Prentice RL, Manson JE, Wu L, Barad D, Barnabei VM, et al. Postmenopausal hormone therapy and risk of cardiovascular disease by age and years since menopause. JAMA. 2007;297(13):1465–77.

11. Clarkson TB, Melendez GC, Appt SE. Timing hypothesis for postmenopausal hormone therapy: its origin, current status, and future. Menopause. 2013;20(3):342–53.
12. Clarkson TB. Estrogen effects on arteries vary with stage of reproductive life and extent of subclinical atherosclerosis progression. Menopause. 2007;14(3 Pt 1):373–84.
13. Gierach GL, Johnson BD, Bairey Merz CN, Kelsey SF, Bittner V, Olson MB, et al. Hypertension, menopause, and coronary artery disease risk in the Women's Ischemia Syndrome Evaluation (WISE) Study. J Am Coll Cardiol. 2006;47(3 Suppl):S50–8.
14. Schunkert H, Danser AH, Hense HW, Derkx FH, Kurzinger S, Riegger GA. Effects of estrogen replacement therapy on the renin-angiotensin system in postmenopausal women. Circulation. 1997;95(1):39–45.
15. Yanes LL, Romero DG, Iliescu R, Zhang H, Davis D, Reckelhoff JF. Postmenopausal hypertension: role of the renin-angiotensin system. Hypertension. 2010;56(3):359–63.
16. Vongpatanasin W. Autonomic regulation of blood pressure in menopause. Semin Reprod Med. 2009;27(4):338–45.
17. Freedman RR. Menopausal hot flashes: mechanisms, endocrinology, treatment. J Steroid Biochem Mol Biol. 2014;142:115–20.
18. Maranon RO, Reckelhoff JF. Mechanisms responsible for postmenopausal hypertension in a rat model: roles of the renal sympathetic nervous system and the renin-angiotensin system. Physiol Rep. 2016;4(2):e12669.
19. Hart EC, Charkoudian N. Sympathetic neural regulation of blood pressure: influences of sex and aging. Physiology. 2014;29(1):8–15.
20. van der Schouw YT, Grobbee DE. Menopausal complaints, oestrogens, and heart disease risk: an explanation for discrepant findings on the benefits of post-menopausal hormone therapy. Eur Heart J. 2005;26(14):1358–61.
21. Gast GC, Grobbee DE, Pop VJ, Keyzer JJ, Wijnands-van Gent CJ, Samsioe GN, et al. Menopausal complaints are associated with cardiovascular risk factors. Hypertension. 2008;51(6):1492–8.
22. Gast GC, Pop VJ, Samsioe GN, Grobbee DE, Nilsson PM, Keyzer JJ, et al. Vasomotor menopausal symptoms are associated with increased risk of coronary heart disease. Menopause. 2011;18(2):146–51.
23. Jackson EA, El Khoudary SR, Crawford SL, Matthews K, Joffe H, Chae C, et al. Hot flash frequency and blood pressure: data from the study of Women's Health Across the Nation. J Womens Health. 2016;25(12):1204–9.
24. Thurston RC, Sutton-Tyrrell K, Everson-Rose SA, Hess R, Matthews KA. Hot flashes and subclinical cardiovascular disease: findings from the Study of Women's Health Across the Nation Heart Study. Circulation. 2008;118(12):1234–40.
25. Thurston RC, Sutton-Tyrrell K, Everson-Rose SA, Hess R, Powell LH, Matthews KA. Hot flashes and carotid intima media thickness among midlife women. Menopause. 2011;18(4): 352–8.
26. Thurston RC, Christie IC, Matthews KA. Hot flashes and cardiac vagal control during women's daily lives. Menopause. 2012;19(4):406–12.
27. Hoikkala H, Haapalahti P, Viitasalo M, Vaananen H, Sovijarvi AR, Ylikorkala O, et al. Association between vasomotor hot flashes and heart rate variability in recently postmenopausal women. Menopause. 2010;17(2):315–20.
28. Barnes JN, Hart EC, Curry TB, Nicholson WT, Eisenach JH, Wallin BG, et al. Aging enhances autonomic support of blood pressure in women. Hypertension. 2014;63(2):303–8.
29. Thurston RC, El Khoudary SR, Sutton-Tyrrell K, Crandall CJ, Sternfeld B, Joffe H, et al. Vasomotor symptoms and insulin resistance in the study of women's health across the nation. J Clin Endocrinol Metab. 2012;97(10):3487–94.
30. Szmuilowicz ED, Manson JE, Rossouw JE, Howard BV, Margolis KL, Greep NC, et al. Vasomotor symptoms and cardiovascular events in postmenopausal women. Menopause. 2011;18(6):603–10.
31. Stearns V, Ullmer L, Lopez JF, Smith Y, Isaacs C, Hayes D. Hot flushes. Lancet. 2002;360(9348):1851–61.

32. Collen AC, Manhem K, Sverrisdottir YB. Sympathetic nerve activity in women 40 years after a hypertensive pregnancy. J Hypertens. 2012;30(6):1203–10.
33. Drost JT, van der Schouw YT, Herber-Gast GC, Maas AH. More vasomotor symptoms in menopause among women with a history of hypertensive pregnancy diseases compared with women with normotensive pregnancies. Menopause. 2013;20(10):1006–11.
34. De Vos M, Devroey P, Fauser BC. Primary ovarian insufficiency. Lancet. 2010;376(9744):911–21.
35. Coulam CB, Adamson SC, Annegers JF. Incidence of premature ovarian failure. Obstet Gynecol. 1986;67(4):604–6.
36. Rosenberg L, Hennekens CH, Rosner B, Belanger C, Rothman KJ, Speizer FE. Early menopause and the risk of myocardial infarction. Am J Obstet Gynecol. 1981;139(1):47–51.
37. Jacobsen BK, Heuch I, Kvale G. Age at natural menopause and all-cause mortality: a 37-year follow-up of 19,731 Norwegian women. Am J Epidemiol. 2003;157(10):923–9.
38. Lubiszewska B, Kruk M, Broda G, Ksiezycka E, Piotrowski W, Kurjata P, et al. The impact of early menopause on risk of coronary artery disease (PREmature Coronary Artery Disease In Women—PRECADIW case-control study). Eur J Prev Cardiol. 2012;19(1):95–101.
39. Muka T, Oliver-Williams C, Kunutsor S, Laven JS, Fauser BC, Chowdhury R, et al. Association of age at onset of menopause and time since onset of menopause with cardiovascular outcomes, intermediate vascular traits, and all-cause mortality: a systematic review and meta-analysis. JAMA Cardiol. 2016;1(7):767–76.
40. Atsma F, Bartelink ML, Grobbee DE, van der Schouw YT. Postmenopausal status and early menopause as independent risk factors for cardiovascular disease: a meta-analysis. Menopause. 2006;13(2):265–79.
41. Knauff EA, Westerveld HE, Goverde AJ, Eijkemans MJ, Valkenburg O, van Santbrink EJ, et al. Lipid profile of women with premature ovarian failure. Menopause. 2008;15(5):919–23.
42. Parashar S, Reid KJ, Spertus JA, Shaw LJ, Vaccarino V. Early menopause predicts angina after myocardial infarction. Menopause. 2010;17(5):938–45.
43. Daan NM, Muka T, Koster MP, Roeters van Lennep JE, Lambalk CB, Laven JS, et al. Cardiovascular risk in women with premature ovarian insufficiency compared to premenopausal women at middle age. J Clin Endocrinol Metab. 2016;101(9):3306–15.
44. Roeters van Lennep JE, Heida KY, Bots ML, Hoek A, Collaborators of the Dutch Multidisciplinary Guideline Development Group on Cardiovascular Risk Management After Reproductive D. Cardiovascular disease risk in women with premature ovarian insufficiency: a systematic review and meta analysis. Eur J Prev Cardiol. 2016;23(2):178–86.
45. Stolk L, Perry JR, Chasman DI, He C, Mangino M, Sulem P, et al. Meta-analyses identify 13 loci associated with age at menopause and highlight DNA repair and immune pathways. Nat Genet. 2012;44(3):260–8.
46. Rebbeck TR, Mitra N, Domchek SM, Wan F, Chuai S, Friebel TM, et al. Modification of ovarian cancer risk by BRCA1/2-interacting genes in a multicenter cohort of BRCA1/2 mutation carriers. Cancer Res. 2009;69(14):5801–10.
47. Arts-de Jong M, Maas AH, Massuger LF, Hoogerbrugge N, de Hullu JA. BRCA1/2 mutation carriers are potentially at higher cardiovascular risk. Crit Rev Oncol Hematol. 2014;91(2):159–71.
48. Bae I, Fan S, Meng Q, Rih JK, Kim HJ, Kang HJ, et al. BRCA1 induces antioxidant gene expression and resistance to oxidative stress. Cancer Res. 2004;64(21):7893–909.
49. Fridlich R, Annamalai D, Roy R, Bernheim G, Powell SN. BRCA1 and BRCA2 protect against oxidative DNA damage converted into double-strand breaks during DNA replication. DNA Repair. 2015;30:11–20.
50. Parker WH, Broder MS, Chang E, Feskanich D, Farquhar C, Liu Z, et al. Ovarian conservation at the time of hysterectomy and long-term health outcomes in the nurses' health study. Obstet Gynecol. 2009;113(5):1027–37.
51. Howard BV, Kuller L, Langer R, Manson JE, Allen C, Assaf A, et al. Risk of cardiovascular disease by hysterectomy status, with and without oophorectomy: the Women's Health Initiative Observational Study. Circulation. 2005;111(12):1462–70.

52. Ingelsson E, Lundholm C, Johansson AL, Altman D. Hysterectomy and risk of cardiovascular disease: a population-based cohort study. Eur Heart J. 2011;32(6):745–50.
53. Mu F, Rich-Edwards J, Rimm EB, Spiegelman D, Missmer SA. Endometriosis and risk of coronary heart disease. Circ Cardiovasc Qual Outcomes. 2016;9(3):257–64.
54. Moreau KL, Hildreth KL, Meditz AL, Deane KD, Kohrt WM. Endothelial function is impaired across the stages of the menopause transition in healthy women. J Clin Endocrinol Metab. 2012;97(12):4692–700.
55. Bechlioulis A, Kalantaridou SN, Naka KK, Chatzikyriakidou A, Calis KA, Makrigiannakis A, et al. Endothelial function, but not carotid intima-media thickness, is affected early in menopause and is associated with severity of hot flushes. J Clin Endocrinol Metab. 2010;95(3):1199–206.
56. Robinson JG, Wallace R, Limacher M, Ren H, Cochrane B, Wassertheil-Smoller S, et al. Cardiovascular risk in women with non-specific chest pain (from the Women's Health Initiative Hormone Trials). Am J Cardiol. 2008;102(6):693–9.
57. Gulati M, Cooper-DeHoff RM, McClure C, Johnson BD, Shaw LJ, Handberg EM, et al. Adverse cardiovascular outcomes in women with nonobstructive coronary artery disease: a report from the Women's Ischemia Syndrome Evaluation Study and the St James Women Take Heart Project. Arch Intern Med. 2009;169(9):843–50.
58. Messner B, Bernhard D. Smoking and cardiovascular disease: mechanisms of endothelial dysfunction and early atherogenesis. Arterioscler Thromb Vasc Biol. 2014;34(3):509–15.
59. Matsuzawa Y, Guddeti RR, Kwon TG, Lerman LO, Lerman A. Treating coronary disease and the impact of endothelial dysfunction. Prog Cardiovasc Dis. 2015;57(5):431–42.
60. Flammer AJ, Anderson T, Celermajer DS, Creager MA, Deanfield J, Ganz P, et al. The assessment of endothelial function: from research into clinical practice. Circulation. 2012;126(6):753–67.
61. Mitchell GF, Hwang SJ, Vasan RS, Larson MG, Pencina MJ, Hamburg NM, et al. Arterial stiffness and cardiovascular events: the Framingham Heart Study. Circulation. 2010;121(4):505–11.
62. Mattace-Raso FU, van der Cammen TJ, Hofman A, van Popele NM, Bos ML, Schalekamp MA, et al. Arterial stiffness and risk of coronary heart disease and stroke: the Rotterdam Study. Circulation. 2006;113(5):657–63.
63. Ong P, Athanasiadis A, Sechtem U. Patterns of coronary vasomotor responses to intracoronary acetylcholine provocation. Heart. 2013;99(17):1288–95.
64. Anderson TJ, Uehata A, Gerhard MD, Meredith IT, Knab S, Delagrange D, et al. Close relation of endothelial function in the human coronary and peripheral circulations. J Am Coll Cardiol. 1995;26(5):1235–41.
65. Sade LE. Vascular function tests in women with no obstructive CAD: a few pieces of the puzzle. JACC Cardiovasc Imaging. 2016;9(4):418–20.
66. Cutler JA, Sorlie PD, Wolz M, Thom T, Fields LE, Roccella EJ. Trends in hypertension prevalence, awareness, treatment, and control rates in United States adults between 1988–1994 and 1999–2004. Hypertension. 2008;52(5):818–27.
67. Hage FG, Mansur SJ, Xing D, Oparil S. Hypertension in women. Kidney Int Suppl. 2013;3(4):352–6.
68. Ljungman C, Kahan T, Schioler L, Hjerpe P, Hasselstrom J, Wettermark B, et al. Gender differences in antihypertensive drug treatment: results from the Swedish Primary Care Cardiovascular Database (SPCCD). J Am Soc Hypertens. 2014;8(12):882–90.
69. Burt VL, Whelton P, Roccella EJ, Brown C, Cutler JA, Higgins M, et al. Prevalence of hypertension in the US adult population. Results from the Third National Health and Nutrition Examination Survey, 1988–1991. Hypertension. 1995;25(3):305–13.
70. Wassertheil-Smoller S, Anderson G, Psaty BM, Black HR, Manson J, Wong N, et al. Hypertension and its treatment in postmenopausal women: baseline data from the Women's Health Initiative. Hypertension. 2000;36(5):780–9.
71. Staessen J, Bulpitt CJ, Fagard R, Lijnen P, Amery A. The influence of menopause on blood pressure. J Hum Hypertens. 1989;3(6):427–33.
72. Boggia J, Thijs L, Hansen TW, Li Y, Kikuya M, Bjorklund-Bodegard K, et al. Ambulatory blood pressure monitoring in 9357 subjects from 11 populations highlights missed opportunities for cardiovascular prevention in women. Hypertension. 2011;57(3):397–405.

73. Vasan RS, Larson MG, Leip EP, Evans JC, O'Donnell CJ, Kannel WB, et al. Impact of high-normal blood pressure on the risk of cardiovascular disease. N Engl J Med. 2001;345(18):1291–7.
74. O'Brien E, Parati G, Stergiou G, Asmar R, Beilin L, Bilo G, et al. European Society of Hypertension position paper on ambulatory blood pressure monitoring. J Hypertens. 2013;31(9):1731–68.
75. Franklin SS, Thijs L, Hansen TW, O'Brien E, Staessen JA. White-coat hypertension: new insights from recent studies. Hypertension. 2013;62(6):982–7.
76. Margolis KL, Asche SE, Bergdall AR, Dehmer SP, Groen SE, Kadrmas HM, et al. Effect of home blood pressure telemonitoring and pharmacist management on blood pressure control: a cluster randomized clinical trial. JAMA. 2013;310(1):46–56.
77. McManus RJ, Mant J, Haque MS, Bray EP, Bryan S, Greenfield SM, et al. Effect of self-monitoring and medication self-titration on systolic blood pressure in hypertensive patients at high risk of cardiovascular disease: the TASMIN-SR randomized clinical trial. JAMA. 2014;312(8):799–808.
78. James PA, Oparil S, Carter BL, Cushman WC, Dennison-Himmelfarb C, Handler J, et al. 2014 evidence-based guideline for the management of high blood pressure in adults: report from the panel members appointed to the Eighth Joint National Committee (JNC 8). JAMA. 2014;311(5):507–20.
79. SPRINT Research Group, Wright Jr JT, Williamson JD, Whelton PK, Snyder JK, Sink KM, et al. A randomized trial of intensive versus standard blood-pressure control. N Engl J Med. 2015;373(22):2103–16.
80. Egan BM, Li J, Wagner CS. Systolic Blood Pressure Intervention Trial (SPRINT) and target systolic blood pressure in future hypertension guidelines. Hypertension. 2016;68(2):318–23.
81. Lopez-Jaramillo P, Coca A, Sanchez R, Zanchetti A. Hypertension guidelines: is it time to reappraise blood pressure thresholds and targets? Position statement of the Latin American Society of Hypertension. Hypertension. 2016;68(2):257–62.
82. Wenger NK, Ferdinand KC, Bairey Merz CN, Walsh MN, Gulati M, Pepine CJ, et al. Women, hypertension, and the systolic blood pressure intervention trial. Am J Med. 2016;129(10):1030–6.
83. Franklin SS, Gustin W, Wong ND, Larson MG, Weber MA, Kannel WB, et al. Hemodynamic patterns of age-related changes in blood pressure. The Framingham Heart Study. Circulation. 1997;96(1):308–15.
84. Denton KM, Hilliard LM, Tare M. Sex-related differences in hypertension: seek and ye shall find. Hypertension. 2013;62(4):674–7.
85. Sandberg K, Ji H. Sex differences in primary hypertension. Biol Sex Differ. 2012;3(1):7.
86. Staessen JA, van der Heijden-Spek JJ, Safar ME, Den Hond E, Gasowski J, Fagard RH, et al. Menopause and the characteristics of the large arteries in a population study. J Hum Hypertens. 2001;15(8):511–8.
87. Cadeddu C, Franconi F, Cassisa L, Campesi I, Pepe A, Cugusi L, et al. Arterial hypertension in the female world: pathophysiology and therapy. J Cardiovasc Med. 2016;17(4):229–36.
88. Reckelhoff JF, Fortepiani LA. Novel mechanisms responsible for postmenopausal hypertension. Hypertension. 2004;43(5):918–23.
89. Coylewright M, Reckelhoff JF, Ouyang P. Menopause and hypertension: an age-old debate. Hypertension. 2008;51(4):952–9.
90. Khalil RA. Sex hormones as potential modulators of vascular function in hypertension. Hypertension. 2005;46(2):249–54.
91. Reckelhoff JF. Gender differences in the regulation of blood pressure. Hypertension. 2001;37(5):1199–208.
92. Ashraf MS, Vongpatanasin W. Estrogen and hypertension. Curr Hypertens Rep. 2006;8(5):368–76.
93. Pechere-Bertschi A, Burnier M. Gonadal steroids, salt-sensitivity and renal function. Curr Opin Nephrol Hypertens. 2007;16(1):16–21.

94. Tominaga T, Suzuki H, Ogata Y, Matsukawa S, Saruta T. The role of sex hormones and sodium intake in postmenopausal hypertension. J Hum Hypertens. 1991;5(6):495–500.
95. Kim JM, Kim TH, Lee HH, Lee SH, Wang T. Postmenopausal hypertension and sodium sensitivity. J Menopausal Med. 2014;20(1):1–6.
96. Pechere-Bertschi A, Burnier M. Female sex hormones, salt, and blood pressure regulation. Am J Hypertens. 2004;17(10):994–1001.
97. Mancia G, Fagard R, Narkiewicz K, Redon J, Zanchetti A, Bohm M, et al. 2013 ESH/ESC guidelines for the management of arterial hypertension: the Task Force for the Management of Arterial Hypertension of the European Society of Hypertension (ESH) and of the European Society of Cardiology (ESC). Eur Heart J. 2013;34(28):2159–219.
98. Drost JT, Arpaci G, Ottervanger JP, de Boer MJ, van Eyck J, van der Schouw YT, et al. Cardiovascular risk factors in women 10 years post early preeclampsia: the Preeclampsia Risk EValuation in FEMales study (PREVFEM). Eur J Prev Cardiol. 2012;19(5):1138–44.
99. Regnault V, Thomas F, Safar ME, Osborne-Pellegrin M, Khalil RA, Pannier B, et al. Sex difference in cardiovascular risk: role of pulse pressure amplification. J Am Coll Cardiol. 2012;59(20):1771–7.
100. Regitz-Zagrosek V, Brokat S, Tschope C. Role of gender in heart failure with normal left ventricular ejection fraction. Prog Cardiovasc Dis. 2007;49(4):241–51.
101. Coutinho T. Arterial stiffness and its clinical implications in women. Can J Cardiol. 2014;30(7):756–64.
102. Cleland JG, Swedberg K, Follath F, Komajda M, Cohen-Solal A, Aguilar JC, et al. The EuroHeart Failure survey programme—a survey on the quality of care among patients with heart failure in Europe. Part 1: patient characteristics and diagnosis. Eur Heart J. 2003;24(5):442–63.
103. Borlaug BA, Paulus WJ. Heart failure with preserved ejection fraction: pathophysiology, diagnosis, and treatment. Eur Heart J. 2011;32(6):670–9.
104. Merz AA, Cheng S. Sex differences in cardiovascular ageing. Heart. 2016;102(11):825–31.
105. Maas AH, Franke HR. Women's health in menopause with a focus on hypertension. Neth Heart J. 2009;17(2):68–72.
106. Davies PF. Hemodynamic shear stress and the endothelium in cardiovascular pathophysiology. Nat Clin Pract Cardiovasc Med. 2009;6(1):16–26.
107. Brandes RP. Endothelial dysfunction and hypertension. Hypertension. 2014;64(5):924–8.
108. Oparil S. Women and hypertension: what did we learn from the Women's Health Initiative? Cardiol Rev. 2006;14(6):267–75.
109. Gerber LM, Sievert LL, Warren K, Pickering TG, Schwartz JE. Hot flashes are associated with increased ambulatory systolic blood pressure. Menopause. 2007;14(2):308–15.
110. Ikeda H, Inoue T, Uemura S, Kaibara R, Tanaka H, Node K. Effects of candesartan for middle-aged and elderly women with hypertension and menopausal-like symptoms. Hypertens Res. 2006;29(12):1007–12.
111. Oelkers WH. Drospirenone in combination with estrogens: for contraception and hormone replacement therapy. Climacteric. 2005;8(Suppl 3):19–27.
112. Rautaharju PM, Kooperberg C, Larson JC, LaCroix A. Electrocardiographic predictors of incident congestive heart failure and all-cause mortality in postmenopausal women: the Women's Health Initiative. Circulation. 2006;113(4):481–9.
113. Farmer RD, Lawrenson RA, Thompson CR, Kennedy JG, Hambleton IR. Population-based study of risk of venous thromboembolism associated with various oral contraceptives. Lancet. 1997;349(9045):83–8.
114. van Hylckama VA, Helmerhorst FM, Vandenbroucke JP, Doggen CJ, Rosendaal FR. The venous thrombotic risk of oral contraceptives, effects of oestrogen dose and progestogen type: results of the MEGA case-control study. BMJ. 2009;339:b2921.
115. Lidegaard O, Lokkegaard E, Svendsen AL, Agger C. Hormonal contraception and risk of venous thromboembolism: national follow-up study. BMJ. 2009;339:b2890.
116. Shufelt CL, Bairey Merz CN. Contraceptive hormone use and cardiovascular disease. J Am Coll Cardiol. 2009;53(3):221–31.

117. Pomp ER, Rosendaal FR, Doggen CJ. Smoking increases the risk of venous thrombosis and acts synergistically with oral contraceptive use. Am J Hematol. 2008;83(2):97–102.
118. Tanis BC, van den Bosch MA, Kemmeren JM, Cats VM, Helmerhorst FM, Algra A, et al. Oral contraceptives and the risk of myocardial infarction. N Engl J Med. 2001;345(25):1787–93.
119. Cibula D, Gompel A, Mueck AO, La Vecchia C, Hannaford PC, Skouby SO, et al. Hormonal contraception and risk of cancer. Hum Reprod Update. 2010;16(6):631–50.
120. Merz CN, Johnson BD, Berga S, Braunstein G, Reis SE, Bittner V, et al. Past oral contraceptive use and angiographic coronary artery disease in postmenopausal women: data from the National Heart, Lung, and Blood Institute-sponsored Women's Ischemia Syndrome Evaluation. Fertil Steril. 2006;85(5):1425–31.
121. Weill A, Dalichampt M, Raguideau F, Ricordeau P, Blotiere PO, Rudant J, et al. Low dose oestrogen combined oral contraception and risk of pulmonary embolism, stroke, and myocardial infarction in five million French women: cohort study. BMJ. 2016;353:i2002.
122. Roos-Hesselink JW, Cornette J, Sliwa K, Pieper PG, Veldtman GR, Johnson MR. Contraception and cardiovascular disease. Eur Heart J. 2015;36(27):1728–34, 34a–34b.
123. Kaunitz AM. Clinical practice. Hormonal contraception in women of older reproductive age. N Engl J Med. 2008;358(12):1262–70.
124. Martinelli I, Lensing AW, Middeldorp S, Levi M, Beyer-Westendorf J, van Bellen B, et al. Recurrent venous thromboembolism and abnormal uterine bleeding with anticoagulant and hormone therapy use. Blood. 2016;127(11):1417–25.
125. Maas AH, Euler M, Bongers MY, Rolden HJ, Grutters JP, Ulrich L, et al. Practice points in gynecardiology: Abnormal uterine bleeding in premenopausal women taking oral anticoagulant or antiplatelet therapy. Maturitas. 2015;82(4):355–9.
126. Oldgren J, Wallentin L, Alexander JH, James S, Jonelid B, Steg G, et al. New oral anticoagulants in addition to single or dual antiplatelet therapy after an acute coronary syndrome: a systematic review and meta-analysis. Eur Heart J. 2013;34(22):1670–80.
127. Dans AL, Connolly SJ, Wallentin L, Yang S, Nakamya J, Brueckmann M, et al. Concomitant use of antiplatelet therapy with dabigatran or warfarin in the Randomized Evaluation of Long-Term Anticoagulation Therapy (RE-LY) trial. Circulation. 2013;127(5):634–40.
128. Stampfer MJ, Colditz GA. Estrogen replacement therapy and coronary heart disease: a quantitative assessment of the epidemiologic evidence. Prev Med. 1991;20(1):47–63.
129. Grodstein F, Stampfer MJ, Manson JE, Colditz GA, Willett WC, Rosner B, et al. Postmenopausal estrogen and progestin use and the risk of cardiovascular disease. N Engl J Med. 1996;335(7):453–61.
130. Rossouw JE, Anderson GL, Prentice RL, LaCroix AZ, Kooperberg C, Stefanick ML, et al. Risks and benefits of estrogen plus progestin in healthy postmenopausal women: principal results From the Women's Health Initiative randomized controlled trial. JAMA. 2002;288(3):321–33.
131. Salpeter SR, Cheng J, Thabane L, Buckley NS, Salpeter EE. Bayesian meta-analysis of hormone therapy and mortality in younger postmenopausal women. Am J Med. 2009;122(11):1016–22. e1
132. Schierbeck LL, Rejnmark L, Tofteng CL, Stilgren L, Eiken P, Mosekilde L, et al. Effect of hormone replacement therapy on cardiovascular events in recently postmenopausal women: randomised trial. BMJ. 2012;345:e6409.
133. Maas AH, van der Schouw YT, Grobbee DE, van der Graaf Y. Rise and fall of hormone therapy in postmenopausal women with cardiovascular disease. Menopause. 2004;11(2):228–35.
134. Harman SM, Black DM, Naftolin F, Brinton EA, Budoff MJ, Cedars MI, et al. Arterial imaging outcomes and cardiovascular risk factors in recently menopausal women: a randomized trial. Ann Intern Med. 2014;161(4):249–60.

135. Hodis HN, Mack WJ, Henderson VW, Shoupe D, Budoff MJ, Hwang-Levine J, et al. Vascular effects of early versus late postmenopausal treatment with estradiol. N Engl J Med. 2016;374(13):1221–31.
136. Bergendal A, Kieler H, Sundstrom A, Hirschberg AL, Kocoska-Maras L. Risk of venous thromboembolism associated with local and systemic use of hormone therapy in peri- and postmenopausal women and in relation to type and route of administration. Menopause. 2016;23(6):593–9.
137. Canonico M, Oger E, Plu-Bureau G, Conard J, Meyer G, Levesque H, et al. Hormone therapy and venous thromboembolism among postmenopausal women: impact of the route of estrogen administration and progestogens: the ESTHER study. Circulation. 2007;115(7):840–5.
138. Gleason CE, Dowling NM, Wharton W, Manson JE, Miller VM, Atwood CS, et al. Effects of hormone therapy on cognition and mood in recently postmenopausal women: findings from the randomized, controlled KEEPS-Cognitive and Affective Study. PLoS Med. 2015;12(6):e1001833; discussion e.
139. Shumaker SA, Legault C, Rapp SR, Thal L, Wallace RB, Ockene JK, et al. Estrogen plus progestin and the incidence of dementia and mild cognitive impairment in postmenopausal women: the Women's Health Initiative Memory Study: a randomized controlled trial. JAMA. 2003;289(20):2651–62.
140. Shumaker SA, Legault C, Kuller L, Rapp SR, Thal L, Lane DS, et al. Conjugated equine estrogens and incidence of probable dementia and mild cognitive impairment in postmenopausal women: Women's Health Initiative Memory Study. JAMA. 2004;291(24):2947–58.
141. Rees MC. HRT in premature menopause. BMJ. 2008;337:a1668.
142. North American Menopause Society. The 2012 hormone therapy position statement of: the North American Menopause Society. Menopause. 2012;19(3):257–71.
143. Manson JE, Kaunitz AM. Menopause management—getting clinical care back on track. N Engl J Med. 2016;374(9):803–6.
144. Geukes M, van Aalst MP, Nauta MC, Oosterhof H. The impact of menopausal symptoms on work ability. Menopause. 2012;19(3):278–82.
145. Sarrel PM. Women, work, and menopause. Menopause. 2012;19(3):250–2.
146. Neves ECM, Birkhauser M, Samsioe G, Lambrinoudaki I, Palacios S, Borrego RS, et al. EMAS position statement: the ten point guide to the integral management of menopausal health. Maturitas. 2015;81(1):88–92.
147. de Villiers TJ, Hall JE, Pinkerton JV, Perez SC, Rees M, Yang C, et al. Revised global consensus statement on menopausal hormone therapy. Maturitas. 2016;91:153–5.
148. Mintziori G, Lambrinoudaki I, Goulis DG, Ceausu I, Depypere H, Erel CT, et al. EMAS position statement: Non-hormonal management of menopausal vasomotor symptoms. Maturitas. 2015;81(3):410–3.

Chapter 6
Heart Failure in Women: Is There a Typical Female Type?

Arantxa Barandiarán Aizpurua and Vanessa van Empel

Abstract Patients with heart failure (HF) with preserved ejection fraction (HFpEF) make up 50% of all cases of HF and they are typically female, older, have a history of hypertension, and share multiple co-morbidities including obesity, diabetes and renal insufficiency. Complaints of reduced exercise tolerance and dyspnea on exertion are often attributed to 'healthy' aging, and not due to disease, leaving a significant percentage of the HFpEF population under-diagnosed. The aetiology is complex, heterogeneous and to a large extent unclarified. The appropriate diagnostic criteria and treatment options are still a challenge and under development.

Keywords Diastolic dysfunction • Dyspnea • Echocardiography • Endothelial dysfunction • Fibrosis • Heart failure with preserved ejection fraction (HFpEF) • Heart failure with reduced ejection fraction (HFrEF) • Inflammation • Myocardial stiffness

Introduction

Cardiologists are more and more aware that the manifestations of ischemic heart disease (IHD) are different in men and women. This is also the case for heart failure (HF). Although the lifetime risk to develop HF at age 55 years is similar for men and women, respectively 33% and 28%, there are striking sex-differences in the prevalence of the different types of HF [1]. Evidently HF caused by peripartum cardiomyopathy (PPCM) is exclusively present in women, but HF with reduced ejection fraction (HFrEF), usually following obstructive coronary artery disease (CAD), is far more prevalent in men. Women however are predominantly affected by heart failure with preserved ejection fraction (HFpEF), which is the focus of the current chapter [2]. Peripartum cardiomyopathy will be discussed in Chap. 8.

A. Barandiarán Aizpurua, M.D. • V. van Empel, M.D., Ph.D. (✉)
Department of Cardiology, Maastricht University Medical Centre, Maastricht, The Netherlands
e-mail: Vanessa.van.empel@mumc.nl

A.H.E.M. Maas, C.N. Bairey Merz (eds.), *Manual of Gynecardiology*,
DOI 10.1007/978-3-319-54960-6_6

Gender Differences in Myocardial Remodelling with Ageing

Healthy female hearts are smaller compared to men, and women have higher heart rates [3]. However, not only healthy hearts show sex differences, also myocardial remodelling in response to stress is sex-specific. With aging the LV volume increases modestly in men, but not in women, additionally age-related increase in cardiovascular stiffness is more pronounced in women [4, 5]. In response to pressure overload, such as seen in aortic stenosis, females develop concentric hypertrophy with smaller internal cavity and relatively larger wall thickness compared to men, who in general develop more eccentric hypertrophy [6]. In addition, women also preserve better ejection fraction and myocardial contractility than men during pressure overload [7]. This is also the case in HF patients; female HFpEF patients have a higher LV ejection fraction and demonstrate more LV diastolic and systolic stiffness than men, which may explain their greater predisposition for HFpEF [3]. Sex-specific myocardial remodelling contribute to differences in regulation of fibrosis and inflammation, but the exact mechanism remains unclear [8].

Heart Failure with Preserved Ejection Fraction

Background

HFpEF patients make up 50% of all cases of HF [2]. Their main symptoms are reduced exercise capacity and dyspnea on exertion. Previously, this type of HF was called diastolic heart failure, however this term was abandoned because it did not cover the scope of abnormalities that are seen in HFpEF [9]. HFpEF patients are typically female, older, have a history of hypertension, and share multiple comorbidities including obesity, diabetes and renal insufficiency [2]. Among people >65 years of age presenting to primary care with breathlessness on exertion, one in six will have unrecognized HF (mainly HFpEF) [10]. The prognosis of HFpEF is poor and comparable to that of HF with reduced ejection fraction (HFrEF). The annual mortality of HFpEF is estimated at 10–30% [2, 11]. Approximately 60% of patients die from cardiovascular disease (CVD), mainly to HF itself or to sudden cardiac death. Patients who need to be hospitalized for HF have the highest risk of death. Surprisingly, 40% of mortality is contributed to non-cardiac causes, which is significant higher in patients with HFpEF than in HFrEF [12, 13]. Although the number of hospital admissions for HFrEF and HFpEF are equal, HFpEF patients are hospitalized more often for non-cardiac reasons (Table 6.1).

HFpEF is a complex heterogeneous entity, of which the underlying pathophysiology remains still largely unclear. Over the last decade multiple studies have attributed a role for inflammation and endothelial dysfunction in the pathophysiology of HFpEF [14]. However, despite these new insights this has not yet resulted into appropriate treatment options. Standard HF drugs, such as beta-blockers, ACE-inhibitors and mineralocorticoid antagonists, although proven to be effective in HFrEF, thus far failed to improve outcomes in HFpEF [15].

Table 6.1 Diagnostic criteria for heart failure with preserved ejection fraction

1. Symptoms and/or signs	
Symptoms	Signs
Breathlessness, orthopnea, paroxysmal nocturnal dyspnea, reduced exercise tolerance, fatigue, tiredness	Elevated jugular venous pressure, hepatojugular reflux, third heart sound, peripheral edema, pulmonary crepitations
2. Structural or functional abnormalities	
Structural	Functional
Left venticular hypertrophy, enlarged left atrial volume index	Diastolic dysfunction
3. Elevated levels of natriuretic peptide	

Diagnostic Pathway

The evaluation and diagnosis of a patient suspected of HFpEF remains challenging. Complaints of reduced exercise tolerance and dyspnea on exertion is often attributed to 'healthy' aging, and not due to disease, leaving a significant percentage of the HFpEF population under-diagnosed. Secondly, diagnostic criteria of HFpEF, and cut-off values for diastolic function, can be difficult to interpret and remain a topic of debate. The current criteria to diagnose HFpEF include [1] presence of symptoms and/or signs of HF [2]; normal LV ejection fraction (LVEF $\geq$ 50%) [3]; elevated levels of natriuretic peptides and [4] relevant structural heart disease (LV hypertrophy/LA enlargement) or diastolic dysfunction [15]. Initial assessment of HFpEF therefore includes clinical assessment of symptoms or signs of HF in combination with laboratory measurements and an echocardiography. As previous studies have shown that echocardiographic measures to assess diastolic dysfunction correlate poorly with actual LV filling pressures and lack accuracy, it may be helpful to perform right heart catheterisation to better evaluate left ventricular filling pressures [16, 17]. Additionally, some pathophysiological features of HFpEF may not be evident at rest. Considering that many of the diagnostic echocardiographic parameters used are load dependent and that symptoms principally occur during activity one should consider exercise testing, either stress-echocardiography or, preferably, an invasive assessment of the haemodynamic response to exercise if echocardiography at rest is inconclusive [18].

Pathophysiology

A central pathophysiologic feature of HFpEF appears to be an increase in the left ventricular end-diastolic pressure (LVEDD). Both vascular and myocardial stiffness may lead to an increase of the LVEDD. Vascular stiffness, caused by ageing and co-morbidities, hinders the diastolic filling [9]. Another important clinical manifestation of vascular stiffness is hypertension, which often goes hand in hand with HFpEF. Due to stiffness of the myocardium, the heart can no longer "relax" in the diastolic phase, thus the LVEDD is relatively high compared to the amount of blood in the ventricle. Factors that contribute to the myocardial stiffness by fibrosis formation are changes in the extracellular matrix, changes in the myocyte intrinsic stiffness, microvascular dysfunction and metabolic abnormalities [19]. Myocardial stiffness is further augmented by the presence of left ventricular hypertrophy, which occurs in response to prolonged hypertension. MRI studies show that the heart not only stiffens due to hypertrophy, but also by the presence of fibrosis [20].

Fibrosis of the Myocardium

In HFpEF patients, fibrosis is present both in the myocardium as well as in the vessels, which contributes to the deterioration of the diastolic and the systolic function [21, 22]. Fibrosis formation is caused by changes in amount of collagen deposition in the extracellular matrix [22]. Analyses from endomyocardial biopsies demonstrate the collagen synthesis is increased and enzymes that break down collagen are reduced [23, 24]. As a result, we see a pattern of diffuse fibrosis, as opposed to after a myocardial infarction where very localized fibrosis is present. This diffuse fibrosis is caused by, among other things, the activation of TGF-β (transforming growth factor-β) in response to the increased inflammation of the microvascular endothelium [19]. There are sex-specific patterns in regulation of fibrosis in response pressure overload [8]. How this contributes to the predisposition of females to HFpEF remains to be investigated.

Role of Inflammation

Several co-morbidities, which frequently occur in HFpEF, such as diabetes and obesity, cause a chronic low-grade systemic inflammation [25]. This inflammation induces endothelial dysfunction, which is subsequently associated with increased oxidative stress [26]. Although these processes are described both for HFrEF and HFpEF, endothelial dysfunction is more prevalent in HFpEF, even when adjusted for age, sex, the presence of diabetes and hypertension [27]. This suggests that endothelial dysfunction is not merely a result of multiple co-morbidities, but is specifically related to the pathophysiology of HFpEF. Furthermore, endothelial dysfunction is negatively associated with the prognosis of HFpEF [28]. An increased oxidative stress induces diastolic stiffness of the myocyte by an increase in cyclic GMP (guanosinemonofostaat), and ultimately a change in the titin protein, which is a component of the cytoskeleton of the cardiomyocyte [29].

Management of HFpEF

The standard drug therapy for HF such as beta-blockers, ACE inhibitors/angiotensin receptor antagonists (ARBs) or mineralocorticoid antagonists have not shown any beneficial effect in patients with HFpEF [15]. These drugs have been extensively studied in several clinical trials, and provide no improvement in survival, exercise tolerance, functional class or quality of life. Diuretics are recommended if fluid retention is present, and although they may reduce symptoms, the prognosis is not altered [15]. The reasons for these negative results remain unclear. As described earlier in this chapter, it remains a challenge to diagnose HFpEF and consequently the various studies have used different inclusion and exclusion criteria. This results in a very large variety of different types and degrees of HFpEF [30]. One of the reasons for the negative results lies therefore, at least partly, in the fact that HFpEF is not a uniform disease. Due to the presence of numerous co-morbidities, the HFpEF population represents a very heterogeneous group, wherein it is not unlikely that specific sub-groups may still benefit from certain HF medications [31]. In the future, a better characterization of the different subgroups of HFpEF patients will also provide valuable information for more effective treatment. This should result in a personalized treatment, based on the specific characteristics of the disease, instead of the current one-size-fits-all approach.

Because of the negative and neutral findings of recent trials, the emphasis of treatment in HFpEF is currently focused on treatment of the various co-morbidities, such as optimal regulation of blood pressure and strict regulation of glucose levels. Most drugs that are used in patients with HFrEF are safe for HFpEF patients, and most of the drugs that should be avoided in HFrEF, should also be avoided in HFpEF, with the exception of verapamil and diltiazem [15]. These calcium blockers can be given safely to HFpEF patients.

Besides medical therapy, exercise training is an important part of the treatment of heart failure, also in HFpEF. Various studies in HFpEF patients report an improvement in exercise tolerance after exercise training; for instance the multi-centre Ex-DHF-P study, which included HFpEF patients with NYHA class 2-3, showed that 32 sessions in which a combined aerobic and strength training improved exercise tolerance, diastolic function and quality of life [32]. Whether there is an impact on survival or the number of hospitalizations is unknown yet.

New Developments

Spironolacton has shown to decrease mortality in HFrEF and could be a promising therapy for HFpEF [33]. Spironolactone exerts its effect by a competitive antagonism with the intracellular aldosterone receptor. Aldosterone plays a role in hypertension, endothelial dysfunction and myocardial fibrosis, which are all processes involved in the onset of HFpEF. Intervention in this system therefore seems attractive. Previous studies already showed that patients with hypertension develop less LV hypertrophy when treated with spironolactone [34, 35]. However the TOPCAT study, a large international randomized, placebo-controlled trial, failed to show beneficial effect of spironolactone treatment on the combined endpoint of mortality and hospitalization in patients with HFpEF [36]. However, the results are somewhat more complex as there was a large difference in event rates in the placebo group among the different geographical areas. A post-hoc analysis showed that when patients from Russia and Georgia (approximately 45% of all patients) were excluded from the analysis, there was a positive effect with regard to fewer hospital admissions for heart failure [37]. It was therefore suspected that these countries enrolled too many 'unreal' HFpEF patients and that spironolactone may still need to get a place in the treatment of HFpEF.

Phosphodiesterase-5 inhibitors (PDE-5) intervene in the sGC NO-cGMP-signaling pathway (see figure). Increased cGMP activates cGMP-dependent protein kinases, which work favourably on ventricular hypertrophy, diastolic relaxation and stiffness. Inhibition of PDE 5 leads to an accumulation of intracellular cGMP, and therefore could work beneficial. Animal studies show that sildenafil, a PDE-5 inhibitor, affects the cardiomyocyte remodelling. Sildenafil reduced progression of ventricular remodelling and dysfunction and suppressed fibrosis formation and left ventricular hypertrophy [38, 39]. Additionally, in a small, randomized trial of 44 patients with HFpEF and (slightly) increased right ventricular pressures, sildenafil improved hemodynamics, RV function, and also quality of life compared to placebo [40]. However, a multi-centre randomized study with 216 HFpEF patients, showed no difference in exercise tolerance or clinical status after 24 weeks of treatment with sildenafil or placebo [41]. Further investigation to evaluate the role of this drug is needed.

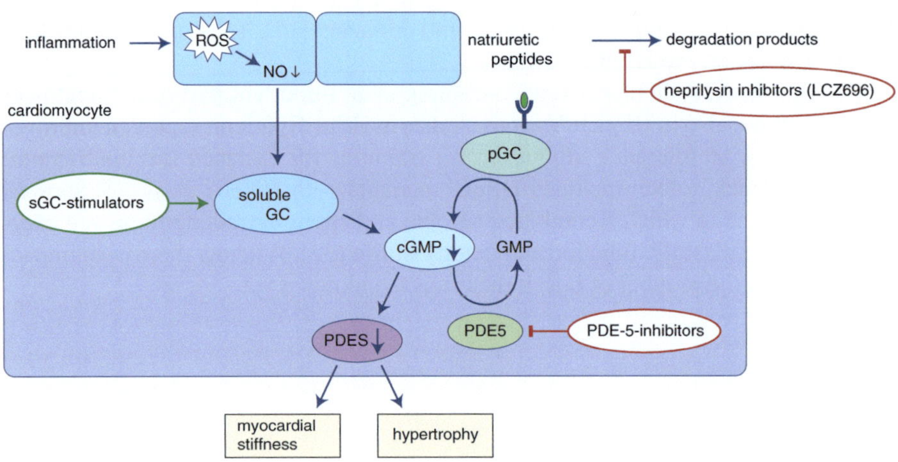

- *Soluble guanylate cyclase (sGC-) stimulators* also intervene in the NO-sGC-cGMP signaling pathway, just like PDE-5 inhibitors. sGC stimulators directly stimulate the NO-soluble guanylate cyclase receptor (sGC), independently of nitric oxide (NO) but also act in synergy with NO to produce anti-aggregatory, anti-proliferative, and vasodilatory effects. The phase II trial soluble guanylate Cyclase stimulator Heart Study (SOCRATES) studies the effect of an oral sGC stimulator (vericiguat) on the change in NT-proBNP and left atrial volume and will further investigate the safety and tolerability [42]. The study is nearing completion and the results of this study will be known in the near future.

- *LCZ696* is an angiotensin-II receptor blocker (valsartan) in combination with a neprilysin-inhibitor (sacubitril). Sacubitril inhibits neprilysin, which degradates vasoactive peptides such as natriuretic peptides, bradykinin and adreno medulline. Thus sacubitril increases the levels of these peptides, resulting in vasodilation, and reduction of the extra-cellular volume. Recent data have shown an impressive effect of LCZ696 at HFrEF [43]. Whether similar results are present in HFpEF, is currently being studied in an ongoing Phase III study. The recent Paramount study, a Phase II study, randomized 301 patients to HFpEF LCZ696 or valsartan [44]. After 36 weeks of treatment, the LCZ696-group showed a reduction in NT-proBNP, as well as left atrium volume compared to the valsartan-group. These data are encouraging in the expectation that LCZ696 might also affect survival and hospitalization in patients with HFpEF.

Case Report

A 76 year-old woman presents at the outpatient cardiology department with dizziness, fatigue and shortness of breath on exertion. These complaints have been present for at least 3 years, but her breathlessness has worsened considerably in recent months. She does not have orthopnea or peripheral edema. She is familiar with hypertension since many years, for which she is treated by her GP, and has no other risk factors for heart disease.

On physical examination, her blood pressure was 155/83 mmHg with an irregular heart rate of 60 beats/min. Her BMI was 30.1 kg/m^2. The central venous pressure was not elevated, and at auscultation no heart murmurs were present. Auscultation of the lungs revealed minimal bilateral basal crackles. She had no peripheral edema. The ECG showed atrial fibrillation of 58 beats/min. Echocardiography showed a normal left ventricular (LV) diameter, a normal left systolic ventricular function (ejection fraction 62%), mild LV hypertrophy (LV mass index 105 g/m^2) and a vastly enlarged left atrium (LA volume index 46 mL/m^2). No significant valve abnormalities. She has signs of diastolic dysfunction with elevated filling pressure (E/e '16) and normal right ventricular pressures and function. The laboratory tests are normal, except for a low ferritin indicating a lack of iron.

This 76 year-old woman, with dyspnea on exertion and NYHA functional class III, has classical clinical features of heart failure with preserved ejection fraction (HFpEF).

References

1. Bleumink GS, Knetsch AM, Sturkenboom MC, Straus SM, Hofman A, Deckers JW, Witteman JC, Stricker BH. Quantifying the heart failure epidemic: prevalence, incidence rate, lifetime risk and prognosis of heart failure. The Rotterdam Study. Eur Heart J. 2004;25:1614–9.
2. Owan TE, Hodge DO, Herges RM, Jacobsen SJ, Roger VL, Redfield MM. Trends in prevalence and outcome of heart failure with preserved ejection fraction. N Engl J Med. 2006;355:251–9.

3. Gori M, Lam CS, Gupta DK, Santos AB, Cheng S, Shah AM, Claggett B, Zile MR, Kraigher-Krainer E, Pieske B, Voors AA, Packer M, Bransford T, Lefkowitz M, McMurray JJ, Solomon SD, Investigators P. Sex-specific cardiovascular structure and function in heart failure with preserved ejection fraction. Eur J Heart Fail. 2014;16:535–42.
4. Redfield MM, Jacobsen SJ, Borlaug BA, Rodeheffer RJ, Kass DA. Age- and gender-related ventricular-vascular stiffening: a community-based study. Circulation. 2005;112:2254–62.
5. Regitz-Zagrosek V, Brokat S, Tschope C. Role of gender in heart failure with normal left ventricular ejection fraction. Prog Cardiovasc Dis. 2007;49:241–51.
6. Cramariuc D, Rieck AE, Staal EM, Wachtell K, Eriksen E, Rossebo AB, Gerdts E. Factors influencing left ventricular structure and stress-corrected systolic function in men and women with asymptomatic aortic valve stenosis (a SEAS substudy). Am J Cardiol. 2008;101:510–5.
7. Villari B, Campbell SE, Schneider J, Vassalli G, Chiariello M, Hess OM. Sex-dependent differences in left ventricular function and structure in chronic pressure overload. Eur Heart J. 1995;16:1410–9.
8. Kararigas G, Dworatzek E, Petrov G, Summer H, Schulze TM, Baczko I, Knosalla C, Golz S, Hetzer R, Regitz-Zagrosek V. Sex-dependent regulation of fibrosis and inflammation in human left ventricular remodelling under pressure overload. Eur J Heart Fail. 2014;16:1160–7.
9. Borlaug BA. The pathophysiology of heart failure with preserved ejection fraction. Nat Rev Cardiol. 2014;11:507–15.
10. Rutten FH, Cramer MJ, Grobbee DE, Sachs AP, Kirkels JH, Lammers JW, Hoes AW. Unrecognized heart failure in elderly patients with stable chronic obstructive pulmonary disease. Eur Heart J. 2005;26:1887–94.
11. Martinez-Selles M, Doughty RN, Poppe K, Whalley GA, Earle N, Tribouilloy C, McMurray JJ, Swedberg K, Kober L, Berry C, Squire I, Meta-Analysis Global Group In Chronic Heart Failure. Gender and survival in patients with heart failure: interactions with diabetes and aetiology. Results from the MAGGIC individual patient meta-analysis. Eur J Heart Fail. 2012;14:473–9.
12. Ather S, Chan W, Bozkurt B, Aguilar D, Ramasubbu K, Zachariah AA, Wehrens XH, Deswal A. Impact of noncardiac comorbidities on morbidity and mortality in a predominantly male population with heart failure and preserved versus reduced ejection fraction. J Am Coll Cardiol. 2012;59:998–1005.
13. Quiroz R, Doros G, Shaw P, Liang CS, Gauthier DF, Sam F. Comparison of characteristics and outcomes of patients with heart failure preserved ejection fraction versus reduced left ventricular ejection fraction in an urban cohort. Am J Cardiol. 2014;113:691–6.
14. van Empel V, Brunner-La Rocca HP. Inflammation in HFpEF: key or circumstantial? Int J Cardiol. 2015;189:259–63.
15. Ponikowski P, Voors AA, Anker SD, Bueno H, Cleland JG, Coats AJ, Falk V, Gonzalez-Juanatey JR, Harjola VP, Jankowska EA, Jessup M, Linde C, Nihoyannopoulos P, Parissis JT, Pieske B, Riley JP, Rosano GM, Ruilope LM, Ruschitzka F, Rutten FH, van der Meer P, Authors/Task Force M, Document R. 2016 ESC Guidelines for the diagnosis and treatment of acute and chronic heart failure: The Task Force for the diagnosis and treatment of acute and chronic heart failure of the European Society of Cardiology (ESC). Developed with the special contribution of the Heart Failure Association (HFA) of the ESC. Eur J Heart Fail. 2016;18:891–975.
16. Brunner-La Rocca HP, Attenhofer CH, Jenni R. Can the extent of change of the left ventricular doppler inflow pattern during the valsalva maneuver predict an elevated left ventricular end-diastolic pressure? Echocardiography. 1998;15:211–8.
17. Swanson KL, Utz JP, Krowka MJ. Doppler echocardiography-right heart catheterization relationships in patients with idiopathic pulmonary fibrosis and suspected pulmonary hypertension. Med Sci Monit. 2008;14:CR177–82.
18. van Empel VP, Kaye DM. Integration of exercise evaluation into the algorithm for evaluation of patients with suspected heart failure with preserved ejection fraction. Int J Cardiol. 2013;168:716–22.
19. Paulus WJ, Tschope C. A novel paradigm for heart failure with preserved ejection fraction: comorbidities drive myocardial dysfunction and remodeling through coronary microvascular endothelial inflammation. J Am Coll Cardiol. 2013;62:263–71.

20. Su MY, Lin LY, Tseng YH, Chang CC, Wu CK, Lin JL, Tseng WY. CMR-verified diffuse myocardial fibrosis is associated with diastolic dysfunction in HFpEF. JACC Cardiovasc Imaging. 2014;7:991–7.
21. van Heerebeek L, Borbely A, Niessen HW, Bronzwaer JG, van der Velden J, Stienen GJ, Linke WA, Laarman GJ, Paulus WJ. Myocardial structure and function differ in systolic and diastolic heart failure. Circulation. 2006;113:1966–73.
22. Kasner M, Westermann D, Lopez B, Gaub R, Escher F, Kuhl U, Schultheiss HP, Tschope C. Diastolic tissue Doppler indexes correlate with the degree of collagen expression and cross-linking in heart failure and normal ejection fraction. J Am Coll Cardiol. 2011; 57:977–85.
23. Westermann D, Lindner D, Kasner M, Zietsch C, Savvatis K, Escher F, von Schlippenbach J, Skurk C, Steendijk P, Riad A, Poller W, Schultheiss HP, Tschope C. Cardiac inflammation contributes to changes in the extracellular matrix in patients with heart failure and normal ejection fraction. Circ Heart Fail. 2011;4:44–52.
24. van Heerebeek L, Hamdani N, Handoko ML, Falcao-Pires I, Musters RJ, Kupreishvili K, Ijsselmuiden AJ, Schalkwijk CG, Bronzwaer JG, Diamant M, Borbely A, van der Velden J, Stienen GJ, Laarman GJ, Niessen HW, Paulus WJ. Diastolic stiffness of the failing diabetic heart: importance of fibrosis, advanced glycation end products, and myocyte resting tension. Circulation. 2008;117:43–51.
25. Sciarretta S, Ferrucci A, Ciavarella GM, De Paolis P, Venturelli V, Tocci G, De Biase L, Rubattu S, Volpe M. Markers of inflammation and fibrosis are related to cardiovascular damage in hypertensive patients with metabolic syndrome. Am J Hypertens. 2007;20:784–91.
26. van Heerebeek L, Hamdani N, Falcao-Pires I, Leite-Moreira AF, Begieneman MP, Bronzwaer JG, van der Velden J, Stienen GJ, Laarman GJ, Somsen A, Verheugt FW, Niessen HW, Paulus WJ. Low myocardial protein kinase G activity in heart failure with preserved ejection fraction. Circulation. 2012;126:830–9.
27. Mohammed SF, Borlaug BA, Roger VL, Mirzoyev SA, Rodeheffer RJ, Chirinos JA, Redfield MM. Comorbidity and ventricular and vascular structure and function in heart failure with preserved ejection fraction: a community-based study. Circ Heart Fail. 2012;5:710–9.
28. Borlaug BA, Olson TP, Lam CS, Flood KS, Lerman A, Johnson BD, Redfield MM. Global cardiovascular reserve dysfunction in heart failure with preserved ejection fraction. J Am Coll Cardiol. 2010;56:845–54.
29. Borbely A, Falcao-Pires I, van Heerebeek L, Hamdani N, Edes I, Gavina C, Leite-Moreira AF, Bronzwaer JG, Papp Z, van der Velden J, Stienen GJ, Paulus WJ. Hypophosphorylation of the Stiff N2B titin isoform raises cardiomyocyte resting tension in failing human myocardium. Circ Res. 2009;104:780–6.
30. Shah SJ, Kitzman DW, Borlaug BA, van Heerebeek L, Zile MR, Kass DA, Paulus WJ. Phenotype-specific treatment of heart failure with preserved ejection fraction: a multiorgan roadmap. Circulation. 2016;134:73–90.
31. Senni M, Paulus WJ, Gavazzi A, Fraser AG, Diez J, Solomon SD, Smiseth OA, Guazzi M, Lam CS, Maggioni AP, Tschope C, Metra M, Hummel SL, Edelmann F, Ambrosio G, Stewart Coats AJ, Filippatos GS, Gheorghiade M, Anker SD, Levy D, Pfeffer MA, Stough WG, Pieske BM. New strategies for heart failure with preserved ejection fraction: the importance of targeted therapies for heart failure phenotypes. Eur Heart J. 2014;35:2797–815.
32. Edelmann F, Gelbrich G, Dungen HD, Frohling S, Wachter R, Stahrenberg R, Binder L, Topper A, Lashki DJ, Schwarz S, Herrmann-Lingen C, Loffler M, Hasenfuss G, Halle M, Pieske B. Exercise training improves exercise capacity and diastolic function in patients with heart failure with preserved ejection fraction: results of the Ex-DHF (Exercise training in Diastolic Heart Failure) pilot study. J Am Coll Cardiol. 2011;58:1780–91.
33. Pitt B, Zannad F, Remme WJ, Cody R, Castaigne A, Perez A, Palensky J, Wittes J. The effect of spironolactone on morbidity and mortality in patients with severe heart failure. Randomized Aldactone Evaluation Study Investigators. N Engl J Med. 1999;341:709–17.
34. Kurrelmeyer KM, Ashton Y, Xu J, Nagueh SF, Torre-Amione G, Deswal A. Effects of spironolactone treatment in elderly women with heart failure and preserved left ventricular ejection fraction. J Card Fail. 2014;20:560–8.

35. Shah AM, Claggett B, Sweitzer NK, Shah SJ, Deswal A, Anand IS, Fleg JL, Pitt B, Pfeffer MA, Solomon SD. Prognostic importance of changes in cardiac structure and function in heart failure with preserved ejection fraction and the impact of spironolactone. Circ Heart Fail. 2015;8:1052–8.
36. Pitt B, Pfeffer MA, Assmann SF, Boineau R, Anand IS, Claggett B, Clausell N, Desai AS, Diaz R, Fleg JL, Gordeev I, Harty B, Heitner JF, Kenwood CT, Lewis EF, O'Meara E, Probstfield JL, Shaburishvili T, Shah SJ, Solomon SD, Sweitzer NK, Yang S, McKinlay SM, Investigators T. Spironolactone for heart failure with preserved ejection fraction. N Engl J Med. 2014;370:1383–92.
37. Solomon SD, Claggett B, Lewis EF, Desai A, Anand I, Sweitzer NK, O'Meara E, Shah SJ, McKinlay S, Fleg JL, Sopko G, Pitt B, Pfeffer MA, Investigators T. Influence of ejection fraction on outcomes and efficacy of spironolactone in patients with heart failure with preserved ejection fraction. Eur Heart J. 2016;37:455–62.
38. Nagayama T, Hsu S, Zhang M, Koitabashi N, Bedja D, Gabrielson KL, Takimoto E, Kass DA. Sildenafil stops progressive chamber, cellular, and molecular remodeling and improves calcium handling and function in hearts with pre-existing advanced hypertrophy caused by pressure overload. J Am Coll Cardiol. 2009;53:207–15.
39. Takimoto E, Champion HC, Li M, Belardi D, Ren S, Rodriguez ER, Bedja D, Gabrielson KL, Wang Y, Kass DA. Chronic inhibition of cyclic GMP phosphodiesterase 5A prevents and reverses cardiac hypertrophy. Nat Med. 2005;11:214–22.
40. Guazzi M, Vicenzi M, Arena R, Guazzi MD. PDE5 inhibition with sildenafil improves left ventricular diastolic function, cardiac geometry, and clinical status in patients with stable systolic heart failure: results of a 1-year, prospective, randomized, placebo-controlled study. Circ Heart Fail. 2011;4:8–17.
41. Redfield MM, Chen HH, Borlaug BA, Semigran MJ, Lee KL, Lewis G, MM LW, Rouleau JL, Bull DA, Mann DL, Deswal A, Stevenson LW, Givertz MM, Ofili EO, O'Connor CM, Felker GM, Goldsmith SR, Bart BA, SE MN, Ibarra JC, Lin G, Oh JK, Patel MR, Kim RJ, Tracy RP, Velazquez EJ, Anstrom KJ, Hernandez AF, Mascette AM, Braunwald E, Trial RELAX. Effect of phosphodiesterase-5 inhibition on exercise capacity and clinical status in heart failure with preserved ejection fraction: a randomized clinical trial. JAMA. 2013;309:1268–77.
42. Pieske B, Butler J, Filippatos G, Lam C, Maggioni AP, Ponikowski P, Shah S, Solomon S, Kraigher-Krainer E, Samano ET, Scalise AV, Muller K, Roessig L, Gheorghiade M, Investigators S and Coordinators. Rationale and design of the SOluble guanylate Cyclase stimulatoR in heArT failurE Studies (SOCRATES). Eur J Heart Fail. 2014;16:1026–38.
43. Jhund PS, Fu M, Bayram E, Chen CH, Negrusz-Kawecka M, Rosenthal A, Desai AS, Lefkowitz MP, Rizkala AR, Rouleau JL, Shi VC, Solomon SD, Swedberg K, Zile MR, JJ MM, Packer M, Investigators P-H and Committees. Efficacy and safety of LCZ696 (sacubitril-valsartan) according to age: insights from PARADIGM-HF. Eur Heart J. 2015;36:2576–84.
44. Solomon SD, Zile M, Pieske B, Voors A, Shah A, Kraigher-Krainer E, Shi V, Bransford T, Takeuchi M, Gong J, Lefkowitz M, Packer M, McMurray JJ, Prospective comparison of AwARBoMOhfwpefI. The angiotensin receptor neprilysin inhibitor LCZ696 in heart failure with preserved ejection fraction: a phase 2 double-blind randomised controlled trial. Lancet. 2012;380:1387–95.

Chapter 7
Cardiotoxicity During and After Breast Cancer Treatment

Angela H.E.M. Maas

Abstract As cardiovascular diseases (CVD) are the main cause of death in women worldwide, they are also frequently present in breast cancer (BC) patients and in late survivors. Radiation therapy, chemotherapy, immunotherapy and angiogenic therapy may induce cardiotoxicity and vascular damage. In the rapidly evolving field of cardio-oncology it is recommended that pre-existing CVD risk factors should be assessed in all BC patients and aggressively managed, starting at the time of treatment (or even before) and continuing throughout survivorship. The use of advanced cardiac imaging techniques improves earlier detection of cardiac damage and heart failure, enabling a more timely treatment.

Keywords Anthracyclines • Blood pressure • BRCA 1/2 mutation carriers • Breast cancer • Cardiotoxicity • Cardio-oncology • Chemotherapy • Ejection fraction • Immunotherapy • Systolic heart failure • Radiation therapy • Risk factors • Trastuzumab

Introduction

In Western populations one out of eight women will develop breast cancer (BC). Due to improved screening modalities and the development of novel cancer treatments, including targeted and immunologic therapies, 5 year BC survival rates are more than 90%. Ten-year survival rates for invasive BC is now approximately 83% (www.seer.cancer.gov). Despite these impressive advancements in survival, cardiovascular toxicity is increasingly observed as a serious complication of treatment. This has led to the rapid evolving field of cardio-oncology with a bread focus not only on myocardial toxicity, but also on vascular disease, accelerated onset of hypertension and arrhythmias. New strategies are currently being developed to better preserve and restore cardiovascular health in patients with cancer and cancers survivors, for which an optimal interdisciplinary collaboration and understanding is needed [1, 2].

A.H.E.M. Maas, M.D., Ph.D.
Department of Cardiology, Women's Cardiac Health Program,
Radboud University Medical Center, Nijmegen, The Netherlands
e-mail: angela.maas@radboudumc.nl

A.H.E.M. Maas, C.N. Bairey Merz (eds.), *Manual of Gynecardiology*,
DOI 10.1007/978-3-319-54960-6_7

Cardiovascular Risk in Breast Cancer Patients

As cardiovascular diseases (CVD) are the main cause of death in women worldwide, they are also frequently present in BC patients and in late survivors (Fig. 7.1). In a population of 415 postmenopausal women with hormone receptor (HR) positive early BC the 10-year predicted CVD risk was equivalent to or higher than BC recurrence risk [3]. Risk factors like obesity, diabetes and hypertension are important in the occurrence of both CVD and BC [4–7]. Women with unhealthy lifestyle behavior, CVD risk factors and genetic factors are more susceptible for cardiotoxicity during BC therapy [8, 9]. This concept is also known as the 'multiple-hit' hypothesis. Preliminary data also suggest that cancer itself may induce subclinical myocardial damage before any treatment has been started [10]. Despite the individual differences in CVD risk profile, the various classifications/stages of BC and the variety of BC treatment regimens that are needed, a tailored patient approach with early and late

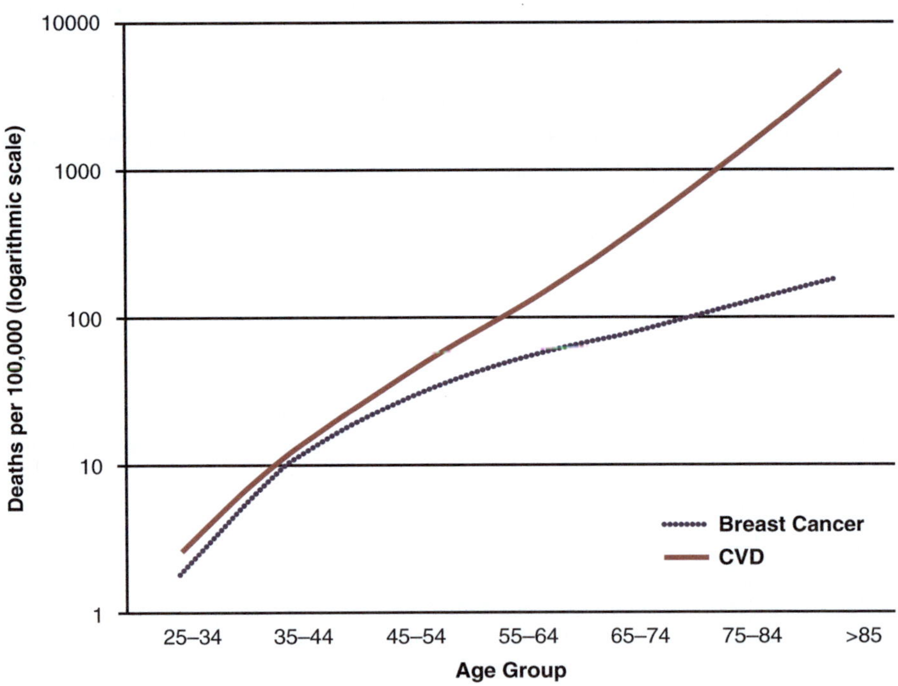

Fig. 7.1 CVD and breast cancer deaths in women. Source: US Centers for Disease Control and Prevention [1999–2013]

cardio-surveillance is not yet standard routine care (Fig. 7.2) [11]. This may result in (too) late referral for cardiac treatment, as illustrated in the patient case. In 2016 the ESC has released a first position paper on cancer treatments and cardiovascular toxicity [12].

Woman 56 years with heart failure, caused by repeated chemotherapy and trastuzumab.

Medical History

- 13 years ago: BC Left-sided (infiltrating ductal CA, 4 cm, ER+,0/14 L-nodes pos)
  Radiotherapy, 5 x FEC chemotherapy and Tamoxifen (5 yrs)
- 9 years later: T4 BC Right-sided, ER-, PR-, Her2Neu +++. Invasive ductal CA.
  Neo-adjuvant 2 x FEC chemo+Carboplatin/Paclitaxel and Trastuzumab
- After 1 year: chemo stopped, because of extravasation right arm. Ablation right breast performed.
  Trastuzumab continued
- 2 years later: metastases cervical right sided. Continuation of Paclitaxel + Trastuzumab.
  PET-CT-scan: complete remission
  6 months later: 50 Gy radiotherapy neck right sided.
  Trastuzumab stopped, because LVEF < 42% (no HF treatment started)

  6 months later: hospitalization with HF and pneumonia . ACE inhibitor, and B blocker started.
  New ECHO: LVEF 22%, dilated LV, secondary MI (gr 2+/6), TI, atrial dilatation.

  Cardiologist: advises to implant ICD. Patient refuses and consults other cardiologist: no ICD, update of HF medication before her holiday leave. During her last year of life her EF remained stable at 22%, with acceptable functional class II NYHA . She died of metastatic BC.

- Comments:: HF medication should have been started at the first signs of LV decline, to improve her quality of life. .
  There is no evidence for ICD use in patients with HFrEF caused by cardiotoxicity.

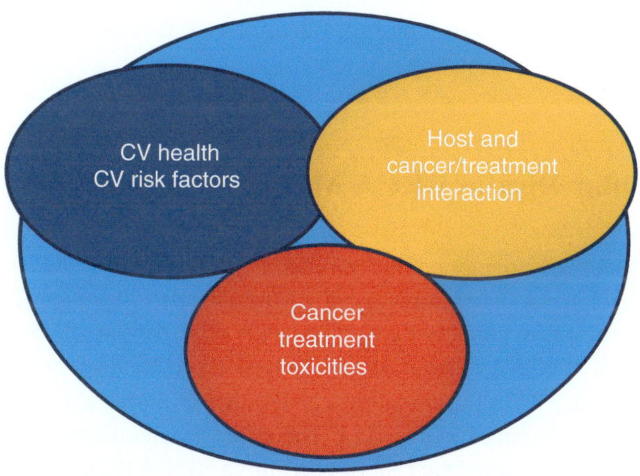

Fig. 7.2 Patient surveillance in treatment for breast cancer

Table 7.1 Baseline risk factors for cardiotoxicity in breast cancer treatment

Demographic and other CVD risk factors	• Age >50 years for trastuzumab
	• Age >65 years for anthracyclines
Lifestyle risk factors	• Smoking
	• High alcohol intake
	• Obesity
	• Sedentary lifestyle
Current heart disease	• Heart failure (HFpEF or HFrEF)
	• Asymptomatic LV dysfunction (LVEF <50% or high NT-proBNP)
	• Evidence of ischemic heart disease (previous ACS, CABG, PCI, angina)
	• Moderate/severe valvular heart disease with LVH or LV impairment
	• Hypertensive heart disease with LVH
	• Cardiomyopathy (dilated, hypertrophic or restrictive)
	• Cardiac sarcoidosis with myocardial involvement
	• Cardiac arrhythmias (e.g. AF, ventricular tachycardias)
Previous cardiotoxic cancer treatment	• Prior anthracycline use
	• Prior radiotherapy chest or mediastinum

Adapted from: Zamorano JL et al. Eur Heart J 2016 [12]
ACS acute coronary syndrome, *AF* atrial fibrillation, *CABG* coronary artery bypass graft, *CVD* cardiovascular disease, *HFpEF* heart failure with preserved ejection fraction, *HFrEF* heart failure with reduced ejection fraction, *LVH* left ventricular hypertrophy, *NT-proBNP* N-terminal Pro-B-type natriuretic peptide, *PCI* percutaneous coronary intervention

In this paper it is recommended that pre-existing CVD risk factors should be assessed and aggressively managed, starting at the time of treatment (or even before) and continuing throughout survivorship. Baseline risk factors for cardiotoxicity are depicted in Table 7.1.

Cardiovascular Risk in BRCA Mutation Carriers

Over the past decades an increasing number of women have been identified with hereditary BC, related to mutations in one of the two BRCA genes. The cumulative risk in BRCA1 mutation carriers by age 70 is 57–65% for breast and 39% for ovarian cancer and in BRCA2 carriers 45–49% and 10–18% respectively [13]. It has been suggested that BRCA1/2 mutation carriers are at increased risk of CVD compared to the general population [14, 15]. The exact mechanisms have not been elucidated yet, however the intrinsic risk of carrying a BRCA1/2 mutation, exposure to preventive risk reducing salpingo-oophorectomy (RRSO) before 40–45 years of age, chemotherapy and radiation therapy may add to a higher CVD risk [16]. In BRCA1/2-knockout mice, a higher susceptibility towards doxorubicin-induced cardiotoxicity has been reported [17]. However, a prospective study in 39 BRCA1/2 mutation carriers compared to 42 sporadic BC patients did not show an increased risk of anthracycline-induced cardiotoxicity in BRCA1/2 mutation carriers [18].

Risk of Radiation Therapy for Breast Cancer

Radiation therapy has been reported to increase the longterm risk of death due to CVD, even after 20 years of follow-up [19]. This risk is especially present for left-sided BC patients as with older radiation techniques part of the heart might be included in the irradiated volumes. In an older Swedish cohort of BC patients it was found that women treated with radiation therapy for left-sided BC had more ischemic heart disease (IHD) than women treated for right-sided BC, especially in the mid-left anterior descending artery and diagonal branches [20]. In a population based case-control study absolute radiation risks for ischemic heart disease (IHD) were greater in women with preexisting CVD risk factors than in those without [21]. The increased risk for coronary events started within the first 5 years after radiotherapy and continued for three decades thereafter. It is unknown yet to which extent radiation therapy induces coronary microvascular dysfunction (CMD). Current smoking increases the sensitivity of myocardial cells to the ionizing effects of radiation therapy, enhancing the risk for fibrosis and IHD [7]. The use of breath-hold techniques for left-sided BC patients is currently more often applied to reduce the individual heart dose of radiation [22, 23]. This technique may also be protective in right-sided BC patients who need loco-regional treatment (including the internal mammary lymph nodes) [24].

Cardiotoxicity of Chemotherapy for Breast Cancer

The cardiotoxic effects of anti-neoplastic agents can be divided into irreversible cardiomyocyte loss (type I) and reversible (type II) myocardial damage [25]. Type I is caused by anthracyclines, such as doxorubicin and epirubicin, and leads to cardiomyocyte apoptosis and necrosis. The harmful effects are cumulative and dose-dependent, with an interindividual range in toxic threshold depending on age (>65 years), renal failure, specific genetic polymorphisms, presence of hypertension, previous radiotherapy and combined use of type II agents [12, 26]. Subclinical LV deterioration occurs in 10–50% of treated patients, with a mean decline of 10% in LV function when compared to pre-treatment values, especially in the first year after treatment [27, 28]. This early asymptomatic loss of LV function can progress over time (years) to symptomatic heart failure (HF), which is most frequently seen in elderly women above 65 years of age. Of note is that subclinical HF may remain undiagnosed (for years), whereas symptoms of tiredness and dyspnea at effort are attributed to previous BC and ageing.

Immuno- and Targeted Therapies

Trastuzumab is a monoclonal antibody indicated in >20% of BC patients who are positive for the human epidermal growth factor receptor 2 (HER2) and in women with metastatic BC. The use of trastuzumab has increased over the past 15 years and is associated with an absolute 14% higher incidence rate for HF with reduced ejection fraction (HFrEF) or cardiomyopathy over 3 years of follow-up [29]. Although still debated, its cardiotoxic effects on LV function are assumed to be reversible (type II) and not related to cumulative dose but to the number of treatment sessions (see patient case) [30, 31]. Determinants of cardiotoxicity with trastuzumab are concomitant or prior treatment with anthracyclines, higher age, and the presence of hypertension. Trastuzumab cardiotoxicity usually manifests early during treatment [31]. In BC-trials, the incidence of symptomatic HF in trastuzumab-treated patients was 2–4% and the incidence of cardiac dysfunction was 3–19% [32–34]. In most BC registries treatment with trastuzumab is (temporarily) interrupted when ejection fraction (EF) falls below 45% [34]. Although not proven yet, early administration of HF drugs, such as ACE and ARBs, is likely to limit LV deterioration [28]. Currently, novel anti-HER2 targeted therapies are on the market (pertuzumab, lapatinib), which are potentially safer for the myocardium but less well investigated [35].

Cardiovascular Risk with Anti-angiogenic and Endocrine Therapies

The use of vascular endothelial growth factors (VEGF) inhibitors, such as bevacizumab for metastatic BC has increased over the past years. Nearly all patients who are treated with VEGF signaling inhibitors have an increase in blood pressure, often within 1 week of treatment [36]. The overall incidence of hypertension is reported to be 20–25% [37]. In a low percentage of patients (1–2%) signs if LV dysfunction and HF are described [38]. Given the high prevalence of hypertension in the ageing female population, adequate monitoring and management of blood pressure is needed when anti-VEGF agents are administered.

Endocrine therapy with the selective estrogen receptor modulator (SERM) tamoxifen (TAM) has been used for over decades and has a very low CVD risk [39, 40]. It is approved as adjuvant therapy and palliative therapy for hormone receptor positive primary and metastatic BC. In patients at increased thrombotic and CVD risk, tamoxifen may increase the occurrence of VTE and stroke [41]. In a meta-analysis it was recently found that aromatase inhibitors (AI) (exemestane, anastrozole, letrozole) are superior to TAM as adjuvant hormonal therapy for postmenopausal ER-positive BC [42]. However, AI's are associated with increased risk of developing CVD especially with longer treatment durations [43, 44]. Conflicting data have been reported on adverse effects of AI's on lipid profiles, which may add to a higher CVD risk [45].

Optimal Cardiac Surveillance and Treatment During/After BC Therapy

The first step to identify patients at increased risk for cardiotoxicity during BC therapy is to assess their baseline CVD risk (see Table 7.1) [12]. It remains to be determined however, which determinants are most important to predict future cardiotoxicity.

Whereas BC treatment has evolved into highly patient-tailored treatment strategies, the concurrent use of cardiac evaluation tools that can accurately assess both cardiac function and structure is presently lacking in the cardiac monitoring of BC patients with the use of routine echocardiography or radionuclide angiography. It may be more appropriate to use new ultrasound techniques with 3D possibilities, strain imaging and cardiac magnetic resonance (MRI), which are safe for the patients and reveal more earlier signs of LV damage [46–48]. Cardiac MRI is complementary to echocardiography and allows for unique and non-invasive insights into myocardial structure such as the tissue relaxation properties and the presence of diffuse fibrosis [49]. In Table 7.2 the currently available diagnostic tools are described.

Thus far it is still debated whether preventive use of ACE inhibitors, ARBs and b-blockers is indicated before anthracycline treatment has started, when baseline EF is normal [12]. Cardiotoxic effects of trastuzumab can be reduced by a drug-free interval after initial chemotherapy [32, 50]. It is advised to temporarily interrupt

Table 7.2 Diagnostic tools for the detection of cardiotoxicity

Technique	Diagnostic criteria	Advantages	Major limitations
Echocardiography: 3D-based LVEF 2D Simpson's LVEF GLS	LVEF > 10 percentage points decrease from baseline suggestive for cardiotoxicity. GLS >15% relative percentage reduction from baseline suggestive of cardiotoxicity.	Wide available No radiation Assessment other structural abnormalities	Inter-observer variability Image quality GLS technical requirements
Nuclear cardiac imaging (MUGA)	LVEF > 10 percentage points decrease from baseline suggestive for cardiotoxicity. LVEF < 50% suggestive of cardiotoxicity.	Reproducibility	Cumulative radiation exposure Limited structural and functional cardiac information
Cardiac magnetic resonance (MRI)	Alternative when other imaging modalities are non-diagnostic. Promising in detection early signs of cardiotoxicity.	Reproducibility Early detection diffuse fibrosis with T1/T2 mapping	Limited availability Time consuming
Cardiac biomarkers Troponin 1 hs-Troponin 1 BNP NT-proBNP	Indicators for potential benefit HF therapy	Reproducibility Availability High-sensitivity	Significance of subtle rise unknown Variations with different assays Routine use needs to be determined

Adapted from Zamorano JL et al. [12]
ACE angiotensin converting enzyme inhibitors, *BNP* B-type natriuretic peptide, *GLS* global longitudinal strain, *LV* left ventricular, *LVEF* left ventricular ejection fraction, *MUGA* multigated radionuclide angiography, *NT-proBNP* N-terminal fragment B-type natriuretic peptide

trastuzumab therapy when EF falls below 45% or when there is a drop of >10% in LVEF from baseline. Several studies have confirmed the beneficial effects of HF medication such as ACE inhibitors, ARBs and (additional) b-blockers when subclinical or overt HF occurs during BC treatment and more preventive studies are on the way [28, 51, 52]. Arrhythmias, especially atrial fibrillation (AF) can occur at all stages of BC treatment and need to be treated with antiarrhythmic drugs/b-blockers and antithrombotic medication, with considerations on quality of life, life expectancy and potential (bleeding) risks. There is no evidence as yet that the use of a defibrillator (ICD) prolongs life when sever HF due to cardiotoxicity occurs (see patient case).

Key Issues Cardio-surveillance During/After BC Treatment

- Assess individual baseline CVD risk before BC treatment
- Initiate HF medication when LVEF decreases >10% (ACE or ARB, and B-blocker) or LVEF <45%.
- Consider temporarily interruption of trastuzumab if EF <45% or >10% decrease in baseline LVEF
- Continue HF medication when EF reduction persists after treatment
- Monitor/treat blood pressure with use VEGF -inhibitors
- Long-term follow-up LV function advised after signs of cadiotoxicity during treatment
- Maintain a healthy lifestyle, as far as possible, during and after BC treatment

References

1. Barac A, et al. Cardiovascular health of patients with cancer and cancer survivors: a roadmap to the next level. J Am Coll Cardiol. 2015;65(25):2739–46.
2. Moslehi JJ. Cardiovascular toxic effects of targeted cancer therapies. N Engl J Med. 2016;375(15):1457–67.
3. Bardia A, et al. Comparison of breast cancer recurrence risk and cardiovascular disease incidence risk among postmenopausal women with breast cancer. Breast Cancer Res Treat. 2012;131(3):907–14.
4. Calle EE, et al. Overweight, obesity, and mortality from cancer in a prospectively studied cohort of U.S. adults. N Engl J Med. 2003;348(17):1625–38.
5. Larsson SC, Mantzoros CS, Wolk A. Diabetes mellitus and risk of breast cancer: a meta-analysis. Int J Cancer. 2007;121(4):856–62.
6. Xue F, Michels KB. Diabetes, metabolic syndrome, and breast cancer: a review of the current evidence. Am J Clin Nutr. 2007;86(3):s823–35.
7. Hooning MJ, et al. Long-term risk of cardiovascular disease in 10-year survivors of breast cancer. J Natl Cancer Inst. 2007;99(5):365–75.
8. Jones LW, et al. Early breast cancer therapy and cardiovascular injury. J Am Coll Cardiol. 2007;50(15):1435–41.
9. Lal H, Kolaja KL, Force T. Cancer genetics and the cardiotoxicity of the therapeutics. J Am Coll Cardiol. 2013;61(3):267–74.

10. Pavo N, et al. Cardiovascular biomarkers in patients with cancer and their association with all-cause mortality. Heart. 2015;101(23):1874–80.
11. Maas AH, et al. Cardiovascular surveillance in breast cancer treatment: a more individualized approach is needed. Maturitas. 2016;89:58–62.
12. Zamorano JL, et al. 2016 ESC Position Paper on cancer treatments and cardiovascular toxicity developed under the auspices of the ESC Committee for practice guidelines: the Task Force for cancer treatments and cardiovascular toxicity of the European Society of Cardiology (ESC). Eur Heart J. 2016;37(36):2768–801.
13. Antoniou A, et al. Average risks of breast and ovarian cancer associated with BRCA1 or BRCA2 mutations detected in case series unselected for family history: a combined analysis of 22 studies. Am J Hum Genet. 2003;72(5):1117–30.
14. Arts-de Jong M, et al. BRCA1/2 mutation carriers are potentially at higher cardiovascular risk. Crit Rev Oncol Hematol. 2014;91(2):159–71.
15. Mai PL, et al. Potential excess mortality in BRCA1/2 mutation carriers beyond breast, ovarian, prostate, and pancreatic cancers, and melanoma. PLoS One. 2009;4(3):e4812.
16. van Westerop LL, et al. Cardiovascular risk of BRCA1/2 mutation carriers: a review. Maturitas. 2016;91:135–9.
17. Singh KK, et al. BRCA2 protein deficiency exaggerates doxorubicin-induced cardiomyocyte apoptosis and cardiac failure. J Biol Chem. 2012;287(9):6604–14.
18. Barac A, et al. Cardiac function in BRCA1/2 mutation carriers with history of breast cancer treated with anthracyclines. Breast Cancer Res Treat. 2016;155(2):285–93.
19. Bouillon K, et al. Long-term cardiovascular mortality after radiotherapy for breast cancer. J Am Coll Cardiol. 2011;57(4):445–52.
20. Nilsson G, et al. Distribution of coronary artery stenosis after radiation for breast cancer. J Clin Oncol. 2012;30(4):380–6.
21. Darby SC, et al. Risk of ischemic heart disease in women after radiotherapy for breast cancer. N Engl J Med. 2013;368(11):987–98.
22. Swanson T, et al. Six-year experience routinely using moderate deep inspiration breath-hold for the reduction of cardiac dose in left-sided breast irradiation for patients with early-stage or locally advanced breast cancer. Am J Clin Oncol. 2013;36(1):24–30.
23. Mast ME, et al. Left-sided breast cancer radiotherapy with and without breath-hold: does IMRT reduce the cardiac dose even further? Radiother Oncol. 2013;108(2):248–53.
24. Essers M, et al. Should breathing adapted radiotherapy also be applied for right-sided breast irradiation? Acta Oncol. 2016;55(4):460–5.
25. Suter TM, Ewer MS. Cancer drugs and the heart: importance and management. Eur Heart J. 2013;34(15):1102–11.
26. Lenneman CG, Sawyer DB. Cardio-oncology: an update on cardiotoxicity of cancer-related treatment. Circ Res. 2016;118(6):1008–20.
27. Takemura G, Fujiwara H. Doxorubicin-induced cardiomyopathy from the cardiotoxic mechanisms to management. Prog Cardiovasc Dis. 2007;49(5):330–52.
28. Cardinale D, et al. Early detection of anthracycline cardiotoxicity and improvement with heart failure therapy. Circulation. 2015;131(22):1981–8.
29. Chen J, et al. Incidence of heart failure or cardiomyopathy after adjuvant trastuzumab therapy for breast cancer. J Am Coll Cardiol. 2012;60(24):2504–12.
30. Procter M, et al. Longer-term assessment of trastuzumab-related cardiac adverse events in the Herceptin Adjuvant (HERA) trial. J Clin Oncol. 2010;28(21):3422–8.
31. Farolfi A, et al. Trastuzumab-induced cardiotoxicity in early breast cancer patients: a retrospective study of possible risk and protective factors. Heart. 2013;99(9):634–9.
32. Slamon D, et al. Adjuvant trastuzumab in HER2-positive breast cancer. N Engl J Med. 2011;365(14):1273–83.
33. Romond EH, et al. Trastuzumab plus adjuvant chemotherapy for operable HER2-positive breast cancer. N Engl J Med. 2005;353(16):1673–84.
34. Suter TM, et al. Trastuzumab-associated cardiac adverse effects in the Herceptin Adjuvant trial. J Clin Oncol. 2007;25(25):3859–65.

35. Swain SM, et al. Pertuzumab, trastuzumab, and docetaxel in HER2-positive metastatic breast cancer. N Engl J Med. 2015;372(8):724–34.
36. Chen HX, Cleck JN. Adverse effects of anticancer agents that target the VEGF pathway. Nat Rev Clin Oncol. 2009;6(8):465–77.
37. Li W, et al. Vascular and metabolic implications of novel targeted cancer therapies: focus on kinase inhibitors. J Am Coll Cardiol. 2015;66(10):1160–78.
38. Cameron D, et al. Adjuvant bevacizumab-containing therapy in triple-negative breast cancer (BEATRICE): primary results of a randomised, phase 3 trial. Lancet Oncol. 2013;14(10):933–42.
39. Bonanni B, et al. Effect of tamoxifen at low doses on ultrasensitive C-reactive protein in healthy women. J Thromb Haemost. 2003;1(10):2149–52.
40. Pinkerton JV, Thomas S. Use of SERMs for treatment in postmenopausal women. J Steroid Biochem Mol Biol. 2014;142:142–54.
41. Davies C, et al. Long-term effects of continuing adjuvant tamoxifen to 10 years versus stopping at 5 years after diagnosis of oestrogen receptor-positive breast cancer: ATLAS, a randomised trial. Lancet. 2013;381(9869):805–16.
42. Ryden L, et al. Aromatase inhibitors alone or sequentially combined with tamoxifen in postmenopausal early breast cancer compared with tamoxifen or placebo – meta-analyses on efficacy and adverse events based on randomized clinical trials. Breast. 2016;26:106–14.
43. Amir E, et al. Toxicity of adjuvant endocrine therapy in postmenopausal breast cancer patients: a systematic review and meta-analysis. J Natl Cancer Inst. 2011;103(17):1299–309.
44. Chlebowski RT, et al. Benefit/risk for adjuvant breast cancer therapy with tamoxifen or aromatase inhibitor use by age, and race/ethnicity. Breast Cancer Res Treat. 2015;154(3):609–16.
45. Lintermans A, Neven P. Safety of aromatase inhibitor therapy in breast cancer. Expert Opin Drug Saf. 2015;14(8):1201–11.
46. Kerkhove D, et al. How to monitor cardiac toxicity of chemotherapy: time is muscle! Heart. 2014;100(15):1208–17.
47. Thavendiranathan P, et al. Reproducibility of echocardiographic techniques for sequential assessment of left ventricular ejection fraction and volumes: application to patients undergoing cancer chemotherapy. J Am Coll Cardiol. 2013;61(1):77–84.
48. Walker J, et al. Role of three-dimensional echocardiography in breast cancer: comparison with two-dimensional echocardiography, multiple-gated acquisition scans, and cardiac magnetic resonance imaging. J Clin Oncol. 2010;28(21):3429–36.
49. Plana JC, et al. Expert consensus for multimodality imaging evaluation of adult patients during and after cancer therapy: a report from the American Society of Echocardiography and the European Association of Cardiovascular Imaging. Eur Heart J Cardiovasc Imaging. 2014;15(10):1063–93.
50. Curigliano G, et al. Cardiovascular toxicity induced by chemotherapy, targeted agents and radiotherapy: ESMO clinical practice guidelines. Ann Oncol. 2012;23(Suppl 7):vii155–66.
51. Gulati G, et al. Prevention of cardiac dysfunction during adjuvant breast cancer therapy (PRADA): a 2 × 2 factorial, randomized, placebo-controlled, double-blind clinical trial of candesartan and metoprolol. Eur Heart J. 2016;37(21):1671–80.
52. Seicean S, et al. Cardioprotective effect of beta-adrenoceptor blockade in patients with breast cancer undergoing chemotherapy: follow-up study of heart failure. Circ Heart Fail. 2013;6(3):420–6.

Chapter 8
Cardiomyopathies in Women

Vera Regitz-Zagrosek, Denise Hilfiker-Kleiner, and Tobias Pfeffer

Abstract Peripartum cardiomyopathy (PPCM) is a potentially threatening disease in low and middle income countries, where healthcare systems and supervision during pregnancy are not well controlled and doctors are unaware of the disease. Symptoms and signs are typical for systolic HF and may develop rapidly, leading to severe acute systolic failure, ventricular arrhythmias or sudden cardiac death. Inhibiting prolactin secretion with Bromocriptine may offer a novel specific therapeutic option. Dilated cardiomyopathy (DCM) and hypertrophic cardiomyopathy (HCM), and probably also non-compaction and arrhythmogenic right ventricular CM have a greater prevalence in men than in women. This chapter contains expert information on sex differences in myocardial adaptation of the human heart.

Keywords Arrhythmias • Bromocriptine • Cardiac resynchronization therapy (CRT) • Dilated cardiomyopathy (DCM) • Gender myocardial adaptation • Genetics • Heart failure • Heart transplantation • Hypertrophic cardiomyopathy (HCM) • Idiopathic dilated cardiomyopathy (IDC) • LV-assisted device (LVAD) • Peripartum cardiomyopathy (PPCM) • Pregnancy • Prolactin • Systolic heart failure

Peripartum Cardiomyopathy

Introduction

Peripartum cardiomyopathy (PPCM) occurs in all parts of the world [1]. The incidence varies strongly in different parts of the world, emphasizing the involvement of genetic and/or cultural factors. Known predisposing factors are age >30 years,

V. Regitz-Zagrosek, M.D., Ph.D. (✉)
Institute of Gender in Medicine, Center for Cardiovascular Research, Charité, Universitätsmedizin Berlin, Berlin, Germany
e-mail: vera.regitz-zagrosek@charite.de

D. Hilfiker-Kleiner, Ph.D. • T. Pfeffer, M.D.
Center for Cardiology, Angiology and Molecular Cardiology, Medizinische Hochschule Hannover, Hannover, Germany
e-mail: hilfiker.denise@mh-hannover.de

A.H.E.M. Maas, C.N. Bairey Merz (eds.), *Manual of Gynecardiology*,
DOI 10.1007/978-3-319-54960-6_8

multiparity and multiple childbirths, family history, ethnicity, genetic variants, pregnancy induced hypertension and prolonged use of beta-agonists. The aetiology of PPCM is uncertain and probably inhomogenous. Inflammation and autoimmune processes may play a role.

Epidemiological studies reveal that the incidence in Africa (1 in 100 to 1 in 1000 pregnancies) and Haiti (1 in 299 pregnancies) is very high. Other countries like Europe, United States report rising rates of PPCM (in the USA from 1 in 4350 in 1993 to 1 in 2.229 in 2002). The genetic background as well as lifestyle may contribute to PPCM. Furthermore, familial clustering of PPCM has been observed especially in families with both familial and sporadic idiopathic dilated cardiomyopathy (IDC) and that the presence of truncating gene variants in TTN is the most prevalent genetic predisposition for each of these disorders [2]. The combination of specific genetic conditions with the pathophysiological burden induced by late pregnancy may be a trigger for the disease.

In late pregnancy neo-angiogenesis is limited due to inhibition of Vascular Endothelial Growth Factor (VEGF) signaling by circulating soluble fms-like tyrosine kinase (sFLT) [3]. Furthermore, hemodynamic stress of late pregnancy may enhance stress to the heart and may lead to the increased production of free radicals that may now activate proteases such as Cathepsin D. This can cleave the nursing hormone prolactin into an antiangiogenic and into a pro-apoptotic fragment, which is probably a major cause of the disease in a number of patients [4]. Prolactin is synthesized at high levels around delivery and can be suppressed by established drugs like bromocriptine. Administration of bromocriptine in experimental models was able to prevent PPCM and first clinical studies are promising suggesting that the therapy is also effective in patients and suggesting that this pathophysiological mechanism indeed plays a major role and offers a clue to its treatment.

Clinical Problem

The clinical problem of PPCM is high. Families, patients and doctors are confronted with an acutely occurring life threatening disease. It occurs in a setting where a major cardiovascular illness is often not suspected. This is particularly threatening in low and middle income countries, where healthcare systems and supervision during pregnancy are not well controlled and doctors are unaware of the disease. Since the syndrome may develop very acutely and acute heart failure (HF) may develop very fast, extremely rapid action may be required. Patients with rapidly developing acute HF should be transferred to specialized care centers to make sure that all necessary therapeutic modalities are available. Caution is also needed when PPCM develops with atypical clinical symptoms, with syncope, thromboembolism or severe renal or liver failure and the connection to the cardiovascular disease is not evident. PPCM develops more frequently in multipara. Particularly in developing countries the severe acute illness of the mother leaves families alone and puts also the younger siblings into danger.

Diagnostic Pathway

Unfortunately, there are no specific tests to confirm PPCM. It therefore remains a diagnosis of exclusion, which is suggested by a number of signs and symptoms. Most typical is the time of manifestation, in last month before and up to 6 months after delivery. Symptoms and signs are typical for systolic HF and may develop rapidly, leading to severe acute systolic failure, ventricular arrhythmias or sudden cardiac death [1, 4, 5]. Many of these symptoms are considered more or less normal during pregnancy and there is only a gradual difference between complaints that are judged to be normal during pregnancy and those of PPCM. Therefore doctors have to be suspicious if dyspnea and edema in pregnancy are more pronounced than they should be. It is most important, to differentiate aggravation of pre-existing heart disease by pregnancy-mediated hemodynamic changes from PPCM. Unusual manifestations, as mentioned above, may also be the dominant sign. Therefore doctors must assure that not hidden signs of HF are underestimated during pregnancy or postpartum. Complex ventricular arrhythmias and sudden cardiac arrest as first manifestations are also described, but are, as other ECG changes, non-specific findings.

Echocardiography is the diagnostic method of choice. Systolic dysfunction is always present, ventricular dilatation is usually present but may also be absent [6]. Using sex-based normal values is important for correct estimation of ventricular size. Diastolic function will be impaired but is not a hallmark of the disease. Right ventricular function is important for prognosis [7]. Atrial and ventricular thrombi must be identified, for which magnetic resonance imaging (MRI) is a most sensitive method.

The biomarkers natriuretic peptides (BNP or NT-proBNP) are usually elevated according to the severity of HF sFlt-1, which is now developed into a diagnostic tool for preeclampsia, may be elevated but is not a reliable biomarker for PPCM [3]. Cathepsin D, 16-kDa prolactin, mircroRNA-146a, Interferon-γ, asymmetric dimethylarginine should be altered based on pathophysiological considerations and are being tested for their use in PPCM, but not yet ready for use in clinical practice [8].

Treatment Options and Advise

Treatment in PPCM is the same as for dilating cardiomyopathy (DCM), but ACE-inhibitors and Angiotensin-1 receptor blockers (ARB) are contraindicated because of possible renal and other fetotoxicity [4]. Diuretics can be used but physicians should be aware that they reduce placental perfusion and may have negative impact on fetal development [4]. Beta blockers may be used, of which most experience exists with metoprolol. Care should be taken to expect rapid progression of HF and to consult specialized centers early. The guidelines for the management of acute HF should be followed and devices, pacemakers or mechanical circulatory support may be used. If HF persists or progresses despite optimal medical therapy, the use of mechanical circulatory support (MCS), cardiac resynchronization therapy (CRT) or LV-assisted device (LVAD) can be considered [5, 9]. These measures should be discussed with specialists. If MCS is not possible or not desirable for individual reasons or for patients who do not recover after 6–12 months on MCS, cardiac transplantation may be a possibility. Patients with PPCM have a similar prognosis after transplantation as patients with DCM [5]. However, the prognosis of PPCM is different from DCM. More than 50% of patients will have a significant improvement in LV function over the first 6 months after diagnosis [4]. This high rate of spontaneous recovery must be considered when decisions are made [10].

Based on specific pathophysiology and specific disease mechanisms some treatment options beyond the standard therapy of HF are arising. Vascular mediators (relaxin-2, sFlt1) may contribute to the development of PPCM and impair subsequent myocardial recovery [11, 12]. Furthermore, cleavage of the lactating hormone prolactin into anti-angiogenic and pro-apoptotic fragments may contribute to PPCM [13]. Inhibiting prolactin secretion with Bromocriptine may offer a novel specific therapeutic option [1, 4, 5, 14]. A recent small prospective randomized pilot study supports the hypothesis that the addition of bromocriptine to standard HF therapy has beneficial effects on ventricular ejection fraction and clinical outcome in women with acute severe PPCM [15]. Larger trials are underway [16]. See the patient case.

Patient. Peripartum Cardiomyopathy

One week after a complication free delivery of her third child, a 35 year old woman presented with dyspnoea in the emergency ward. Her heart rate was 103/bpm and blood pressure was 123/74 mmHg. Clinical laboratory showed high blood levels of NT-proBNP (1387 ng/l) and moderately increased s-cTroponin T (31 ng/l) while S-CK and S-CKM were in normal range. Haemoglobin was low (106 g/l). ECG revealed sinus rhythm and a LBBB. Echocardiography showed severely decreased left ventricular systolic dysfunction with an LVEF of 13% (MRI 13%, with dilated LV (LVEDD 6.7 cm) and moderate to severe mitral valve regurgitation. MRI displayed no signs of late enhancement. Anamnese revealed that dyspnoea had started already two weeks before delivery and became worse afterwards. Her general physician prescribed a cortisone inhaler to ease dyspnoea symptoms. The patient was diagnosed with PPCM at hospitalization. Treatment was started with standard medication of heart failure (HF) (beta-blocker, ARB, diuretics, mineralocorticoid receptor antagonist and ivabradine) and with the prolactin blocker bromocriptine (2.5-5.0 mg for 8 weeks) in combination with Vitamin K antaginists. Due to her severe HF she obtained a wearable cardioverter defibrillator (WCD) for primary prevention of sudden cardiac death. After 6 months the patient reported overall better clinical status with no dyspnoea. Echocardiography showed moderate recovery to an LVEF of 27% however, with further LV dilatation (LVEDD 7.6 cm). MRI displayed late enhancement inferior at the insertion of the RV. NT-poBNP was still moderately elevated (369 ng/l) while all other cardiac enzymes were normal. The WCD report showed sinus tachycardia's in the follow up and a CRTD system with ICD function was implanted. Bromocriptine was added again to the therapy. Follow-up monitoring showed slow but continuous recovery to an LVEF of 50% with normal ventricle dimensions after 2 years.

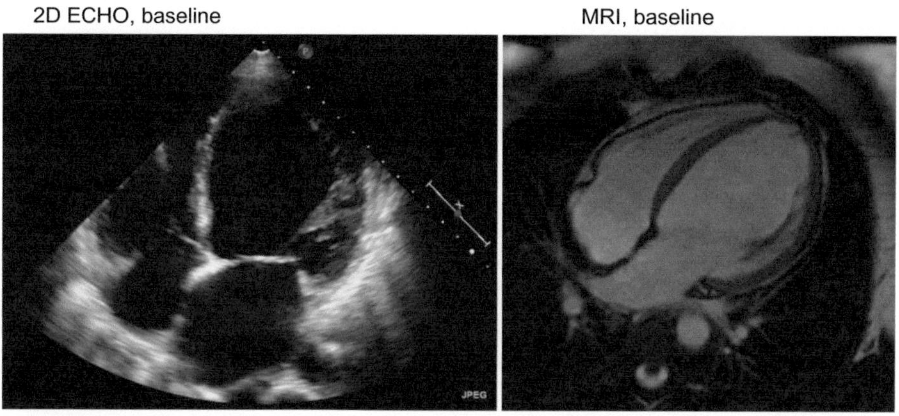

Echocardiography shows severe HF with systolic LV dysfunction and LV dilatation at diagnosis.

MRI revealed no late enhancement at diagnosis

As soon as the baby is delivered, and the patient is hemodynamically stable, standard therapy for HF can be applied. Due to high metabolic demand and fluid intake during nursing it may be considered to stop lactation and breast feeding in PPCM patients with severe illness, after weighing all arguments in favor of breast feeding. As outlined below, bromocriptine is recommended for ablactation because of potential beneficial side effects on PPCM [13, 17]. In patients with PPCM, a subsequent pregnancy carries a recurrence risk of 30–50% [10, 18]. When ejection fraction has not normalized a subsequent pregnancy should be discouraged. Even if ejection fraction is restored to normal, there is still a need for counseling for recurrence risk.

Table (s) with treatment guidelines

Therapy/disease manifestation	ACEI, ARB, ß-blockers	Diuretics	Digitalis, levosimendan, nitrates, hydralazine	Others
Manifestation before partum	Delete ACEI, ARB	Possible, use with caution	Possible	LMW heparins and coumarins may be considered for anticoagulation
After partum	Delete ACEI, ARB, if breast feeding is planned	Possible	Possible	As above
Severe Heart failure	See above	Possible	Possible	Consider transfer to specialized center, discuss mechanical support

Please refer to recent guidelines for details [4]

Dilated Cardiomyopathy

Introduction

Cardiomyopathies (CM) represent rare, but severe causes of HF. Most genetic CM are due to autosomal gene variations and are therefore expected to occur with the same prevalence in women and men. However, dilated cardiomyopathy (DCM) and hypertrophic cardiomyopathy (HCM), and probably also non-compaction and arrhythmogenic right ventricular CM have a greater prevalence in men than in women [19–21]. It has been hypothesized that women are better protected against ventricular dilatation and systolic dysfunction than men or, compensation for the genetic defect in these syndromes appears to be more efficient in women. Therefore, genetic defects lead more rarely to manifest disease in women than in men [22].

Clinical Problem and Pathophysiology

Dilated cardiomyopathies manifest as acute or chronic HF. Pathophysiology is based on functional and morphological alterations of the left and or right ventricle and the response of the periphery. Sex-specific adaptation of the heart will lead to more dilated eccentric ventricles in men and smaller, more hypertrophic ventricles in women [22] (Fig. 8.1). However, this has not yet been fully analyzed in the human

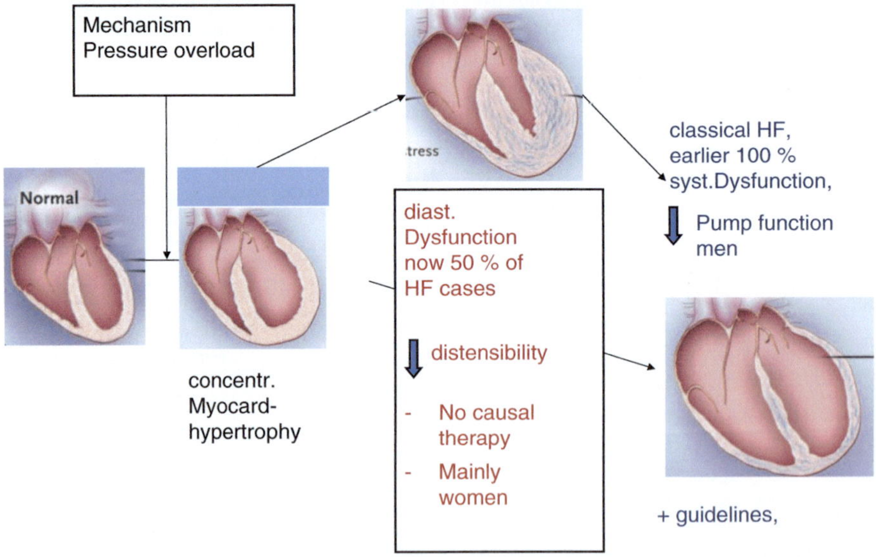

Fig. 8.1 Different mechanisms of myocardial adaptation in the male and in the female human heart. Adapted from European Heart Journal, Regitz-Zagrosek 2016 [26]

and no sex-specific normal values exist. Metabolic switches also differ among women and men. Men exhibit a stronger downregulation of fatty acid oxidation [23]. In animal models, significant sex differences are found for different types of CM induced by different genetic lesions. In most of the genetic CM models, male mice appear more sensitive to genetic interventions than females, and exhibit higher mortality, more severe hypertrophy and more functional impairment. Some of these models mimic human CM. In some models, the severe phenotype in the males could be prevented by estrogen administration [24]. A number of disease genes, most of them affecting cytoskeletal and sarcomere composition, for DCM have been identified, without difference between women and men [2]. A number of cases remains unexplained so far. Diagnosis of genetic components is particularly important, when younger women and men with a desire for children are affected. Specialists for genetic counseling should be involved in management of these patients.

Dilated cardiomyopathy may occur in pregnancy. The clinical manifestation and diagnostic criteria resemble the non-pregnant disease manifestation. They differ from PPCM by the time of manifestation. DCM is often unmasked during the first or second trimester when the hemodynamic load is increasing. Preexisting DCM may exhibit marked deterioration during pregnancy [4]. Patients with LVEF <40%, a predictor of high pregnancy risk, should be monitored in a tertiary care centre. Worsening of DCM during pregnancy may occur and in patients with very severe disease, abortion should be discussed.

Diagnostic Pathway

Diagnosis is based on the clinical signs and symptoms of heart failure—dyspnea, fatigue and exercise intolerance—and alterations of ventricular morphology and function after exclusion of a specific cause for HF. No sex-specific guidelines exist. First diagnosis is usually made by echocardiography, according to the guidelines. Volumes are enlarged, ventricular walls are thin, systolic function and in most cases also diastolic function is decreased. Ventricular, atrial and vascular diameters should be normalized to body surface area to correct for different body sizes in women and men. Coronary angiography and myocardial biopsy may be needed to exclude specific causes of HF, such as coronary, valvular or inflammatory disease. In the ECG, a number of different arrhythmias may be visible. Heart rate-corrected QTc intervals are usually longer in women than in men, putting them into greater danger for ventricular arrhythmias. Atrial fibrillation is a more frequent event in men, but has a greater negative impact on the prognosis in women [25].

The most important biomarker is NT-BNP. Its increase is associated with adverse prognosis. Some studies have claimed that sex-specific normal values should be considered, but this has not been convincingly worked out. High-sensitive Troponin is emerging as a novel biomarker and it appears that women have lower normal values than men [26]. Its sex-specific predictive value in DCM has not yet been clarified.

Treatment

Medical Therapy

Standard therapy for HF is used for treatment of DCM. Even though some sex differences are described for the effects and adverse effects of medical therapy this has not yet let to sex-specific recommendations in the guidelines. Mortality under digitalis treatment was higher in women than in men in a post-hoc analysis of the largest randomized prospective trial on digitalis in HF [27]. Women with HF also have a higher rate of adverse drug events than men especially with diuretics, anticoagulants, digoxin and ACEI [26]. Since DCM may occur in pregnancy, specific problems arise when pregnant women are concerned. In this case, ACEI and ARB must be withdrawn, Diuretics and antithrombotic drugs must be used with more caution, as described above for PPCM.

Cardiac Resynchronization Therapy (CRT)

Resynchronization therapy is an emerging new option for treatment of DCM and HF. So far, women are poorly represented in clinical trials for cardiac resynchronization therapy (CRT) [28–30]. Surprisingly, women experienced more benefit from CRT than men [30, 31] and even earlier indications for its use in women have been discussed. In a recent FDA meta-analysis, three major clinical trials with mild HF suggested an indication for CRT in women with a shorter QRS-duration than in men [32].

Ventricular Assist Device (VAD)

There are no sex differences in the recommendations. However, just based on body size, less women qualified for device therapy in recent years. A severe survival deficit in women after device implantation was identified by registry analysis of the international society of heart and lung transplantation (ISHLT). This is now being changed with miniaturization of the devices. If women and men were compared independent of the device type and clinical state at presentation is taken into account survival benefit for both genders seems to be similar [33]. Referral of women in more severe disease state in earlier studies may explain some of the survival disadvantages described.

Heart Transplantation

More men than women undergo the demanding procedure of heart transplantation. Women are more frequently donors whereas men are more frequently recipients. In a large cohort of patients with idiopathic DCM at the German Heart Institute less than 20% were women, suggesting a referral bias against women. Women referred

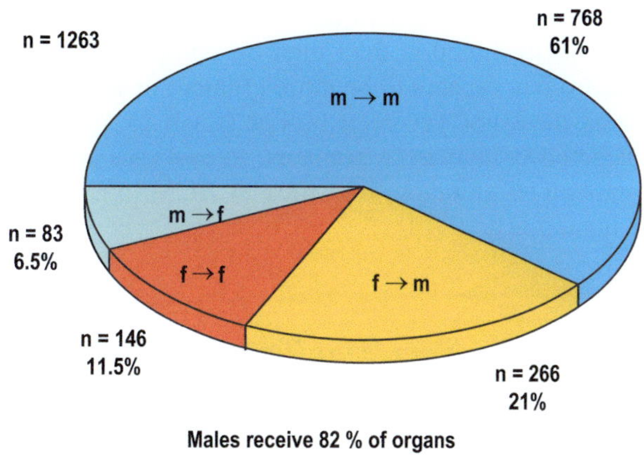

Fig. 8.2 Donor recipient relation in heart transplantation. Women are more frequently donors, men are more frequently recipients. Adapted from European Heart Journal, Regitz-Zagrosek 2016 [26]

for transplantation were more frequently in NYHA III-IV than men, had lower exercise tolerance, respiratory efficiency and kidney function. Women referred for transplantation also had a significantly lower incidence of diabetes than men, notwithstanding the same prevalence of diabetes in women and men with heart failure. We conclude that women are referred at a more advanced disease state and relative contraindications such as diabetes are taken more seriously in women [25]. An international multicenter prospective study on referral for heart transplantation, organ allocation and survival appears mandatory. See Fig. 8.2.

Outcomes

In general, women have better clinical outcomes than men, even though they have poorer quality of life [34]. In most cases of DCM, women appear to survive better than men. Thus it has been suggested that women have more efficient compensatory mechanisms to compensate stress. Less profibrotic changes in the heart and a better metabolic adaptation may play a role there [19, 20]. These observations may pave the way for new therapeutic developments [35, 36].

Hypertrophic Cardiomyopathy

Introduction

Hypertrophic cardiomyopathy (HCM), and probably also non-compaction and arrhythmogenic right ventricular CM have a greater prevalence in men than in women [19–21]. This is astonishing, since they are transmitted by autosomal variants that occur with the same frequency in women and men [26]. As in DCM, it has been hypothesized that women are better protected against fibrosis and ventricular dysfunction than men or, compensation for the genetic defect in these syndromes appears to be more efficient in women [22]. Sex specific survival patterns have not yet been broken down to specific HCM mutations, which are detected in increasing numbers. Phenotypes also depend on genotypes. In a case with a TNI mutation, transition of HCM to DCM has been described in a young woman [37].

Clinical Problem, Manifestation in Pregnancy

Severe problems in HCM arise from the fact that they most often manifest in young adults. In men, they often cause sudden death in active sportsmen and it is not clear why this is not the case in women. Clinical features of HCM are frequently more severe in men than in women, if with the same genetic variant. We described a family where the mother, apparently clinically unsuspicious and undiagnosed transmitted the assumed disease gene, a variant in the MYBPC3, to three sons that underwent heart transplantation or pacemaker implantation at young age (Fig. 8.3). Genetic diagnosis is the same for women and men. Diagnosis of genetic components is particularly important, when younger women with a desire for children are affected. An experienced counselor should be involved in these cases.

HCM is common and frequently diagnosed for the first time in pregnancy [4]. Women with HCM usually tolerate pregnancy well. Increased risk exists in those who are symptomatic before pregnancy, those with significant diastolic dysfunction and in those with a high outflow tract gradient or with arrhythmias. They need

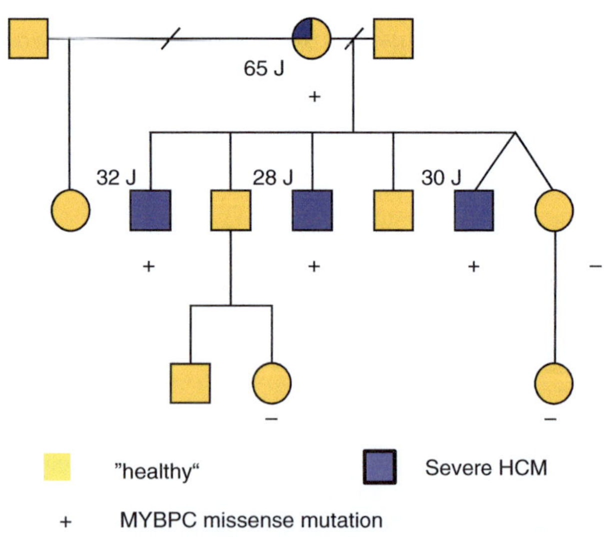

Fig. 8.3 Family tree in HCM family. The IVS711G.A mutation, introducing a frame shift leading to a premature stop codon in exon 9, led to a severe disease manifestation before age 30, severe hypertrophy (TASH or myectomy two times) and symptomatic arrhythmia (one ICD) in three brothers, but to a less severe phenotype in their mother [42]

specialized obstetrical care [38–40]. Syncope may occur during physical activity as a response to outflow tract obstruction. Echocardiography is the diagnostic tool of choice, as in non-pregnant women.

Diagnostic Pathway

Clinical signs, chest pain at exercise, syncope, palpitations are diagnostic hints. Most patients tolerate exercise very well, particularly in early stages. First diagnosis is usually made by echocardiography. MRI now gives a more comprehensive feature of ventricular morphology and/or thrombi. For indications for invasive therapy, exercise studies with measurement of pulmonary artery pressure or wedge pressure are helpful. No sex specific normal values exist. Careful screening for ventricular arrhythmia is mandatory.

Treatment in Pregnant and Non-pregnant Women

Treatment follows guidelines without specific recommendations for women and men. Beta blockers, and Ca-antagonists are the drugs of choice. Atrial fibrillation should be managed according to guidelines. Ablation therapy may be used in cases of severe septal hypertrophy. Search for ventricular arrhythmia is mandatory.

If HCM occurs in pregnancy, prognosis is favorable. β-Blockers should be considered in all pregnant HCM patients. Verapamil can be used as a second choice when β-blockers are not tolerated (be aware of causing AV block in the fetus). Cardioversion should be considered for persistent atrial fibrillation which is poorly tolerated. Patients with a past history or family history of sudden death need close surveillance [41]. Delivery should be planned and performed under β-blocker protection. Most patients can carry through a normal delivery. Epidural anesthesia is not recommended because of its vasodilator effects.

Acknowledgement I thank Arne Kühne for excellent management of the references and Martina Rudek and Sarah Lisa Müller for editorial support. The work was supported by grants from DZHK and from EU FP 7 (RADOX and EUGenMed).

References

1. Sliwa K, Hilfiker-Kleiner D, Mebazaa A, et al. EURObservational Research Programme: a worldwide registry on peripartum cardiomyopathy (PPCM) in conjunction with the Heart Failure Association of the European Society of Cardiology Working Group on PPCM. Eur J Heart Fail. 2014;16(5):583–91.

2. Ware JS, Li J, Mazaika E, et al. Shared genetic predisposition in peripartum and dilated cardiomyopathies. N Engl J Med. 2016;374(3):233–41.
3. Zeisler H, Llurba E, Chantraine F, et al. Predictive value of the sFlt-1:PlGF ratio in women with suspected preeclampsia. N Engl J Med. 2016;374(1):13–22.
4. Regitz-Zagrosek V, Blomstrom Lundqvist C, Borghi C, et al. ESC guidelines on the management of cardiovascular diseases during pregnancy: the Task Force on the Management of Cardiovascular Diseases during Pregnancy of the European Society of Cardiology (ESC). Eur Heart J. 2011;32(24):3147–97.
5. Bauersachs J, Arrigo M, Hilfiker-Kleiner D, et al. Current management of patients with severe acute peripartum cardiomyopathy: practical guidance from the Heart Failure Association of the European Society of Cardiology Study Group on peripartum cardiomyopathy. Eur J Heart Fail. 2016;18(9):1096–105.
6. Briasoulis A, Mocanu M, Marinescu K, et al. Longitudinal systolic strain profiles and outcomes in peripartum cardiomyopathy. Echocardiography. 2016;33(9):1354–60.
7. Blauwet LA, Delgado-Montero A, Ryo K, et al. Right ventricular function in peripartum cardiomyopathy at presentation is associated with subsequent left ventricular recovery and clinical outcomes. Circ Heart Fail. 2016;9(5):e002756.
8. Hilfiker-Kleiner D, Haghikia A, Nonhoff J, Bauersachs J. Peripartum cardiomyopathy: current management and future perspectives. Eur Heart J. 2015;36(18):1090–7.
9. Laliberte B, Reed BN, Ather A, et al. Safe and effective use of pharmacologic and device therapy for peripartum cardiomyopathy. Pharmacotherapy. 2016;36(9):955–70.
10. Habli M, O'Brien T, Nowack E, Khoury S, Barton JR, Sibai B. Peripartum cardiomyopathy: prognostic factors for long-term maternal outcome. Am J Obstet Gynecol. 2008;199(4):415 e1–5.
11. Damp J, Givertz MM, Semigran M, et al. Relaxin-2 and soluble Flt1 levels in peripartum cardiomyopathy: results of the multicenter IPAC study. JACC Heart fail. 2016;4(5):380–8.
12. Raleigh JM, Toldo S, Das A, Abbate A, Salloum FN. Relaxin' the heart: a novel therapeutic modality. J Cardiovasc Pharmacol Ther. 2016;21(4):353–62.
13. Hilfiker-Kleiner D, Kaminski K, Podewski E, et al. A cathepsin D-cleaved 16 kDa form of prolactin mediates postpartum cardiomyopathy. Cell. 2007;128(3):589–600.
14. Habedank D, Kuhnle Y, Elgeti T, Dudenhausen JW, Haverkamp W, Dietz R. Recovery from peripartum cardiomyopathy after treatment with bromocriptine. Eur J Heart Fail. 2008;10(11): 1149–51.
15. Sliwa K, Blauwet L, Tibazarwa K, et al. Evaluation of bromocriptine in the treatment of acute severe peripartum cardiomyopathy: a proof-of-concept pilot study. Circulation. 2010;121(13): 1465–73.
16. Haghikia A, Podewski E, Berliner D, et al. Rationale and design of a randomized, controlled multicentre clinical trial to evaluate the effect of bromocriptine on left ventricular function in women with peripartum cardiomyopathy. Clin Res Cardiol. 2015;104(11):911–7.
17. Sliwa K, Hilfiker-Kleiner D, Petrie MC, et al. Current state of knowledge on aetiology, diagnosis, management, and therapy of peripartum cardiomyopathy: a position statement from the Heart Failure Association of the European Society of Cardiology Working Group on peripartum cardiomyopathy. Eur J Heart Fail. 2010;12(8):767–78.
18. Sliwa K, Fett J, Elkayam U. Peripartum cardiomyopathy. Lancet. 2006;368(9536):687–93.
19. Bagger JP, Baandrup U, Rasmussen K, Moller M, Vesterlund T. Cardiomyopathy in western Denmark. Br Heart J. 1984;52(3):327–31.
20. Gillum RF. Idiopathic cardiomyopathy in the United States, 1970-1982. Am Heart J. 1986;111(4):752–5.
21. Codd MB, Sugrue DD, Gersh BJ, Melton 3rd LJ. Epidemiology of idiopathic dilated and hypertrophic cardiomyopathy. A population-based study in Olmsted County, Minnesota, 1975-1984. Circulation. 1989;80(3):564–72.
22. Regitz-Zagrosek V, Kararigas G. Mechanistic pathways of sex differences in cardiovascular disease. Physiol Rev. 2017;97(1):1–37.

23. Kadkhodayan A, Lin CH, Coggan AR, et al. Sex affects myocardial blood flow and fatty acid substrate metabolism in humans with nonischemic heart failure. J Nucl Cardiol. 2016. PMID: 27048307.
24. Regitz-Zagrosek V. Therapeutic implications of the gender-specific aspects of cardiovascular disease. Nat Rev Drug Discov. 2006;5(5):425–38.
25. Regitz-Zagrosek V, Petrov G, Lehmkuhl E, et al. Heart transplantation in women with dilated cardiomyopathy. Transplantation. 2010;89(2):236–44.
26. EUGenMed Cardiovascular Clinical Study Group, Regitz-Zagrosek V, Oertelt-Prigione S, et al. Gender in cardiovascular diseases: impact on clinical manifestations, management, and outcomes. Eur Heart J. 2016;37(1):24–34.
27. Rathore SS, Wang Y, Krumholz HM. Sex-based differences in the effect of digoxin for the treatment of heart failure. N Engl J Med. 2002;347(18):1403–11.
28. Yancy CW, Jessup M, Bozkurt B, et al. 2013 ACCF/AHA guideline for the management of heart failure: executive summary: a report of the American College of Cardiology Foundation/American Heart Association Task Force on practice guidelines. Circulation. 2013;128(16):1810–52.
29. Bristow MR, Saxon LA, Boehmer J, et al. Cardiac-resynchronization therapy with or without an implantable defibrillator in advanced chronic heart failure. N Engl J Med. 2004;350(21): 2140–50.
30. Moss AJ, Hall WJ, Cannom DS, et al. Cardiac-resynchronization therapy for the prevention of heart-failure events. N Engl J Med. 2009;361(14):1329–38.
31. Arshad A, Moss AJ, Foster E, et al. Cardiac resynchronization therapy is more effective in women than in men: the MADIT-CRT (Multicenter Automatic Defibrillator Implantation Trial with Cardiac Resynchronization Therapy) trial. J Am Coll Cardiol. 2011;57(7):813–20.
32. Zusterzeel R, Selzman KA, Sanders WE, et al. Cardiac resynchronization therapy in women: US Food and Drug Administration meta-analysis of patient-level data. JAMA Intern Med. 2014;174(8):1340–8.
33. Weymann A, Patil NP, Sabashnikov A, et al. Gender differences in continuous-flow left ventricular assist device therapy as a bridge to transplantation: a risk-adjusted comparison using a propensity score-matching analysis. Artif Organs. 2015;39(3):212–9.
34. Levy D, Kenchaiah S, Larson MG, et al. Long-term trends in the incidence of and survival with heart failure. N Engl J Med. 2002;347(18):1397–402.
35. Regitz-Zagrosek V, Dworatzek E, Kintscher U, Dragun D. Sex and sex hormone-dependent cardiovascular stress responses. Hypertension. 2013;61(2):270–7.
36. Petrov G, Regitz-Zagrosek V, Lehmkuhl E, et al. Regression of myocardial hypertrophy after aortic valve replacement: faster in women? Circulation. 2010;122(11 Suppl):S23–8.
37. Regitz-Zagrosek V, Erdmann J, Wellnhofer E, Raible J, Fleck E. Novel mutation in the alpha-tropomyosin gene and transition from hypertrophic to hypocontractile dilated cardiomyopathy. Circulation. 2000;102(17):E112–6.
38. Autore C, Conte MR, Piccininno M, et al. Risk associated with pregnancy in hypertrophic cardiomyopathy. J Am Coll Cardiol. 2002;40(10):1864–9.
39. Thaman R, Varnava A, Hamid MS, et al. Pregnancy related complications in women with hypertrophic cardiomyopathy. Heart. 2003;89(7):752–6.
40. Shin J, Kim M, Lee J, et al. Pregnancy in hypertrophic cardiomyopathy with severe left ventricular outflow tract obstruction. J Cardiovasc Ultrasound. 2016;24(2):158–62.
41. Ashikhmina E, Farber MK, Mizuguchi KA. Parturients with hypertrophic cardiomyopathy: case series and review of pregnancy outcomes and anesthetic management of labor and delivery. Int J Obstet Anesth. 2015;24(4):344–55.
42. Erdmann J, Raible J, Maki-Abadi J, et al. Spectrum of clinical phenotypes and gene variants in cardiac myosin-binding protein C mutation carriers with hypertrophic cardiomyopathy. J Am Coll Cardiol. 2001;38(2):322–30.

Chapter 9
Heart Valve Disease in Women

Eva Gerdts

Abstract Sex-differences are present in the various types of aortic valve disease and aortic root abnormalities. The typical aortic stenosis (AS) patient with a small aortic root is an elderly woman with atherosclerosis and reduced systemic arterial compliance. Sex-differences in outcomes after transcatheter aortic valve replacement (TAVR) are still debated. Primary mitral regurgitation (MR) is more common among women, while secondary MR is more common among men. Women with severe MR are diagnosed and operated at a later stage than men. This chapter gives an update on current diagnosis and management of women with AS or MR, the most common types of valvular heart disease.

Keywords Aortic root diameter • Aortic stenosis (AS) • Aortic valve disease • Echocardiography • LV adaptation • Mitral regurgitation (MR) • Surgical aortic valve replacement (SAVR) • Transcatheter aortic valve replacement (TAVR) • Transvalvular flow • Valvular heart disease

Introduction

During the past 50 years there has been a dramatic shift in the causes and management of valvular heart disease. In Western societies a marked decline in the incidence of rheumatic valve disease and an increase in age and cancer therapy related degenerative valve disease have occurred in women. Technical development in non-invasive imaging methods like echocardiography, cardiac magnetic resonance imaging (cMRI) and computed tomography (CT) has given the possibility of precise, advanced diagnosis of valvular heart disease and its progression over time. Furthermore, new catheter-based treatment of aortic and mitral valve disease has enabled treatment of severe aortic valve stenosis (AS) and mitral valve regurgitation (MR) in elderly women, that could not be treated with conventional open heart surgery. The current chapter gives an update on contemporary diagnosis and management of women with AS or MR, the most common types of valvular heart disease.

E. Gerdts, M.D., Ph.D., F.E.S.C.
Department of Clinical Science, University of Bergen, Bergen, Norway
e-mail: Eva.Gerdts@uib.no

A.H.E.M. Maas, C.N. Bairey Merz (eds.), *Manual of Gynecardiology*,
DOI 10.1007/978-3-319-54960-6_9

Aortic Valve Stenosis

Epidemiology

Degenerative AS is a progressive disease with a spectrum ranging from mild aortic valve thickening without obstruction to left ventricular outflow, termed aortic valve sclerosis, to severe valve calcification with outflow obstruction requiring valve replacement [1, 2]. AS is the most common type of valvular heart disease requiring valve replacement [1, 2]. Epidemiologic data from the Tromsø study in Norway has demonstrated that the prevalence of AS increases with age, being 0.2% in general population <60 years of age, 3.9% among subjects aged 70–79 years and 9.8% among subjects >80 years of age [3]. From the Cardiovascular Health study in the US, it was demonstrated that among subjects over 65 years of age, aortic valve calcification was 50% less common in women than in men, and progression from aortic valve sclerosis to AS was also less common in women [4]. In their study, the association of cardiovascular (CV) risk factors and incident AS was also demonstrated: smoking and hypertension were associated with a 35% respectively 20% increased risk for incident AS [4]. Aortic stenosis due to congenital abnormality is three times more common among men than women [5], while degenerative AS is more common among women with a women to men ratio of 1–0.76 [6].

Diagnosis

In AS progressive calcification of the valve cusps lead to increasing obstruction of left ventricular(LV) outflow tract with secondary left ventricular hypertrophy [1, 2]. In AS patient with concomitant hypertension or obesity, LV hypertrophy may be present even in subjects with mild AS [7, 8]. Presence of left ventricular hypertrophy (LVH) was recently demonstrated as an independent marker of impaired prognosis in AS, independent of the severity of the disease [9]. Aortic stenosis is clinically suspected when a systolic ejection murmur is heard parasternally, typically in the second right intercostal space, and often radiating to the carotid arteries. A severe AS may be suspected from auscultation if the second heart sound is attenuated or absent in subjects >70 years.

Echocardiography is the first line test to confirm the diagnosis and grade the severity of the AS, thereby making the foundation for further management of the individual patient [1, 2]. By echocardiography, peak aortic jet velocity, mean transvalvular gradient and effective valve opening area are used for grading of AS severity [1, 2]. In subjects with small body size, indexation of the valve opening area for body surface area is recommended to avoid overestimation of AS severity, while in obese subjects, such indexation may lead to overestimation of the AS severity [10]. The recommended cut-off values for mild, moderate and severe AS are similar for women and men.

The dimension of the aortic root may significantly impact the accuracy of the severity grading of AS [11]. The impact of a small aortic root on grading of AS is most prominent in milder degree of AS, and diminishes with increasing AS severity [11]. Women have a smaller aortic root dimension than men in normal population [12, 13], and a small aortic root is particularly common among elderly women with AS, and also associated with atherosclerosis in the proximal aorta [12]. In patients with mild AS and a small aortic root dimension, the actual AS severity may be overestimated by 30% if the aortic valve area is not adjusted for post-stenotic pressure recovery. The improved CV risk prediction in AS patients by pressure recovery adjusted aortic valve area (energy loss index) is well demonstrated [14]. However, irrespective of the AS severity, presence of a small aortic root is associated with increased risk for CV events and death in patients with asymptomatic AS [12]. The typical AS patient with a small aortic root is an elderly woman with atherosclerosis and reduced systemic arterial compliance.

In patients with AS, progression rate of the disease does not differ between women and men [15]. However, there is a large variation in individual disease progression rate among AS patients, and in particular comorbidities like diabetes, atherosclerosis and renal disease may all lead to more rapid progression. Serial assessment of disease severity by echocardiography is therefore recommended in the guidelines [2].

As a consequence of AS progression, increasing pressure overload of the LV occurs with compensatory structural changes in LV. Typically, concentric LVH is the most common LV geometric pattern in severe AS [15]. Distinct sex-differences in LV adaptation during progression of AS have been described in patients with severe, symptomatic AS, including women having larger LV wall thicknesses and more concentric LV geometry with smaller internal cavity and larger relative wall thickness than men [16]. However, these differences were not found in patients with moderate, asymptomatic AS [17]. It is well documented that women, independently of LV size, also preserve better LV systolic function than men during progression of AS, whether measured as ejection fraction, midwall function or global longitudinal strain [16–19]. These sex-specific clinical and echocardiographic findings are mirrored by findings in experimental studies in AS, documenting more endocardial fibrosis and abnormal collagen architecture with increased cross-hatching in men [19], and sex-specific activation of pro-fibrotic genes resulting in more interstitial fibrosis in men [20]. Furthermore, a sex- and estrogen-dependent regulation of a fibrosis-related miRNA network was reported in a pressure overload model in mice [21].

While most women with AS may be accurately diagnosed by echocardiography, discordant grading (moderate AS by mean gradient and severe AS by aortic valve area) may occur in up to 30% of individuals [11]. In these patients, low transvalvular flow is often present, whether assessed by stroke volume index <35 mL/m^2 or by trans-aortic flow rate <200 mL/s [1, 22]. In such patients, additional tests including exercise testing, pharmacological stress-echocardiography and multidetector computed tomography (CT) scanning of the aortic valve may be indicated for accurate grading of AS severity and presence of symptoms. Such advanced diagnostic testing in AS is best performed at experienced heart valve centres.

CT of the aortic valve has revealed that calcification is more pronounced in men than in women independent of the severity of the AS [23]. With CT, calcification is measured by Agatston score. Recently, sex specific cut-off values for CT Agatston identifying severe AS (>1200 AU in women and >2000 AU in men) were prognostically validated [24]. These cut-off values may be used for detection of severe AS in patients with low flow and discordantly graded severe AS by conventional echocardiography.

Treatment Options

Aortic stenosis is asymptomatic until severe hemodynamic pressure overload is present. When the cardinal symptoms of angina pectoris, syncope and heart failure appear in patients with severe AS, aortic valve replacement is indicated. It is well recognized that perioperative mortality and complications are higher in women than in men undergoing surgical aortic valve replacement (SAVR) [2]. This has been attributed to higher age and comorbidity burden in women including more hypertension and obesity and the usually smaller body size in women [2]. In contrast, concomitant coronary artery disease and renal impairment are more common in men than in women with AS. Nowadays transcatheter aortic valve replacement (TAVR) may be an option for AS patients who cannot be treated surgically or who have an inacceptable high operative risk [2]. The PARTNER trial recently documented that in high risk patients with AS, treatment with TAVR and SAVR had a comparable 1-year risk for combined mortality and major stroke [25]. A retrospective analysis of the 2-year outcome in the PARTNER trial documented the superior outcome with TAVR in women, in particular when femoral access was used [26]. However, men in the PARTNER trial had a higher prevalence of diabetes, renal impairment and previous coronary artery bypass grafting, all factors that may have impacted the 2-year outcome beyond the type of treatment. A smaller study in patients with severe AS, documented that lack of postoperative regression of LV hypertrophy was particularly associated with reduced survival in women [27]. Therefore, a prospective study designed to assess sex differences in outcome after TAVR is warranted.

Mitral Valve Regurgitation

Epidemiology

In Europe, mitral regurgitation (MR) is the second most common valve disease requiring surgery [2]. Pathological changes in any of the mitral valve components may lead to MR.

Mitral regurgitation may be primary (due to structural disease of the valve itself) or secondary (due to regional or global functional disease in the LV or dilated left atrium) [1, 2]. The most common cause of primary MR in developed countries is a mitral valve prolapse. A mitral valve prolapse results from a disproportion between the valve's connective elements (leaflets, annulus and chordae) and the muscular support (papillary muscle and left ventricular myocardium) [28]. Mitral valve prolapse may be a primary condition or secondary to several disorders, including heritable disorders like the Marfan syndrome or the Ehlers-Danlos syndrome, ostium secundum atrial septal defect, anorexia nervosa or cardiomyopathy [28]. Other causes of primary MR are severe myxomatous degeneration with gross redundancy of both leaflets and the chordal apparatus (Barlow's disease) and fibro-elastic deficiency disease, in which lack of connective tissue leads to chordal rupture or less common causes like connective tissue disorders, rheumatic heart disease, cleft mitral valve, radiation heart disease, annulus calcification or infectious endocarditis [1]. Secondary MR is caused by idiopathic myocardial disease or coronary artery disease. In patients with coronary artery disease, mitral annulus dilatation secondary to post-myocardial infarction remodelling of the LV or ischemic rupture of chordae may occur.

Primary MR is more common among women, while secondary MR is more common among men. Both leaflets and annulus are normally larger in women than in men, probably explaining the somewhat higher prevalence of mild mitral valve prolapse in women [29]. Mitral regurgitation is found in around 20% of adult general population [30]. In the population based Strong Heart Study, presence of MR was independently associated with female sex, older age, lower body mass index, renal dysfunction, as well as with prior myocardial infarction or other mitral valve disease [31].

Diagnosis

A MR is clinically suspected when a holosystolic murmur is heard at the apex of the heart and radiating to the axillary region. The MR must be at least moderate severe to be diagnosed by auscultation. Echocardiography is recommended as first test to diagnose the cause and severity of a MR. There are no sex differences in guideline recommendations for diagnosis or grading of MR [1, 2].

A combination of transthoracic (TTE) and transesophageal (TEE) echocardiography may be necessary to detect the cause of the MR as well as consequences for LV and atrial structure and function and presence of secondary pulmonary hypertension. Three-dimensional TTE is superior to conventional 2-dimensional TTE in visualization of valve structure and function. Three-dimensional TEE is used for guidance during catheter-based mitral valve procedures.

Assessment of MR involves detailed evaluation of its etiology and mechanism. The mechanism of the MR may be described by the Carpentier's classification of leaflet motion: type 1 normal leaflet motion (e.g. annular dilatation, leaflet perforation or mitral valve cleft), type 2 excessive leaflet motion (i.e. chordal elongation or rupture, prolapse) and type 3 restricted leaflet motion (i.e. coronary artery disease, LV dilatation with leaflet tethering) [32]. In patients with type 3 MR due to posterior myocardial infarction, the regurgitation jet is usually eccentric with posterior leaflet tethering. In patients with type 3 MR due to previous anterior myocardial infarction or non-ischemic cardiomyopathy, the regurgitation jet is usually central. Multiple variables with somewhat different criteria are integrated in grading of primary and secondary MR, including qualitative (mitral valve morphology, colour and continuous wave Doppler), semiquantitative (vena contracta width, mitral inflow, pulmonary venous flow), quantitative (regurgitant volume, effective regurgitant orifice area) and supportive measurements (LV and left atrial structure and function and pulmonary arterial pressure).

If a discrepancy between symptoms and MR grading at rest is found, exercise echocardiography is recommended. Cardiac MRI may be used for assessment of LV and left atrial volumes and scar tissue, and may precisely quantify MR volume. Cardiac CT can also be used for accurate assessment of mitral valve anatomy. Advanced diagnostic testing in MR is best performed at experienced heart valve centres.

Treatment

The optimal treatment of a MR is based upon the underlying pathology in the individual patient [32]. Current guidelines do not include sex-specific recommendations [1, 2]. In patients older than 50 years of age with moderate MR, yearly mortality rate is 3% and 6% in those with severe MR with medical treatment [33], while in patients with mild to moderate MR 5-year event-free survival is more than 95%. In patients with mitral valve prolapse, the prolapse location, presence of valvular or annular calcification and the severity of annular dilatation may all affect the feasibility and choice of surgical and transcatheter mitral repair. Novel devices for transcatheter treatment of mitral valve disease are rapidly developing. To date catheter-based reduction of MR may be obtained from MitraClip, direct or indirect annuloplasty and valve replacement.

The effect of surgical treatment of MR is best documented for primary MR [1, 2]. Patients with severe symptomatic MR and left ventricular ejection fraction >30% are generally recommended for surgery. For asymptomatic severe MR, an end-systolic LV dimension >40 mm (>45 mm in European guidelines) and a LV ejection fraction <60% are criteria suggesting referral for surgical treatment [1, 2]. Since women normally have smaller hearts and higher ejection fraction [17], these criteria may lead to underdiagnosis of asymptomatic severe MR in women. From a review of more than 180,000 Medicare beneficiaries, women with MR undergoing mitral valve surgery had lower survival than men, independent of type of valve surgery (mitral repair or replacement, respectively) [34]. The lower survival was attributed to higher preoperative risk in women, in particular heart failure, atrial fibrillation and respiratory failure, all reflecting more longstanding and severe MR at the time of referral for surgical treatment. The authors suggested a physician referral bias, but women seeking medical care at a later stage and lack of sex-specific criteria for the echocardiographic diagnosis of severe MR may also have contributed. Therefore, a prospective study of modern MR treatment using sex-specific criteria for diagnosis of severe MR is spoken for.

Key Issues Valvular Heart Disease in Women

- Congenital aortic stenosis (AS) occurs more often in men, while degenerative AS is more prevalent in women
- The typical AS patient with a small aortic root is an elderly woman with atherosclerosis and reduced systemic arterial compliance
- Women preserve better LV systolic function than men during progression of AS
- Men have more calcification of the aortic valve than women, independent of the severity of AS
- Perioperative mortality and complications of aortic valve surgery are higher in women than in men
- Gender differences in outcomes after transcatheter aortic valve replacement are still debated
- Primary mitral regurgitation (MR) is more common among women, while secondary MR is more common among men
- The prevalence of mild MR is higher in women than in men
- Women with severe MR are diagnosed and operated at a later stage than men

Case 1. Woman with symptomatic aortic valve stenosis

Ann is a 78 year old retired nurse. She has been treated for hypertension for about 25 years, but has otherwise been in good health her entire life. Currently she uses only an ARB. Lately she has suffered from exertional dyspnea, and a systolic murmur was detected when she visited her general practitioner. She is therefore referred to cardiology outpatient clinic.

Clinical examination reveals that she has a systolic ejection murmur, best heard in the second left intercostal space. The murmur radiates to the carotid arteries and the second heart sound is reduced. The blood pressure is 190/70 mmHg, the heart rate regular at 76 bpm. A 12-lead electrocardiogram is taken and demonstrates sinus rhythm, left ventricular hypertrophy by Sokolow-Lyon voltage criterion, and left ventricular strain pattern. Thus, from the clinical examination a symptomatic, severe aortic valve stenosis is suspected.

By echocardiography a severely calcified aortic valve is visualized. Peak jet velocity is 3.8 m/s, mean transvalvular gradient is 34 mmHg, and the effective aortic valve area is 0.80 cm^2. The left ventricle has concentric left ventricular hypertrophy, ejection fraction is 64%, stroke volume is 29 mL/m^2 and the aortic bulbus diameter is 2.9 cm, reflecting a small aortic root. Adjusting the aortic valve area for pressure recovery in the aortic root (energy loss index) gave an estimated valve area of 0.91 cm^2. Spirometry demonstrated normal lung function.

The patient was referred to the heart valve team. Conventional echocardiography gave discordantly graded aortic stenosis severity, and our patient had a low flow, low gradient severe aortic stenosis with normal left ventricular ejection fraction. The heart team recommended additional imaging. A low-dose dobutamine stress echocardiography was performed, demonstrating a fixed aortic stenosis with increase of the peak jet velocity and mean gradient to 4.2 m/s and 44 mmHg, respectively, and a reduction of the effective aortic valve area to 0.74 cm^2. A computed tomography scan of the aortic valve, aorta and coronary arteries was also performed. The aortic valve calcium score was 1600, the ascending aorta was calcified, but there are no significant coronary artery stenoses.

Conclusion: Ann has a low flow low gradient severe aortic stenosis as confirmed by the additional imaging tests, causing her symptoms. She was recommended transcutaneous aortic valve replacement.

Case 2. Woman with mitral valve regurgitation

Mary, 48 years old, is a teacher in primary school. Her favourite leisure time activities are mountain hiking and climbing. Until recently her health was excellent except for an ankle fracture after a fall a couple of years ago. However, the last 5–6 months she has experienced increasing palpitations and a reduction in physical capacity. Since her mother died from a heart attack 59 years old, she is now referred to the cardiology outpatient clinic by her general practitioner.

Clinical examination reveals blood pressure 130/70 mmHg and regular heart beat 64/min. Auscultation reveals a systolic murmur, best heard at apex and radiating to the left axillary region. Pulmonary auscultation is normal, and there is no peripheral oedema. Resting 12-lead electrocardiogram was normal. Echocardiography showed a prolaps and chordal rupture in the P2 segment of the posterior mitral leaflet. The regurgitant jet was graded 3+ by color Doppler, since systolic reverse of pulmonal venous flow was not present. The regurgitant volume was 50%. The left atrium was enlarged with antero-posterior diameter 4.6 cm, and biplane volume 42 mL/m^2. The left ventricle had borderline dimensions with end-systolic diameter 4.0 cm and ejection fraction 64%. The right atrium and ventricle have normal dimensions.

Based upon a trivial tricuspid regurgitation, the systolic pulmonary artery pressure was estimated to 36 mmHg.

The findings were consistent with a moderate to severe primary mitral regurgitation. The patient was referred to the heart valve team for further evaluation. The heart team suggested further imaging. Additional three-dimentional echocardiography and cardiac magnetic resonance imaging was performed, confirming the diagnosis of a localized prolapse with rupture of two chordae in the P2 segment of the posterior mitral leaflet. The left ventricle had borderline size in relation to body size, ejection fraction was normal. An exercise echocardiography was performed. At 125 W load, mitral regurgitant volume had increased to 60% and the systolic pulmonary artery pressure to 60 mmHg. The patient did not develop any symptoms. No signs of ischemia was recorded on the electrocardiogram during exercise. Computed tomography angiography did not reveal coronary stenosis. Ambulatory Holter registration revealed prevalent supraventricular ectopic beats, but no episodes of atrial fibrillation.

Conclusion: Mary had an asymptomatic severe primary mitral regurgitation with enlargement of the left atrium and exercise induced pulmonal hypertension. The valve disease was suitable for repair, and surgical mitral valve repair was recommended.

References

1. Nishimura RA, Otto CM, Bonow RO, Carabello BA, Erwin 3rd JP, Guyton RA, O'Gara PT, Ruiz CE, Skubas NJ, Sorajja P, Sundt 3rd TM, Thomas JD. American College of Cardiology/American Heart Association Task Force on Practice Guidelines. 2014 AHA/ACC guideline for the management of patients with valvular heart disease: executive summary: a report of the American College of Cardiology/American Heart Association Task Force on Practice Guidelines. J Am Coll Cardiol. 2014;63:2438–88.
2. Joint Task Force on the Management of Valvular Heart Disease of the European Society of Cardiology (ESC); European Association for Cardio-Thoracic Surgery (EACTS), Vahanian A, Alfieri O, Andreotti F, Antunes MJ, Barón-Esquivias G, Baumgartner H, Borger MA, Carrel TP, De Bonis M, Evangelista A, Falk V, Iung B, Lancellotti P, Pierard L, Price S, Schäfers HJ, Schuler G, Stepinska J, Swedberg K, Takkenberg J, Von Oppell UO, Windecker S, Zamorano JL, Zembala M. Guidelines on the management of valvular heart disease (version 2012). Eur Heart J. 2012;33:2451–96.
3. Eveborn GW, Schirmer H, Heggelund G, Lunde P, Rasmussen K. The evolving epidemiology of valvular aortic stenosis. the Tromsø study. Heart. 2013;99:396–400.
4. Stewart BF, Siscovick D, Lind BK, Gardin JM, Gottdiener JS, Smith VE, Kitzman DW, Otto CM. Clinical factors associated with calcific aortic valve disease. Cardiovascular Health Study. J Am Coll Cardiol. 1997;29:630–4.
5. Siu SC, Silversides CK. Bicuspid aortic valve disease. J Am Coll Cardiol. 2010;55:2789–800.
6. Davies MJ, Treasure T, Parker DJ. Demographic characteristics of patients undergoing aortic valve replacement for stenosis: relation to valve morphology. Heart. 1996;75(2):174–8.

7. Rieck ÅE, Cramariuc D, Boman K, Gohlke-Bärwolf C, Staal EM, Lønnebakken MT, Rossebø AB, Gerdts E. Hypertension in aortic stenosis: implications for left ventricular structure and cardiovascular events. Hypertension. 2012;60:90–7.
8. Rogge BP, Cramariuc D, Lønnebakken MT, Gohlke-Bärwolf C, Chambers JB, Boman K, Gerdts E. Effect of overweight and obesity on cardiovascular events in asymptomatic aortic stenosis: a SEAS Substudy (Simvastatin ezetimibe in aortic stenosis). J Am Coll Cardiol. 2013;62:1683–90.
9. Gerdts E, Rossebø AB, Pedersen TR, Cioffi G, Lønnebakken MT, Cramariuc D, Rogge BP, Devereux RB. Relation of left ventricular mass to prognosis in initially asymptomatic mild to moderate aortic valve stenosis. Circ Cardiovasc Imaging. 2015;8:e003644.
10. Rogge BP, Gerdts E, Cramariuc D, Bahlmann E, Jander N, Gohlke-Bärwolf C, Pedersen TR, Lønnebakken MT. Impact of obesity and nonobesity on grading the severity of aortic valve stenosis. Am J Cardiol. 2014;113:1532–5.
11. Bahlmann E, Cramariuc D, Gerdts E, Gohlke-Baerwolf C, Nienaber CA, Eriksen E, Wachtell K, Chambers J, Kuck KH, Ray S. Impact of pressure recovery on echocardiographic assessment of asymptomatic aortic stenosis: a SEAS substudy. JACC Cardiovasc Imaging. 2010;3:555–62.
12. Bahlmann E, Cramariuc D, Minners J, Lønnebakken MT, Ray S, Gohlke-Baerwolf C, Nienaber CA, Jander N, Seifert R, Chambers JB, Kuck KH, Gerdts E. Small aortic root in aortic valve stenosis: clinical characteristics and prognostic implications. Eur Heart J Cardiovasc Imaging. 2017;18(4):404–12.
13. Muraru D, Maffessanti F, Kocabay G, Peluso D, Dal Bianco L, Piasentini E, Jose SP, Iliceto S, Badano LP. Ascending aorta diameters measured by echocardiography using both leading edge-to-leading edge and inner edge-to-inner edge conventions in healthy volunteers. Eur Heart J Cardiovasc Imaging. 2014;15:415–22.
14. Bahlmann E, Gerdts E, Cramariuc D, Gohlke-Baerwolf C, Nienaber CA, Wachtell K, Seifert R, Chambers JB, Kuck KH, Ray S. Prognostic value of energy loss index in asymptomatic aortic stenosis. Circulation. 2013;127:1149–56.
15. Cramariuc D, Rogge BP, Lønnebakken MT, Boman K, Bahlmann E, Gohlke-Bärwolf C, Chambers JB, Pedersen TR, Gerdts E. Sex differences in cardiovascular outcome during progression of aortic valve stenosis. Heart. 2015;101:209–14.
16. Douglas PS, Otto CM, Mickel MC, Labovitz A, Reid CL, Davis KB. Gender differences in left ventricle geometry and function in patients undergoing balloon dilatation of the aortic valve for isolated aortic stenosis. NHLBI Balloon Valvuloplasty Registry. Br Heart J. 1995;73:548–54.
17. Cramariuc D, Rieck AE, Staal EM, Wachtell K, Eriksen E, Rossebø AB, Gerdts E. Factors influencing left ventricular structure and stress-corrected systolic function in men and women with asymptomatic aortic valve stenosis (a SEAS substudy). Am J Cardiol. 2008;101:510–5.
18. Carroll JD, Carroll EP, Feldman T, Ward DM, Lang RM, McGaughey D, Karp RB. Sex-associated differences in left ventricular function in aortic stenosis of the elderly. Circulation. 1992;86:1099–107.
19. Villari B, Campbell SE, Schneider J, Vassalli G, Chiariello M, Hess OM. Sex-dependent differences in left ventricular function and structure in chronic pressure overload. Eur Heart J. 1995;16:1410–9.
20. Petrov G, Regitz-Zagrosek V, Lehmkuhl E, Krabatsch T, Dunkel A, Dandel M, Dworatzek E, Mahmoodzadeh S, Schubert C, Becher E, Hampl H, Hetzer R. Regression of myocardial hypertrophy after aortic valve replacement: faster in women? Circulation. 2010;122(11 Suppl):S23–8.
21. Queirós AM, Eschen C, Fliegner D, Kararigas G, Dworatzek E, Westphal C, Sanchez Ruderisch H, Regitz-Zagrosek V. Sex- and estrogen-dependent regulation of a miRNA network in the healthy and hypertrophied heart. Int J Cardiol. 2013;169:331–8.
22. Capoulade R, Le Ven F, Clavel MA, Dumesnil JG, Dahou A, Thébault C, Arsenault M, O'Connor K, Bédard É, Beaudoin J, Sénéchal M, Bernier M, Pibarot P. Echocardiographic predictors of outcomes in adults with aortic stenosis. Heart. 2016;102:934–42.

23. Aggarwal SR, Clavel MA, Messika-Zeitoun D, Cueff C, Malouf J, Araoz PA, Mankad R, Michelena H, Vahanian A, Enriquez-Sarano M. Sex differences in aortic valve calcification measured by multidetector computed tomography in aortic stenosis. Circ Cardiovasc Imaging. 2013;6:40–7.
24. Clavel MA, Pibarot P, Messika-Zeitoun D, Capoulade R, Malouf J, Aggarval S, Araoz PA, Michelena HI, Cueff C, Larose E, Miller JD, Vahanian A, Enriquez-Sarano M. Impact of aortic valve calcification, as measured by MDCT, on survival in patients with aortic stenosis: results of an international registry study. J Am Coll Cardiol. 2014;64:1202–13.
25. Smith CR, Leon MB, Mack MJ, Miller DC, Moses JW, Svensson LG, Tuzcu EM, Webb JG, Fontana GP, Makkar RR, Williams M, Dewey T, Kapadia S, Babaliaros V, Thourani VH, Corso P, Pichard AD, Bavaria JE, Herrmann HC, Akin JJ, Anderson WN, Wang D, Pocock SJ. PARTNER Trial Investigators. Transcatheter versus surgical aortic-valve replacement in high-risk patients. N Engl J Med. 2011;364:2187–98.
26. Williams M, Kodali SK, Hahn RT, Humphries KH, Nkomo VT, Cohen DJ, Douglas PS, Mack M, McAndrew TC, Svensson L, Thourani VH, Tuzcu EM, Weissman NJ, Kirtane AJ, Leon MB. Sex-related differences in outcomes after transcatheter or surgical aortic valve replacement in patients with severe aortic stenosis: insights from the PARTNER Trial (Placement of Aortic Transcatheter Valve). J Am Coll Cardiol. 2014;63:1522–8.
27. Petrov G, Dworatzek E, Schulze TM, Dandel M, Kararigas G, Mahmoodzadeh S, Knosalla C, Hetzer R, Regitz-Zagrosek V. Maladaptive remodeling is associated with impaired survival in women but not in men after aortic valve replacement. JACC Cardiovasc Imaging. 2014;7:1073–80.
28. Devereux RB, Kramer-Fox R, Kligfield P. Mitral valve prolapse: causes, clinical manifestations, and management. Ann Intern Med. 1989;111:305–17.
29. Avierinos JF, Inamo J, Grigioni F, Gersh B, Shub C, Enriquez-Sarano M. Sex differences in morphology and outcomes of mitral valve prolapse. Ann Intern Med. 2008;149:787–95.
30. Devereux RB, Jones EC, Roman MJ, Howard BV, Fabsitz RR, Liu JE, Palmieri V, Welty TK, Lee ET. Prevalence and correlates of mitral valve prolapse in a population-based sample of American Indians: the Strong Heart Study. Am J Med. 2001;111:679–85.
31. Jones EC, Devereux RB, Roman MJ, Liu JE, Fishman D, Lee ET, Welty TK, Fabsitz RR, Howard BV. Prevalence and correlates of mitral regurgitation in a population-based sample (the Strong Heart Study). Am J Cardiol. 2001;87:298–304.
32. Stone GW, Vahanian AS, Adams DH, Abraham WT, Borer JS, Bax JJ, Schofer J, Cutlip DE, Krucoff MW, Blackstone EH, Généreux P, Mack MJ, Siegel RJ, Grayburn PA, Enriquez-Sarano M, Lancellotti P, Filippatos G, Kappetein AP, Mitral Valve Academic Research Consortium (MVARC). Clinical trial design principles and endpoint definitions for transcatheter mitral valve repair and replacement: part 1: clinical trial design principles: a consensus document from the Mitral Valve Academic Research Consortium. J Am Coll Cardiol. 2015;66:278–307.
33. Enriquez-Sarano M, Akins CW, Vahanian A. Mitral regurgitation. Lancet. 2009;373:1382–94.
34. Vassileva CM, McNeely C, Mishkel G, Boley T, Markwell S, Hazelrigg S. Gender differences in long-term survival of Medicare beneficiaries undergoing mitral valve operations. Ann Thorac Surg. 2013;96:1367–73.

Chapter 10
Female Aspects of Electrocardiography and Cardiac Arrhythmias

Angela H.E.M. Maas and Reinder Evertz

Abstract Normograms of the ECG are derived from the standard male patient. Women have a longer duration of the P-wave and PR-interval, while the QRS complex is smaller with a lower voltage. Non-specific ST-T changes are more often present in women than in men and vary by age. Paroxysmal supraventricular tachycardia's (PSVT) are later diagnosed in women than in men. Women with atrial fibrillation (AF) have more symptoms, undergo fewer cardioversions and have a worse quality of life than men. Women more often develop Torsades de pointes (TdP) with some antiarrhythmic drugs. Although implantable defibrillator devices (ICD) therapy in secondary prevention are equally beneficial in both genders, they are less often applied in women. The quality of mammograms may be reduced by the presence of an implanted medical device.

Keywords Anti-arrhythmic drugs • Arrhythmias • Atrial fibrillation (AF) • Atrioventricular nodal re-entrant tachycardias (AVNRT) • Breast tissue • CHA2DS2-VASc risk score • Electrocardiogram (ECG) • Implantable defibrillator devices (ICD) • Mammograms • Menstrual cycle • Novel oral anticoagulants (NOACs) • QT-interval • Sex-hormones • Supraventricular tachycardia (SVT) • Thrombo-embolic risk • Torsade de pointes (TdP)

Introduction

Sex-related differences in electrocardiography and cardiac arrhythmias are present in clinical symptoms, diagnostics, therapeutic options and side-effects of therapy [1]. In most studies from which guidelines for the management of arrhythmias have

A.H.E.M. Maas, M.D., Ph.D. (✉)
Department of Cardiology, Women's Cardiac Health Program,
Radboud University Medical Center, Nijmegen, The Netherlands
e-mail: angela.maas@radboudumc.nl

R. Evertz, M.D.
Department of Cardiology, Radboud University Medical Center, Nijmegen, The Netherlands
e-mail: Reinder.Evertz@radboudumc.nl

A.H.E.M. Maas, C.N. Bairey Merz (eds.), *Manual of Gynecardiology*,
DOI 10.1007/978-3-319-54960-6_10

been developed, women have been importantly underrepresented. As a consequence, many guidelines are still lacking an appropriate gender-sensitive approach [2, 3].

Electrocardiogram in Women

Baseline characteristics of the electrocardiogram (ECG) show several differences between men and women, of which the clinical significance is often unclear. These concern amplitudes and duration as well as repolarization patterns [4]. Normograms of the ECG are derived from the standard male patient. Important factors that affect sex-variations in ECG recordings are related to thorax size and the presence of adipose tissue. Breast tissue in women, dependent on breast size and shape as well as adipose tissue in obese patients, contributes to lower QRS and T-amplitudes with an increase in amplitude of the QRS complex after mastectomy [5, 6]. Breast tissue in women also interferes with correct positioning of the precordial leads affecting the quality of ECG recordings [7, 8]. As initial clinical decision making in acute and chronic settings of cardiac care is to a great extent based on ECGs, it occurs relatively often that these are misinterpreted in female patients. This may lead to unnecessary diagnostic testing and is a serious burden for the expanding costs of healthcare. Moreover, the use of advanced imaging techniques has reduced technical skills of young doctors in ECG reading and interpretation, whereas the ECG is still the cornerstone in the cardiology diagnostic work-up [9, 10].

Women have on average a higher resting heart rate (HR) than men, with a mean of 3–5 beats/min faster HR [11]. This may partly be explained by differences in body habitus and exercise tolerance, but differences in intrinsic electrophysiological properties of the sinus node and autonomic nervous system may also play a role [12]. In premenopausal women, the resting HR is faster in the luteal phase than in the follicular phase of the menstrual cycle [13]. Women have a longer duration of the P-wave and PR-interval, while the QRS complex is smaller with a lower voltage, also after correction for cardiac mass and bodyweight [4, 14].

The corrected QT interval (QTc) is longer (mean 10–20 ms) in women than in men, which is associated with an increased risk of drug-induced QT-prolongation and Torsade de pointes tachycardia [15–17]. During menstrual cycle and pregnancy there is QTc variability, suggesting intrinsic hormonal regulation in female hearts [18]. This may interfere with side effects of medical therapy. During childhood there is no difference in QT interval between boys and girls. During puberty however, QTc shortens in male adolescents, while after 50 years of age most sex-differences in QTc resolve. It is assumed that high testosterone levels shorten QTc during puberty [19]. Estrogens also affect the length of the QT interval by the fast and persistent sodium current and sodium–calcium exchange in myocardial cells [18, 20]. According to the guidelines of the AHA the upper limit of QTc is 450 ms in men and 460 ms in women [21]. In the Copenhagen City ECG study, prolongation of the QTc interval resulted in a worse prognosis in men whereas in women, a very short QTc interval was equivalent in risk to a borderline prolonged QTc interval [22]. The effect of the QTc interval on the absolute risk of cardiovascular

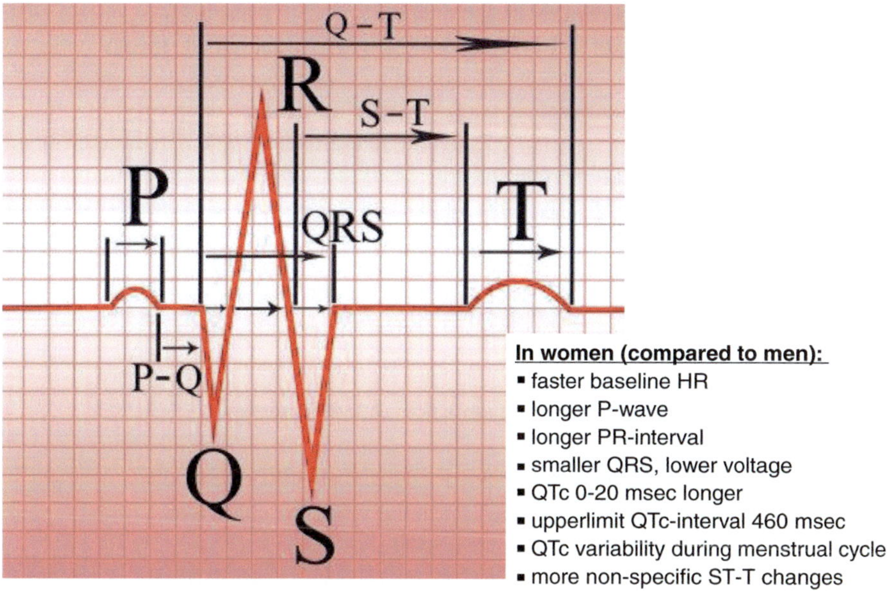

Fig. 10.1 Sex differences in electrocardiography

death was found to be most pronounced in the elderly and in those with known CAD, whereas the effect was negligible for healthy middle-aged women.

Non-specific ST-T changes are more often present in women than in men and vary by age. In a large healthy Dutch population it was shown that sex-dependent differences were apparent for most ECG parameters (www.normalecg.org) [23]. Age trends were present for the QTc interval, QRS axis, and indices of left ventricular hypertrophy. Amplitudes in the left precordial leads showed a substantial increase in the older age groups for women, but not for men. ST J-point amplitudes in adolescent males are distinctly higher than in similarly aged women, dissolving at old age. ST-T deviations may carry important prognostic information for IHD mortality risk, as was shown for both genders in the Copenhagen City ECG study and for postmenopausal women in the Women's Health initiative (WHI) study [24, 25]. In postmenopausal women using hormone therapy unopposed estrogen mildly prolongs myocardial repolarization, which is reversed by progesterone [26]. Figure 10.1 summarizes most important sex-differences in the baseline ECG.

Paroxysmal Supraventricular Tachycardias in Women

Atrioventricular nodal re-entrant tachycardias (AVNRT) occur significantly more often in women than in men, presumably related to hormonal effects on AV conduction [27]. The prevalence of AVNRT in women peaks in the second and third decennium and around menopause. Cyclic hormonal variations in premenopausal women influence the occurrence of AVNRT with a predominance in the luteal phase when progesterone levels are at highest [28, 29]. During pregnancy and after delivery, an increased incidence of supraventricular tachycardia (SVT) and especially AVNRT has been described [30]. For atrioventricular re-entrant tachycardia, using a bypass tract outside the AV node, no difference in incidence between men and woman has been described.

Paroxysmal supraventricular tachycardia's (PSVT) are later diagnosed in women than in men and are often associated with feelings of anxiety, panic and undetermined vibrations in the chest [31]. Symptoms can easily be misinterpreted as being from psychological origin [32]. This may also lead to later referral and eventually even for delay in radiofrequency (RF) ablation in women, such as shown in patient case A.

28-yr old woman with AV nodal re-entry tachycardia

Medical history: attacks of 'hyperventilation' since almost 10 years

Patient history: patient arrives at the emergency department with anxiety, signs of hyperventilation and an uneasy feeling 'of flibbering' inside her chest. She has had these attacks for more than 8 years, usually once a month for 10 minutes, and at previous presentations her ECG had shown no abnormalities. This time, the attack persists longer, over 30 minutes, with feelings of dizzyness, palpitations and a slight sensation of chest pain. She has a healthy lifestyle with a good physical condition.

Physical examination: expression of anxiety, respiratory rate 24/min, RR 105/65 mmHg, pulse 170/min, regular. Body temperature 37.1˚C. Fast and regular heartbeats, with no murmurs at ausculation.

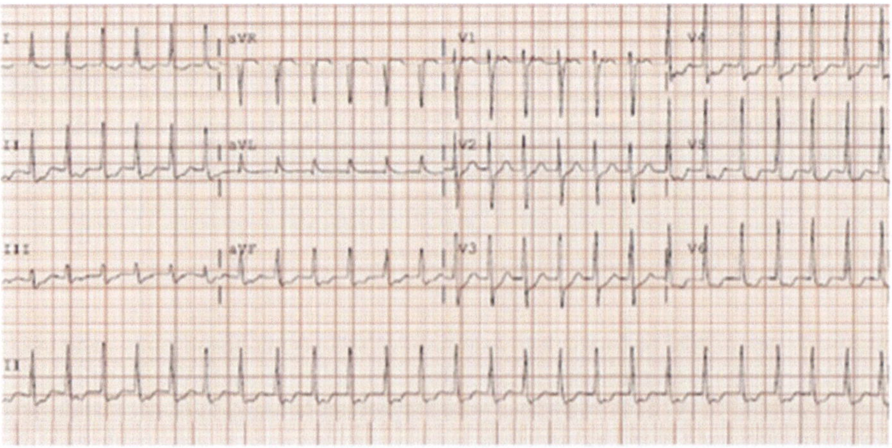

ECHO: no structural cardiac abnormalities

Discussion: an AV nodal re-entry tachycardia is a frequent occurring ectopic supraventricular tachycardia, especially in younger patients with a structural normal heart. Adenosine intravenously is effective in most cases to restore sinusrythm.
In women it may take longer to obtain the diagnosis than in men, with a longer interval before ablation-therapy is performed (ref. 31)

Radboudumc

Sex and Gender Differences in Atrial Fibrillation

Men are at 1.5-fold higher risk than women to develop atrial fibrillation (AF) during lifetime [33]. However, given their longer life-expectancy, the absolute number of women with AF is higher [34]. With the increase in obesity, sedentary lifestyle and hypertension over the past decades, the absolute number of individuals with AF is rising. In the Swedish adult population the prevalence is currently estimated at 2.9%, not counting individuals with 'silent AF', which is comparable with the 3% prevalence as mentioned in the recent 2016 ESC guidelines AF [35, 36]. Atrial fibrillation is independently associated with a twofold increased risk of all-cause mortality in women and a 1.5-fold increase in men [33, 37, 38]. In the Euro Heart Survey on AF it was found that women with AF were generally older, with a lower quality of life, more co-morbidity and more cardiac symptoms compared to men [39, 40]. Women also had more often heart failure (HF) with preserved left ventricular systolic function (HFpEF), and less frequent HF with reduced ejection fraction systolic (HFrEF). In the Outcomes Registry for Better Informed Treatment of Atrial Fibrillation (ORBIT-AF) women with AF had more symptoms and a worse quality of life than men [41].

It has been disputed whether AF is more strongly associated with the risk of stroke and CVD mortality in women than in men [38, 42–45]. In a recent meta-analysis of more than 30 studies in >4.3 million patients, AF was associated with a higher risk of all cause (RR 1,12, 95% CI 1.07–1.17) and an almost twofold CVD mortality in women than in men [46]. Women are also prone to more severe strokes when they do occur [47]. A worse LA function in women than in men with AF contributes to their higher stroke risk [48]. This is closely related to sex-differences in cardiac and arterial remodeling with ageing, with more impaired diastolic dysfunction and arterial stiffening in women compared to men [49, 50]. Nevertheless, women are less likely to receive anticoagulation and undergo fewer cardioversions, AF ablations or pulmonary vein isolations than men [41, 51–54]. Also, women have more peri-procedural complications of AF catheter ablations and a higher recurrence-rate of AF after cardioversion [55, 56].

The CHA2DS2-VASc risk score has included female sex as a risk factor for stroke prevention (Table 10.1). Recommended is to use vitamin K antagonists or

Table 10.1 CHA_2DS_2-VASc risk score for stroke prevention in patients with atrial fibrillation

CHA_2DS_2-VASc risk factor	Points
Signs and symptoms of HF or reduced EF	1
Resting blood pressure > 140/90 or use antihypertensive medication	1
Age ≥ 75 years	2
Diabetes mellitus (fasting glucose >7 mmol/L or insulin/medication)	1
Previous stroke, TIA or thrombo-embolism	2
Previous ACS, peripheral artery disease or aortic plaque	1
Age 65–74	1
Female sex	1

Adapted from: 2016 ESC guidelines atrial fibrillation, ref. [36]
CHA_2DS_2-VASc: Congestive heart failure, Hypertension, Age (2×), Diabetes, Stroke (2×), Vascular disease, Sex
HF heart failure, *EF* ejection fraction, *TIA* transient ischemic attack, *ACS* acute coronary syndrome

novel oral anticoagulants (NOACs) when the risk score is ≥1 for men, and ≥2 for women, balancing the expected stroke reduction, bleeding risk, and patient preference [36]. Of note is that women are underrepresented in the majority of NOAC-trials and that risk of abnormal uterine bleeding in premenopausal women is largely unknown [57, 58].

Ventricular Arrhythmias in Women

In patients with ischemic heart disease (IHD) the risk of sudden cardiac death is more than twofold higher in men than in women [59]. This may importantly be related to the higher obstructive atherosclerosis burden and sex-differences in plaque compositions in men compared to women [60]. The risk for ventricular tachycardias in non-obstructive coronary artery disease (NOCAD) and coronary microvascular disease (CMD), which are important manifestations of IHD in women, is less well studied. It is assumed that the likelihood of ventricular tachycardias is higher during periods of ischemia. Autonomic changes, such as an increase in sympathetic tone, which frequently occurs in women after menopause, enhances the risk for VT/VF [61, 62]. Chronic psychological stress and depression, more often present in women after menopause than in similarly aged men, may further induce autonomic changes. This leads to a higher use of antidepressants, which is also associated with an increased risk for sudden cardiac death (SCD) [63].

In non-ischemic cardiomyopathies (NICM), there is no evidence for any sex difference in arrhythmias or chance for SCD. Recent studies debate whether an implantable cardioverter-defibrillator (ICD) backup is useful in NICM patients [64, 65]. The Brugada syndrome affects men almost 9× more often and more severely than women. Men with Brugada syndrome have more frequently syncope and SCD than women [66, 67]. It is assumed that testosterone-levels in the ion channels play an important role in the observed sex difference [68].

In congenital long QT-syndrome (LQTS), there is an unexplained female prevalence of disease. Women are especially at a higher risk of cardiac events in the period after giving birth, whereas men are more likely to suffer syncope and SCD until puberty [27, 69]. Acquired LQTS is clinically more common than congenital LQTS and is usually seen with electrolyte abnormalities or the use of medications that prolong ventricular repolarization. Nevertheless, about 30% of acquired LQTS appear to be concealed form of congenital LQTS [70]. Women exhibit longer QTc intervals and are more prone to develop Torsades de pointes during administration of some antiarrhythmic drugs [71]. Up to 70% of the cases of medication-induced Torsades de pointes are in women [72]. Especially Vaughn Williams class IA and class III antiarrhythmic drugs (e.g. quinidine and sotalol) enhance the risk for Torsades de pointes. Most important drugs that prolong QT-interval are antihistamines, certain antibiotics and psychopharmaca such a amytriptiline and lithium (www.qtdrugs.org). Class IC antiarrythmic drugs (e.g. flecainide) may also increase the QT interval and therefore increase the risk for Torsades de pointes [73]

Women represent a minority (10–13%) in VT ablation-studies, but are at higher risk for VT recurrence after 1 year. In a recent study in 2062 patients with ischemic and non-ischemic recurrent VT's undergoing ablation, of which 266 (12.9%) were women, it was found that women were younger, with higher ejection fractions and less VT storms than men [74]. In women, the 1-year success rate was lower with significantly higher rates of VT recurrence. More data are needed to distinguish between sex differences in referral patterns, arrhythmia substrate, and treatment bias.

Sex Differences in Pacing, ICD and CRT Therapy

Women more often have sinus node dysfunction and lower rates of AV conduction abnormalities [75]. In the age group above 80, men receive more dual chamber pacing compared to women. Women more peri-procedural complications, such as pneumothorax and hematomas. These complications do not negatively affect survival rates. [76].

It has been debated whether women profit equally from implantable defibrillator devices (ICD) than men [77–79]. In a large meta-analysis in primary prevention studies, no sex difference in mortality was found [80]. Women have fewer ICD-shocks than men and a lower susceptibility to arrhythmia-triggers, which may justify their lower primary ICD implantation rates. Although the benefit for ICD therapy in secondary prevention is similar among men and women, despite they are offered less often ICD therapy [81, 82]. In (additional) cardiac resynchronization therapy (CRT) a recent FDA meta-analysis of three major clinical trials with mild heart failure (HF) confirmed that the indication for CRT in women seems to be at a shorter QRS duration than in men [83, 84]. This has not resulted yet in a sex-specific treatment advise in the latest 2016 ESC guidelines HF [85].

Screening Mammograms in Women with Pacemakers/ICD

Most aging women undergo screening mammograms at regular intervals. The presence of an implanted medical device in the breast may affect the quality of the mammograms [86]. We recently investigated barriers in females and radiographers for mammography and found that increased pain in women and anxiety in both parties were important determinants of lower compression force and suboptimal positioning technique [87]. About 20% of women with devices had serious doubts on attending screening. Despite the very low chance to damage the leads and pacemaker/ICD devices itself, it may be recommended in women with anxiety to undergo mammography at a radiology department in a hospital with possibilities for PM/ICD control afterwards.

Key Issues Electrocardiography and Cardiac Arrhythmias in Women

- Sex-dependent differences are apparent for most ECG parameters (www.normalecg.org)
- Non-specific ST-T changes are more often present in women than in men and may indicate an adverse prognosis
- Paroxysmal supraventricular tachycardia's (PSVT) are later diagnosed in women than in men and are often associated with anxiety, panic and undetermined vibrations
- Women with AF have more symptoms and co-morbidity than men
- Women with AF have a worse prognosis than men (recurrence rate, stroke risk)
- Women with congenital LQTS are at increased risk for adverse events after giving birth
- Adult women have longer QTc interval and are more prone to Torsades de pointes ventricular tachycardias with certain medications (www.qtdrugs.org)
- Image quality of mammograms can be affected by the presence of a device; the risk for lead fracture during these procedures is low.

References

1. Ghani A, Maas AH, Delnoy PP, Ramdat Misier AR, Ottervanger JP, Elvan A. Sex-based differences in cardiac arrhythmias, ICD utilisation and cardiac resynchronisation therapy. Neth Heart J. 2011;19(1):35–40.
2. Camm AJ, Lip GY, De Caterina R, Savelieva I, Atar D, Hohnloser SH, et al. 2012 focused update of the ESC Guidelines for the management of atrial fibrillation: an update of the 2010 ESC Guidelines for the management of atrial fibrillation. Developed with the special contribution of the European Heart Rhythm Association. Eur Heart J. 2012;33(21):2719–47.
3. Priori SG, Blomstrom-Lundqvist C, Mazzanti A, Blom N, Borggrefe M, Camm J, et al. 2015 ESC Guidelines for the management of patients with ventricular arrhythmias and the prevention of sudden cardiac death: the task force for the management of patients with ventricular arrhythmias and the prevention of sudden cardiac death of the European Society of Cardiology

(ESC). Endorsed by: Association for European Paediatric and Congenital Cardiology (AEPC). Eur Heart J. 2015;36(41):2793–867.
4. Smetana P, Malik M. Sex differences in cardiac autonomic regulation and in repolarisation electrocardiography. Pflugers Arch. 2013;465(5):699–717.
5. Alpert MA, Terry BE, Hamm CR, Fan TM, Cohen MV, Massey CV, et al. Effect of weight loss on the ECG of normotensive morbidly obese patients. Chest. 2001;119(2):507–10.
6. LaMonte CS, Freiman AH. The electrocardiogram after mastectomy. Circulation. 1965;32(5):746–54.
7. Macfarlane PW, Colaco R, Stevens K, Reay P, Beckett C, Aitchison T. Precordial electrode placement in women. Neth Heart J. 2003;11(3):118–22.
8. Rautaharju PM, Park L, Rautaharju FS, Crow R. A standardized procedure for locating and documenting ECG chest electrode positions: consideration of the effect of breast tissue on ECG amplitudes in women. J Electrocardiol. 1998;31(1):17–29.
9. Surawicz B. How to increase the accuracy of electrocardiogram's interpretation and stimulate the interest of the interpreters? J Electrocardiol. 2010;43(3):191–3.
10. Yong CM, Froelicher V, Wagner G. The electrocardiogram at a crossroads. Circulation. 2013;128(1):79–82.
11. Liu K, Ballew C, Jacobs Jr DR, Sidney S, Savage PJ, Dyer A, et al. Ethnic differences in blood pressure, pulse rate, and related characteristics in young adults. The CARDIA study. Hypertension. 1989;14(2):218–26.
12. Larsen JA, Kadish AH. Effects of gender on cardiac arrhythmias. J Cardiovasc Electrophysiol. 1998;9(6):655–64.
13. Burke JH, Ehlert FA, Kruse JT, Parker MA, Goldberger JJ, Kadish AH. Gender-specific differences in the QT interval and the effect of autonomic tone and menstrual cycle in healthy adults. Am J Cardiol. 1997;79(2):178–81.
14. Rautaharju PM, Zhang ZM, Gregg RE, Haisty Jr WK, Vitolins MZ, Curtis AB, et al. Normal standards for computer-ECG programs for prognostically and diagnostically important ECG variables derived from a large ethnically diverse female cohort: the Women's Health Initiative (WHI). J Electrocardiol. 2013;46(6):707–16.
15. Pham TV, Rosen MR. Sex, hormones, and repolarization. Cardiovasc Res. 2002;53(3):740–51.
16. Lehmann MH, Hardy S, Archibald D, Quart B, DJ MN. Sex difference in risk of torsade de pointes with d,l-sotalol. Circulation. 1996;94(10):2535–41.
17. Verkerk AO, Wilders R, Tan HL. Gender disparities in torsade de pointes ventricular tachycardia. Neth Hear J. 2007;15(12):405–11.
18. Anneken L, Baumann S, Vigneault P, Biliczki P, Friedrich C, Xiao L, et al. Estradiol regulates human QT-interval: acceleration of cardiac repolarization by enhanced KCNH2 membrane trafficking. Eur Heart J. 2016;37(7):640–50.
19. Rautaharju PM, Zhou SH, Wong S, Calhoun HP, Berenson GS, Prineas R, et al. Sex differences in the evolution of the electrocardiographic QT interval with age. Can J Cardiol. 1992;8(7):690–5.
20. Bernal O, Moro C. Cardiac arrhythmias in women. Rev Esp Cardiol. 2006;59(6):609–18.
21. Rautaharju PM, Surawicz B, Gettes LS, Bailey JJ, Childers R, Deal BJ, et al. AHA/ACCF/HRS recommendations for the standardization and interpretation of the electrocardiogram: part IV: the ST segment, T and U waves, and the QT interval: a scientific statement from the American Heart Association Electrocardiography and Arrhythmias Committee, Council on Clinical Cardiology; the American College of Cardiology Foundation; and the Heart Rhythm Society. Endorsed by the International Society for Computerized Electrocardiology. J Am Coll Cardiol. 2009;53(11):982–91.
22. Nielsen JB, Graff C, Rasmussen PV, Pietersen A, Lind B, Olesen MS, et al. Risk prediction of cardiovascular death based on the QTc interval: evaluating age and gender differences in a large primary care population. Eur Heart J. 2014;35(20):1335–44.
23. Rijnbeek PR, van Herpen G, Bots ML, Man S, Verweij N, Hofman A, et al. Normal values of the electrocardiogram for ages 16–90 years. J Electrocardiol. 2014;47(6):914–21.
24. Rasmussen PV, Nielsen JB, Pietersen A, Graff C, Lind B, Struijk JJ, et al. Electrocardiographic precordial ST-segment deviations and the risk of cardiovascular death: results from the Copenhagen ECG Study. J Am Heart Assoc. 2014;3(3):e000549.

25. Rautaharju PM, Kooperberg C, Larson JC, LaCroix A. Electrocardiographic predictors of incident congestive heart failure and all-cause mortality in postmenopausal women: the Women's Health Initiative. Circulation. 2006;113(4):481–9.
26. Kadish AH, Greenland P, Limacher MC, Frishman WH, Daugherty SA, Schwartz JB. Estrogen and progestin use and the QT interval in postmenopausal women. Ann Noninvasive Electrocardiol. 2004;9(4):366–74.
27. Rivero A, Curtis AB. Sex differences in arrhythmias. Curr Opin Cardiol. 2010;25(1):8–15.
28. Liuba I, Jonsson A, Safstrom K, Walfridsson H. Gender-related differences in patients with atrioventricular nodal reentry tachycardia. Am J Cardiol. 2006;97(3):384–8.
29. Yarnoz MJ, Curtis AB. More reasons why men and women are not the same (gender differences in electrophysiology and arrhythmias). Am J Cardiol. 2008;101(9):1291–6.
30. Tawam M, Levine J, Mendelson M, Goldberger J, Dyer A, Kadish A. Effect of pregnancy on paroxysmal supraventricular tachycardia. Am J Cardiol. 1993;72(11):838–40.
31. Lessmeier TJ, Gamperling D, Johnson-Liddon V, Fromm BS, Steinman RT, Meissner MD, et al. Unrecognized paroxysmal supraventricular tachycardia. Potential for misdiagnosis as panic disorder. Arch Intern Med. 1997;157(5):537–43.
32. Deneke T, Mugge A, Muller P, de Groot JR. Therapeutic implications of gender differences in supraventricular cardiac arrhythmias: lessons of life cannot be learned in a day. Expert Rev Cardiovasc Ther. 2009;7(8):879–82.
33. Benjamin EJ, Wolf PA, D'Agostino RB, Silbershatz H, Kannel WB, Levy D. Impact of atrial fibrillation on the risk of death: the Framingham Heart Study. Circulation. 1998;98(10):946–52.
34. Feinberg WM, Blackshear JL, Laupacis A, Kronmal R, Hart RG. Prevalence, age distribution, and gender of patients with atrial fibrillation. Analysis and implications. Arch Intern Med. 1995;155(5):469–73.
35. Friberg L, Bergfeldt L. Atrial fibrillation prevalence revisited. J Intern Med. 2013;274(5):461–8.
36. Kirchhof P, Benussi S, Kotecha D, Ahlsson A, Atar D, Casadei B, et al. 2016 ESC Guidelines for the management of atrial fibrillation developed in collaboration with EACTS: the task force for the management of atrial fibrillation of the European Society of Cardiology (ESC) developed with the special contribution of the European Heart Rhythm Association (EHRA) of the ESC endorsed by the European Stroke Organisation (ESO). Eur Heart J. 2016;37(38):2893–962.
37. Marijon E, Le Heuzey JY, Connolly S, Yang S, Pogue J, Brueckmann M, et al. Causes of death and influencing factors in patients with atrial fibrillation: a competing-risk analysis from the randomized evaluation of long-term anticoagulant therapy study. Circulation. 2013;128(20):2192–201.
38. Andersson T, Magnuson A, Bryngelsson IL, Frobert O, Henriksson KM, Edvardsson N, et al. Gender-related differences in risk of cardiovascular morbidity and all-cause mortality in patients hospitalized with incident atrial fibrillation without concomitant diseases: a nationwide cohort study of 9519 patients. Int J Cardiol. 2014;177(1):91–9.
39. Dagres N, Nieuwlaat R, Vardas PE, Andresen D, Levy S, Cobbe S, et al. Gender-related differences in presentation, treatment, and outcome of patients with atrial fibrillation in Europe: a report from the Euro Heart Survey on atrial fibrillation. J Am Coll Cardiol. 2007;49(5):572–7.
40. Ko D, Rahman F, Schnabel RB, Yin X, Benjamin EJ, Christophersen IE. Atrial fibrillation in women: epidemiology, pathophysiology, presentation, and prognosis. Nat Rev Cardiol. 2016;13(6):321–32.
41. Piccini JP, Simon DN, Steinberg BA, Thomas L, Allen LA, Fonarow GC, et al. Differences in clinical and functional outcomes of atrial fibrillation in women and men: two-year results from the ORBIT-AF registry. JAMA Cardiol. 2016;1(3):282–91.
42. Chao TF, Liu CJ, Chen SJ, Wang KL, Lin YJ, Chang SL, et al. Atrial fibrillation and the risk of ischemic stroke: does it still matter in patients with a CHA2DS2-VASc score of 0 or 1? Stroke. 2012;43(10):2551–5.
43. Hamaguchi S, Yokoshiki H, Kinugawa S, Tsuchihashi-Makaya M, Yokota T, Takeshita A, et al. Effects of atrial fibrillation on long-term outcomes in patients hospitalized for heart failure in

Japan: a report from the Japanese Cardiac Registry of Heart Failure in Cardiology (JCARE-CARD). Circ J. 2009;73(11):2084–90.
44. Friberg L, Rosenqvist M, Lip GY. Evaluation of risk stratification schemes for ischaemic stroke and bleeding in 182 678 patients with atrial fibrillation: the Swedish Atrial Fibrillation cohort study. Eur Heart J. 2012;33(12):1500–10.
45. Friberg L, Benson L, Rosenqvist M, Lip GY. Assessment of female sex as a risk factor in atrial fibrillation in Sweden: nationwide retrospective cohort study. BMJ. 2012;344:e3522.
46. Emdin CA, Wong CX, Hsiao AJ, Altman DG, Peters SA, Woodward M, et al. Atrial fibrillation as risk factor for cardiovascular disease and death in women compared with men: systematic review and meta-analysis of cohort studies. BMJ. 2016;532:h7013.
47. Nezu T, Hosomi N, Kondo K, Aoki S, Matsumoto M, Kobayashi S, et al. Greater severity of neurological defects in women admitted with atrial fibrillation-related stroke. Circ J. 2016;80(1):250–5.
48. Yoshida K, Obokata M, Kurosawa K, Sorimachi H, Kurabayashi M, Negishi K. Effect of sex differences on the association between stroke risk and left atrial anatomy or mechanics in patients with atrial fibrillation. Circ Cardiovasc Imaging. 2016. PMID: 27729360.
49. Goncalves A, Hung CL, Claggett B, Nochioka K, Cheng S, Kitzman DW, et al. Left atrial structure and function across the spectrum of cardiovascular risk in the elderly: the atherosclerosis risk in communities study. Circ Cardiovasc Imaging. 2016;9(2):e004010.
50. Coutinho T, Borlaug BA, Pellikka PA, Turner ST, Kullo IJ. Sex differences in arterial stiffness and ventricular-arterial interactions. J Am Coll Cardiol. 2013;61(1):96–103.
51. Hsu JC, Maddox TM, Kennedy KF, Katz DF, Marzec LN, Lubitz SA, et al. Oral anticoagulant therapy prescription in patients with atrial fibrillation across the spectrum of stroke risk: insights from the NCDR PINNACLE registry. JAMA Cardiol. 2016;1(1):55–62.
52. Avgil Tsadok M, Gagnon J, Joza J, Behlouli H, Verma A, Essebag V, et al. Temporal trends and sex differences in pulmonary vein isolation for patients with atrial fibrillation. Heart Rhythm. 2015;12(9):1979–86.
53. Shantsila E, Wolff A, Lip GY, Lane DA. Gender differences in stroke prevention in atrial fibrillation in general practice: using the GRASP-AF audit tool. Int J Clin Pract. 2015;69(8):840–5.
54. Roten L, Rimoldi SF, Schwick N, Sakata T, Heimgartner C, Fuhrer J, et al. Gender differences in patients referred for atrial fibrillation management to a tertiary center. Pacing Clin Electrophysiol. 2009;32(5):622–6.
55. Patel D, Mohanty P, Di Biase L, Sanchez JE, Shaheen MH, Burkhardt JD, et al. Outcomes and complications of catheter ablation for atrial fibrillation in females. Heart Rhythm. 2010;7(2):167–72.
56. Rienstra M, Van Veldhuisen DJ, Hagens VE, Ranchor AV, Veeger NJ, Crijns HJ, et al. Gender-related differences in rhythm control treatment in persistent atrial fibrillation: data of the Rate Control Versus Electrical Cardioversion (RACE) study. J Am Coll Cardiol. 2005;46(7):1298–306.
57. Rolden HJ, Grutters JP, van der Wilt GJ, Maas AH. Closing the information gap between clinical and postmarketing trials: the case of dabigatran. Eur Heart J Cardiovasc Pharmacother. 2015;1(3):153–6.
58. Maas AH, Euler M, Bongers MY, Rolden HJ, Grutters JP, Ulrich L, et al. Practice points in gynecardiology: abnormal uterine bleeding in premenopausal women taking oral anticoagulant or antiplatelet therapy. Maturitas. 2015;82(4):355–9.
59. Kannel WB, Wilson PW, D'Agostino RB, Cobb J. Sudden coronary death in women. Am Heart J. 1998;136(2):205–12.
60. Shaw LJ, Bugiardini R, Merz CN. Women and ischemic heart disease: evolving knowledge. J Am Coll Cardiol. 2009;54(17):1561–75.
61. Ripplinger CM, Noujaim SF, Linz D. The nervous heart. Prog Biophys Mol Biol. 2016;120(1–3):199–209.
62. Hart EC, Charkoudian N. Sympathetic neural regulation of blood pressure: influences of sex and aging. Physiology. 2014;29(1):8–15.
63. Whang W, Kubzansky LD, Kawachi I, Rexrode KM, Kroenke CH, Glynn RJ, et al. Depression and risk of sudden cardiac death and coronary heart disease in women: results from the Nurses' Health Study. J Am Coll Cardiol. 2009;53(11):950–8.

64. Kober L, Thune JJ, Nielsen JC, Haarbo J, Videbaek L, Korup E, et al. Defibrillator implantation in patients with nonischemic systolic heart failure. N Engl J Med. 2016;375(13):1221–30.
65. Witt CT, Kronborg MB, Nohr EA, Mortensen PT, Gerdes C, Jensen HK, et al. Adding the implantable cardioverter-defibrillator to cardiac resynchronization therapy is associated with improved long-term survival in ischaemic, but not in non-ischaemic cardiomyopathy. Europace. 2016;18(3):413–9.
66. Sacher F, Meregalli P, Veltmann C, Field ME, Solnon A, Bru P, et al. Are women with severely symptomatic brugada syndrome different from men? J Cardiovasc Electrophysiol. 2008;19(11):1181–5.
67. Jongman JK, Jepkes-Bruin N, Ramdat Misier AR, Beukema WP, Delnoy PP, Oude Lutttikhuis H, et al. Electrical storms in Brugada syndrome successfully treated with isoproterenol infusion and quinidine orally. Neth Hear J. 2007;15(4):151–5.
68. Benito B, Sarkozy A, Mont L, Henkens S, Berruezo A, Tamborero D, et al. Gender differences in clinical manifestations of brugada syndrome. J Am Coll Cardiol. 2008;52(19):1567–73.
69. Rashba EJ, Zareba W, Moss AJ, Hall WJ, Robinson J, Locati EH, et al. Influence of pregnancy on the risk for cardiac events in patients with hereditary long QT syndrome. LQTS investigators. Circulation. 1998;97(5):451–6.
70. Itoh H, Crotti L, Aiba T, Spazzolini C, Denjoy I, Fressart V, et al. The genetics underlying acquired long QT syndrome: impact for genetic screening. Eur Heart J. 2016;37(18):1456–64.
71. Priori SG, Schwartz PJ, Napolitano C, Bloise R, Ronchetti E, Grillo M, et al. Risk stratification in the long-QT syndrome. N Engl J Med. 2003;348(19):1866–74.
72. Makkar RR, Fromm BS, Steinman RT, Meissner MD, Lehmann MH. Female gender as a risk factor for torsades de pointes associated with cardiovascular drugs. JAMA. 1993;270(21):2590–7.
73. Anderson JL, Halperin JL, Albert NM, Bozkurt B, Brindis RG, Curtis LH, DeMets D, Guyton RA, Hochman JS, Kovacs RJ, Ohman EM, Pressler SJ, Sellke FW, Shen WK, Wann LS, Curtis AB, et al. Management of patients with atrial fibrillation (compilation of 2006 ACCF/AHA/ESC and 2011 ACCF/AHA/HRS recommendations): a report of the American College of Cardiology/American Heart Association Task Force on practice guidelines. Circulation. 2013;127(18):1916–26.
74. Frankel DS, Tung R, Santangeli P, Tzou WS, Vaseghi M, Di Biase L, et al. Sex and catheter ablation for ventricular tachycardia: an International Ventricular Tachycardia Ablation Center Collaborative Group Study. JAMA Cardiol. 2016;1(8):938–44.
75. Brunner M, Olschewski M, Geibel A, Bode C, Zehender M. Long-term survival after pacemaker implantation. Prognostic importance of gender and baseline patient characteristics. Eur Heart J. 2004;25(1):88–95.
76. Nowak B, Misselwitz B, Expert committee 'Pacemaker' IoQAH, Erdogan A, Funck R, Irnich W, et al. Do gender differences exist in pacemaker implantation?—results of an obligatory external quality control program. Europace. 2010;12(2):210–5.
77. Russo AM, Poole JE, Mark DB, Anderson J, Hellkamp AS, Lee KL, et al. Primary prevention with defibrillator therapy in women: results from the sudden cardiac death in heart failure trial. J Cardiovasc Electrophysiol. 2008;19(7):720–4.
78. Zareba W, Moss AJ, Jackson Hall W, Wilber DJ, Ruskin JN, McNitt S, et al. Clinical course and implantable cardioverter defibrillator therapy in postinfarction women with severe left ventricular dysfunction. J Cardiovasc Electrophysiol. 2005;16(12):1265–70.
79. Russo AM, Stamato NJ, Lehmann MH, Hafley GE, Lee KL, Pieper K, et al. Influence of gender on arrhythmia characteristics and outcome in the multicenter unsustained tachycardia trial. J Cardiovasc Electrophysiol. 2004;15(9):993–8.
80. Santangeli P, Pelargonio G, Dello Russo A, Casella M, Bisceglia C, Bartoletti S, et al. Gender differences in clinical outcome and primary prevention defibrillator benefit in patients with severe left ventricular dysfunction: a systematic review and meta-analysis. Heart Rhythm. 2010;7(7):876–82.

81. MacFadden DR, Tu JV, Chong A, Austin PC, Lee DS. Evaluating sex differences in population-based utilization of implantable cardioverter-defibrillators: role of cardiac conditions and noncardiac comorbidities. Heart Rhythm. 2009;6(9):1289–96.
82. Curtis LH, Al-Khatib SM, Shea AM, Hammill BG, Hernandez AF, Schulman KA. Sex differences in the use of implantable cardioverter-defibrillators for primary and secondary prevention of sudden cardiac death. JAMA. 2007;298(13):1517–24.
83. Zusterzeel R, Selzman KA, Sanders WE, Canos DA, O'Callaghan KM, Carpenter JL, et al. Cardiac resynchronization therapy in women: US Food and Drug Administration meta-analysis of patient-level data. JAMA Intern Med. 2014;174(8):1340–8.
84. Cheng YJ, Zhang J, Li WJ, Lin XX, Zeng WT, Tang K, et al. More favorable response to cardiac resynchronization therapy in women than in men. Circ Arrhythm Electrophysiol. 2014;7(5):807–15.
85. Ponikowski P, Voors AA, Anker SD, Bueno H, Cleland JG, Coats AJ, et al. 2016 ESC Guidelines for the diagnosis and treatment of acute and chronic heart failure: the task force for the diagnosis and treatment of acute and chronic heart failure of the European Society of Cardiology (ESC) Developed with the special contribution of the Heart Failure Association (HFA) of the ESC. Eur Heart J. 2016;37(27):2129–200.
86. Roelke M, Rubinstein VJ, Kamath S, Krauser D, Ngarmukos T, Parsonnet V. Pacemaker interference with screening mammography. Pacing Clin Electrophysiol. 1999;22(7):1106–7.
87. Paap E, Witjes M, van Landsveld-Verhoeven C, Pijnappel RM, Maas AH, Broeders MJ. Mammography in females with an implanted medical device: impact on image quality, pain and anxiety. Br J Radiol. 2016;89(1066):20160142.

Chapter 11
Cardiac Rehabilitation and Secondary Prevention in Women

Lene Rørholm Pedersen and Eva Prescott

Abstract Physical inactivity is more strongly associated with risk of acute coronary syndromes (ACS) in women than in men. Despite, women and ethnic minorities are less likely to participate in cardiac rehabilitation (CR) programs. Goals for secondary prevention are also less often achieved in women. They also have more depression and anxiety and experience lower quality of life and social support than men. This has an important negative effect on outcomes in ischemic heart disease (IHD). Barriers to CR may be overcome by offering individualized rehabilitation programs that also encompasses home-based cardiac rehabilitation and tele-health based cardiac rehabilitation.

Keywords Cardiac rehabilitation (CR) • Depression • Diet • eHealth • Ethnic minorities • Exercise • Gender bias • Ischemic heart disease (IHD) • Lifestyle • Physical activity • Secondary prevention

Introduction

Secondary prevention is a lifelong process in patients with established cardiovascular disease (CVD). Secondary prevention encompasses participation in a cardiac rehabilitation programme, appropriate medication and lifestyle modification. The effects of such interventions are considerable and have rapid onset: A study following patients after acute coronary syndromes (ACS) found that adaption within the first month after the event of the major recommendations on lifestyle changes (smoking cessation or heart-healthy diet and physical activity), led to an almost 50% reduction in the risk of recurrent events in the next 6 months [1].

L.R. Pedersen, M.D., Ph.D. (✉) • E. Prescott, M.D., D.M.Sc.
Department of Cardiology, Bispebjerg University Hospital, Copenhagen, Denmark
e-mail: lr.pedersen@gmail.com; Eva.Irene.Bossano.Prescott@regionh.dk

A.H.E.M. Maas, C.N. Bairey Merz (eds.), *Manual of Gynecardiology*,
DOI 10.1007/978-3-319-54960-6_11

Recommendations for secondary prevention in women are similar to men, bearing in mind that women overall are older and have more co-morbidity at the time of diagnosing ischemic heart disease (IHD).

Women Participate Less Often in Cardiac Rehabilitation Programmes

Participation in cardiac rehabilitation improves outcome. In a recent meta-analysis comprising 63 studies with almost 15,000 participants and a median follow-up of 12 months, exercise-based cardiac rehabilitation led to 36% reduction in cardiovascular mortality and 18% reduction in risk of hospital re-admission, while the effect on all-cause mortality and ACS was not statistically significant. Also, quality of life was improved [2]. Effects have not been shown to differ between men and women [3, 4]. Cardiac rehabilitation is strongly supported in IHD, chronic heart failure (CHF) and after valve replacement. Unfortunately, uptake is relatively low [3, 5] and even lower in women. This gender difference is seen both in referral and in adherence and is not only explained by women's higher age and greater co-morbidity at the time of presenting with heart disease [5]. A recent meta-analyses comprising 19 observational studies with a total of 241,613 participants found that the participation rate varied hugely from 22 to 74%. Although there was considerable heterogeneity, the overall results indicated that women were 32% less likely to participate in cardiac rehabilitation than their male counterparts [6].

Secondary Prevention Goals Less Often Achieved in Women

Over the latest decades there have been substantial improvements in evidence based intervention post ACS leading to considerably better prognosis in these patients. However, this may not have benefitted men and women equally. The EUROASPIRE (EUROpean Action on Secondary and Primary Prevention through intervention to Reduce Events) survey, which includes data from 24 European countries, has found that whereas pharmacological treatment did not differ between the sexes, women performed worse on the control of most risk factors: women were less likely to have LDL-cholesterol, Hba1C and blood pressure on target, to be non-obese and to perform adequate physical activity. Conversely, men were less likely to be non-smokers and less likely to make dietary changes (Fig. 11.1) [7]. There seemed to be no improvement over time in this gender gap [8]. Similar gender gaps have been reported from the large SWEDEHEART registry [9].

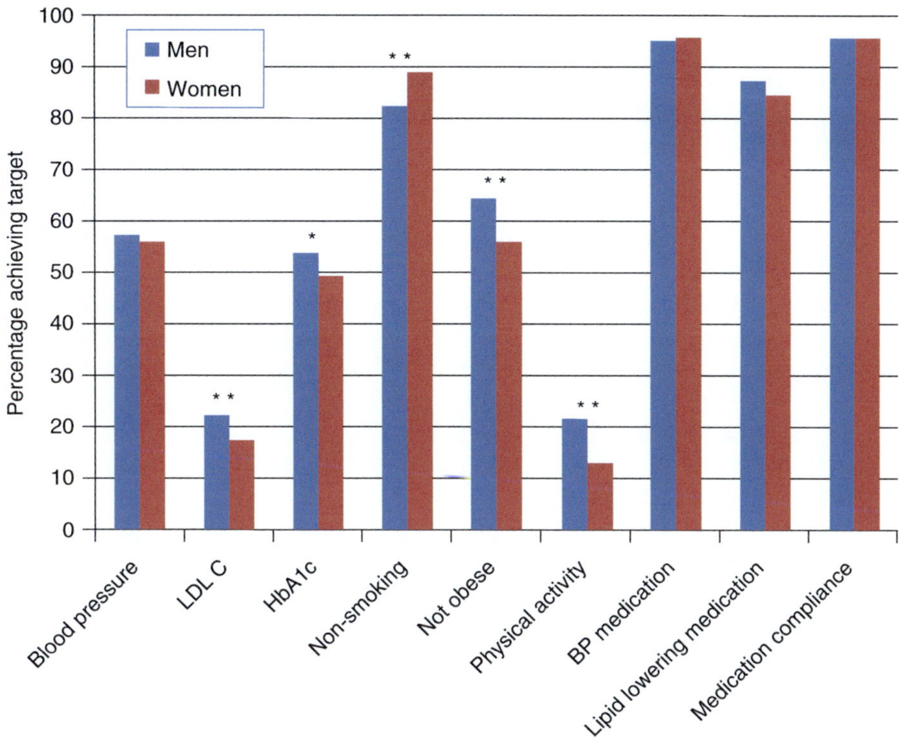

Fig. 11.1 Secondary prevention target achievements among women and men hospitalized for a coronary event in 24 European countries. Data from the EUROASPIRE IV survey, adjusted for age, educational level, index event and country. $^*p < 0.01$, $^{**}p < 0.001$ Data adapted from [7]

Clinical Cases

Case I

Patient

Turkish woman, 67 years referred to cardiac rehabilitation after a non ST elevation ACS 3 months ago. The coronary angiogram showed an 85% mid-LAD stenosis, which was treated with PCI, and diffuse coronary atherosclerosis.

Medical history

Type 2 diabetes

Hypertension

Obesity

Chronic musculoskeletal pain, especially in neck, shoulder and knees after working several years in a cleaning company

Currently

Referral to cardiac rehabilitation has been postponed due to recurrent hospital admissions with chest pain where ACS has been ruled out with normal ECG and normal high-sensitive cardiac troponin. A myocardial scintigraphy has been performed showing no reversible or irreversible ischemia. The patient is sedentary and has never engaged in regular physical activity. After the ACS she rarely leaves the apartment.

Physical exam

Height 163 cm, weight 85 kg, BMI 32 kg/m^2. Waist circumference 97 cm. Blood pressure 150/90 mmHg. Heart rate 62 bpm. No peripheral oedema. Heart auscultation: normal, no murmurs. Lung auscultation: normal, no wheezing.

Laboratory values

Haemoglobin 7.8 mmol/L, LDL 2.3 mmol/L, Hba1c 46 mmol/mol (glucose 7.5 mmol/L).

Echocardiography: LVEF 50%, mild septal hypokinesia, no valvulopathy.

Exercise test: VO_2peak 17.5 mL/kg/min (5 METS).

Other

HADS: score 2 on anxiety, 2 on depression.

Medication

Paracetamol 1 g qid, Metformin 1 g bid, Enalapril 5 mg × sid, Isosorbide mononitrate 60 mg sid, Metoprolol 25 mg bid, Aspirin 75 mg sid, Ticagrelor 90 mg bid, Atorvastatin 40 mg sid.

Comments

This patient has several barriers for physical activity and exercise training since she suffers from musculoskeletal discomfort, is unaccustomed to exercise and still experiences chest pain—though she has no detectable ischaemia. Physical activity should be initiated at low intensity and gradually increased (Fig. 11.2). Resistance training could be added and may relieve her musculoskeletal symptoms. While her diabetes is well-regulated, she is not on target with regard to LDL cholesterol and blood pressure and adjustment of her medical treatment is needed. Due to her overweight and abdominal obesity she should be advised to lose weight and, if available, consult a dietician.

Sociocultural differences in exercise and dietary habits should also be kept in mind and offering a CR program for women may increase likelihood of adherence.

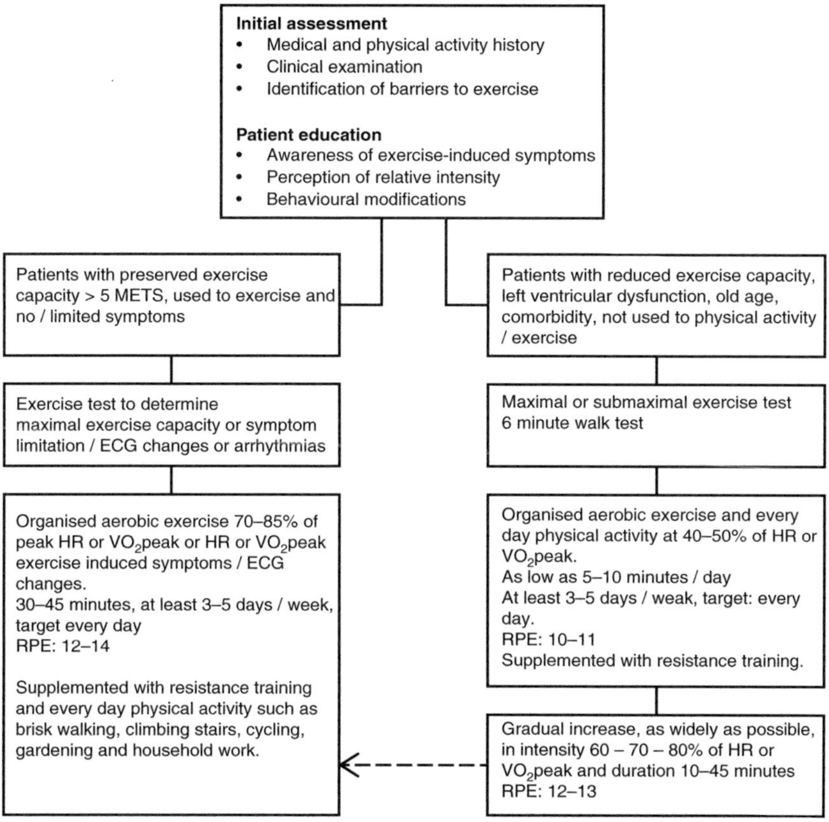

Fig. 11.2 Physical activity and exercise training in patients with CVD referred to cardiac rehabilitation. *METS* metabolic equivalents, *ECG* electrocardiogram, *HR* heart rate, *VO_2peak* peak aerobic capacity, *RPE* rating of perceived exertion/Borg scale. Based on references [10, 14–15]

Case II

Patient

Woman, 42 years, originally referred to cardiac rehabilitation after an ST elevation ACS with revascularization of a 100% LAD stenosis. During the initial hospitalization she was diagnosed with familial hypercholesterolemia with LDL cholesterol of 5.2 mmol/L. A month after the ACS she was re-admitted to hospital after a witnessed out-of-hospital cardiac arrest with ventricular fibrillation and return of spontaneous circulation after 7 min. The CAG showed no new stenosis or stent thrombosis and she had no cognitive deficits. An ICD was implanted as secondary prevention.

She is living with her husband and two children (10 and 13 years old) and has a large social network. Before the ACS she was managing a fulltime job. She had an active life style: Ran 5 km 2–3 times/week and bicycled to work 10 km/day, was a non-smoker and had a BMI 22.3 kg/m^2. Now she is afraid to leave the house and to engage in physical activity for the fear that increasing her heart rate might activate the ICD. She has trouble sleeping and feels tired during the day. Her mood is shifting; she cries and yells at her family "for no reason". She has a hard time accepting her illness since "she was doing all the right things". She does not care about things that used to matter to her.

Physical exam

Weight 65 kg, height 170 cm, BMI 22.5 kg/m^2. Waist circumference 70 cm. Blood pressure 108/88 mmHg. Heart rate 56 bpm. No peripheral oedema. Heart auscultation: normal, no murmurs. Lung auscultation: normal.

Laboratory values

Haemoglobin 8.6 mmol/L, LDL 2.5 mmol/L, Hba1c 45 mmol/mol (glucose 7.4 mmol/L).

Echocardiography: LVEF 45%.

Exercise test: VO_2peak 22.75 mL/kg/min (6.5 METS).

Other

HADS: score 5 on anxiety, 7 on depression.

Medication

Metoprolol 50 mg bid, Enalapril 2.5 mg sid, Atorvastatin 80 mg sid, Aspirin 75 mg sid, Ticagrelor 90 mg bid.

Comments

The patient is young and resourceful with an extensive social network. She was previously healthy and had a healthy lifestyle prior to her ACS. Her LDL-cholesterol has been decreased by >50% but an additional cholesterol-lowering drug (ezetrol) should be considered to further reduce LDL-cholesterol. She has difficulty accepting her illness and shows signs of both anxiety and depression. Though her exercise capacity is reduced after her illness she is used to exercising; however, she is constrained by her fear of inappropriate ICD shock related to exercise.

Initially, supervised exercise sessions can be used to make her feel secure. Adjustment of the ICD and/or training with a heart rate monitor may be appropriate. Exercise at a heart rate 20 bpm below the ICD detection rate has been suggested [10].

A large proportion of cardiac arrest survivors suffer long-term psychological problems such as anxiety. Group-based or individual therapy should be offered to this patient, who also has relatively high HADS scores (Fig. 11.3)

Anxiety	Depression
I feel tense or "wound up" I get a sort of frightened feeling as if something awful is about to happen Worrying thoughts go through my head I can sit at easy and feel relaxed I get a sort of frightened feeling like "butterflies" in the stomach I feel restless as have to be on the move I get sudden feelings of panic	I still enjoy the things I used to enjoy I laugh and see the funny side of things I feel cheerful I feel as if I am slowed down I have lost interest in my appearance I look forward with enjoyment to things I can enjoy a good book or radio or TV program

Fig. 11.3 Hospital Anxiety and Depression Scale (HADS). Each question has graded answers 0–3. The maximal score in each category is 21. Score 0–7 is considered normal, 8–10 borderline abnormal and 11–21 abnormal

Case III

Patient

Woman, 82 years referred to cardiac rehabilitation after recent CABG and biological aortic valve replacement due to symptomatic aortic stenosis.

Medical history

COPD
Type 2 diabetes
Hypertension
Mild renal insufficiency (eGFR 32 mL/min)
Previous gastrointestinal bleeding episode due to angiodysplasia
Myxoedema
Previous hospital admission for depression
Chronic atrial fibrillation

Currently

The patient presents at the outpatient cardiac rehabilitation clinic with her daughter. She complains of dyspnoea, NYHA II, she has no angina, CCS 0.

Her husband, age 90, has dementia and does not leave the home. The patient is the primary caretaker.

Physical exam

Cognitively preserved, height 162 cm, weight 60 kg. BMI 22.9. HR 82 bpm. BP 135/84 mmHg. No peripheral oedema or jugular vein extension. Lung auscultation: normal, no rales or wheezing.

Laboratory values

Haemoglobin 7.6 mmol/L, LDL 1.8 mmol/L, eGFR 32 mL/min, Hba1c 51 mmol/mol (glucose 8.2 mmol/L).

Lung function: FEV_1 64% of predicted.

Echo: LVEF 50%, diastolic dysfunction grade I. The biological valve prosthesis is functioning.

Exercise test: VO_2peak 8.75 mL/kg/min (2.5 METS). Expected for age and gender: 15.7 mL/kg/min.

Other

HADS: score 2 on anxiety, 6 on depression.

Medication

Aspirin 75 mg sid, metoprolol 100 mg sid, metformin 500 mg bid, atorvastatin 80 mg sid, Levothyroxin 100 mcg sid, pantoprazole 20 mg sid, budesonide 320/formoterol 9 mcg bid inh.

Comments

This is a fragile, elderly female patient whose main problem is dyspnea most likely due to the underlying COPD and loss of fitness after a long inactive period prior to and after the operation. She is also at risk of recurrent depression. Her risk factors (cholesterol, blood pressure and diabetes) are under control.

The patient is in need of aerobic and resistance training as well as patient education on the nature of her disease and medication. She is, however, not able to present at the outpatient clinic several times per week because of her husband's illness and therefore prefers no cardiac rehabilitation. Home-based or tele-monitored cardiac rehabilitation could be an option for this patient. She should be offered psychosocial support through individual or group-based therapy and follow-up.

Treatment Options/Advice

Physical Activity

Physical activity and exercise training is central in cardiac rehabilitation. Cardiorespiratory fitness is a strong predictor of cardiac mortality in women with IHD referred for cardiac rehabilitation. For each 1 mL/kg/min increase in initial peak oxygen uptake (VO_2peak) cardiac mortality decreased by 10% [11]. Women have low levels of physical activity which are lower than men. In the EUROASPIRE trial only 31% of women with IHD reported vigorous physical activity for 20 min once or more than once a week while this applied for 43% of men [12]. Physical inactivity is more strongly associated with risk of ACS in women than in men [13]. In order to improve cardiorespiratory fitness aerobic endurance training is recommended [14–15].

Patients referred to cardiac rehabilitation vary considerably with respect to age, co-morbidity, symptoms, readiness to change behaviour, prior training habits and cardiorespiratory fitness as exemplified in the clinical cases. Thus, exercise programmes should be tailored for each participant [10, 14, 15, 16]. Both American and European guidelines stress the importance of an individual risk assessment in patients referred to cardiac rehabilitation based on medical and physical activity history, clinical examination and, if possible, an exercise test to assess exercise capacity and symptoms or arrhythmias related to physical activity [10, 15–16]. Patients with preserved exercise capacity, who are accustomed to physical activity and have no symptoms, can resume every day physical activity and aerobic exercise training at moderate intensity for 30–60 min/day. Otherwise, physical activity should be started at <50% of maximal exercise capacity and gradually increased as widely as possible respecting the patients physical ability as outlined in Fig. 11.2 [10, 14–16]. Resistance training, adapted to the individual patient, can supplement the aerobic exercise training [14, 15].

An assessment of relative intensity can be used to facilitate individualized exercise programmes, by taking into account the patients physical capacity, and to monitor an exercise session [14]. Percentage of maximal heart rate or VO_2peak determined using a cardiopulmonary exercise test is widely used. However, in patients treated with beta-blockers, suffering from chronotropic incompetence or atrial fibrillation, or with a pacemaker heart rate driven exercise may be difficult. In these cases rate of perceived exertion (RPE, Borg Scale [17]) [14].

Weight Loss

Obesity is a modifiable, independent risk factor for CVD [18] and abdominal obesity and visceral adipose tissue in particular, is a predictor of mortality in IHD even at normal range BMI [19]. Premenopausal women tend to accumulate adipose tissue in the hip region and have less visceral adipose tissue than men; however, this differences is diminished after menopause [20]. Weight loss has been demonstrated to improve cardiovascular risk factors such as hypertension, dyslipidemia and insulin resistance. [15] Weight loss or weight maintenance is recommended as secondary prevention in both American and European guidelines and should be obtained by diet, exercise and behaviour modifications aiming at a body mass index between 20 and 25 kg/m^2 and waist circumference <80 cm in women [16, 21].

The beneficial effects of weight loss in secondary prevention of CVD have been debated in relation to the so-called "obesity paradox" suggesting a protective effect of overweight in patients with CVD [22]. However, abdominal obesity and cardiorespiratory fitness may influence the relation between adiposity and prognosis in the obesity paradox [19, 23]. A recent review and meta-analysis [24] distinguishing between intentional weight loss associated with lifestyle changes and observational weight loss with a less well-defined aetiology described in epidemiological studies showed that observational weight loss was associated with more adverse cardiovascular events while intentional weight loss was associated with fewer events.

Diet

The dietary patterns recommended in the European guidelines of CVD prevention resemble the Mediterranean diet. The recommendations are a daily intake of 30–45 g of fibre, preferably from whole grain, 30 g of unsalted nuts, ≥200 g of fruit and ≥200 g of vegetables. In addition, fish 1–2 times/week one of which to be oily fish. Saturated fatty acids should account for <10% of total energy intake and trans unsaturated fatty acids should be avoided. Sugar-sweetened soft drinks should be avoided and alcoholic beverages should be ≤1 glass/day. Women in general are more likely to adhere to a heart-healthy diet than men.

Psychosocial Stress

Women with IHD seem to struggle more with depression and anxiety and experience lower quality of life and social support than men [25]. Lifetime risk of depression is as high as 20% with twice the risk in women compared to men. Among patients with established IHD the prevalence of depression is high although with considerable variation across studies and women again have twice the risk of men of developing depression [26]. IHD patients who develop or have persistent depression or depressive symptoms have poorer outcomes. Meta-analyses indicate a hazard ratio of 1.49 for depressive symptoms and 2.69 for clinical depression [27]. This has been corroborated in registry studies following patients with a diagnosis of depression [26]. The subsequent morbidity and mortality risk associated with depression is similar in men and women but due to the higher prevalence, depression has more impact on female prognosis. Medical treatment of depression has not been shown to improve cardiovascular prognosis perhaps because of the limited effect of the medication and spontaneous recovery. Conversely, the association may partly be explained by lack of lifestyle changes: A study indicated that the excess risk in patients scoring high on depression scales could largely be explained by lack of physical activity [28] and randomized trials have indicated that exercise is efficient treatment of depression while [29] also addressing cardiovascular risk directly. Both the European Society of Cardiology and the American Heart Association guidelines recommend screening and addressing depression in patients with IHD [30].

While clinical depression is universally recognized as a risk factor for IHD and poorer prognosis, the evidence for anxiety is less unequivocal. Recent guidelines have concluded that anxiety is an independent risk factor for development of IHD and for prognosis following development of IHD with relative risk ranging from 1.2 to 1.7. A recent meta-analysis confirmed that anxiety was associated with increased morbidity and mortality risk in patients with IHD with a relative risk of 1.59 based on 13 studies with 9499 patients included. However, the evidence was not as strong as for depression and adjusted analyses indicated that the association was at least partly be explained by confounders [31]. No gender differences were reported in outcome but as for depression, the prevalence of anxiety and panic disorders is twice as high in women as in men with an overall mean of 10% of patients with CVD suffering from anxiety disorders [32].

Persistent exposure to stress may lead to symptoms of burn-out and exhaustion. High levels of self-perceived mental stress over prolonged periods of time was found be associated with increased risk of incident IHD in a meta-analysis of six studies (HR 1.27) [33]. Vital exhaustion is a construct developed by Appels et al. to capture the symptoms of fatigue and depression that were often seen in patients admitted for ACS [34]. Later several prospective studies have confirmed an association between this construct and risk of IHD and CHF with a dose-response relationship. A recent meta-analysis confirmed an adjusted HR of 1.50 (95% CI 1.22–1.85) for developing IHD and of 2.03 (95% CI 1.54–2.68) for recurrent events in patients with IHD. [35] Vital exhaustion seems to be overlapping with the somatic dimension of depression. Similar to depression and anxiety, women score higher on the vital exhaustion scale than men while the excess risk associated with the condition is similar across the two sexes [36, 37].

While medical treatment of depression has been disappointing in terms of improving IHD prognosis, there are several other potential interventions to address these psychosocial stressors. Exercise is one such treatment option. In observational studies more physically active persons score lower on depression and randomized trials have shown effect of structured exercise on depression. In IHD patients, exercise has also been shown to alleviate depressive symptoms in addition to the other well-known beneficial effects of exercise on cardiovascular risk [36, 38, 39]. Structured stress management programmes have been shown to reduce emotional distress and improve a number of cardiovascular risk factors in small studies. An American study of 134 patients with stable IHD found that both stress management and exercise alleviated symptoms and had beneficial effects cardiovascular risk markers when compared to usual care [40]. A randomized Swedish study comparing cognitive behavioural therapy focusing on stress management with conventional care in 372 patients with IHD found a 41% lower rate of recurrent cardiovascular events (P = 0.002) [41]. In a study of 237 women with IHD randomized to a group-based program of relaxation techniques, self-monitoring and cognitive restructuring with an emphasis on self-care and coping with stress exposure from family and work, the intervention was associated with an OR of 0.33 for adverse cardiovascular outcomes [42]. These studies need to be confirmed in larger, multicentre designs.

Addressing Barriers to Cardiac Rehabilitation

Women attend cardiac rehabilitation less often than men, for which there are several reasons. Automated referral seems to overcome bias in referral and diminishes inequality in access to cardiac rehabilitation. However, often the barrier may lie in the patient herself, e.g. due to age, co-morbidity or family and social obligations (as in case III). These barriers may be overcome by offering individualized rehabilitation that also encompasses home-based cardiac rehabilitation and tele-health based cardiac rehabilitation. Home-based cardiac rehabilitation has been shown to be equal to centre-based cardiac rehabilitation in terms of improving clinical and quality of life outcomes while mortality outcomes are not available [43]. Tele-health is a field under rapid development and strong evidence is not yet available. This method of delivering cardiac rehabilitation seems to provide a future option which may ensure high quality individualized cardiac rehabilitation also for patients living in more remote areas, patients with transportation barriers or patients who for other reasons have difficulties in attending centre-based cardiac rehabilitation. Two American studies have shown that cardiac rehabilitation use is lower for racial or ethnic minorities. The reported barriers for participation were driven by finances and reimbursement, misaligned health care priorities and need of the patient and bias in referral. [44, 45] For ethnic minorities general differences in health beliefs, family structure, dietary habits and traditions for leisure-time physical activity especially among women play a major role.

Conclusions

- Women participate less often in CR programmes, due to both referral and patient bias
- Psychosocial distress is twice as common in women as in men and is associated with adverse IHD outcomes
- Women are less likely to achieve most secondary prevention goals than men
- Women are less physically active than men and exercise training should be tailored for each participant.

References

1. Chow CK, Jolly S, Rao-Melacini P, Fox KAA, Anand SS, Yusuf S. Association of diet, exercise, and smoking modification with risk of early cardiovascular events after acute coronary syndromes. Circulation. 2010;121:750–8.
2. Anderson L, Oldridge N, Thompson DR, Zwisler AD, Rees K, Martin N, Taylor RS. Exercise-based cardiac rehabilitation for coronary heart disease. J Am Coll Cardiol. 2016;67:1–12.
3. Doll JA, Hellkamp A, Thomas L, Ho PM, Kontos MC, Whooley MA, Boyden TF, Peterson ED, Wang TY. Effectiveness of cardiac rehabilitation among older patients after acute myocardial infarction. Am Heart J. 2015;170:855–64.
4. Sagar VA, Davies EJ, Briscoe S, Coats AJS, Dalal HM, Lough F, Rees K, Singh S, Taylor RS. Exercise-based rehabilitation for heart failure: systematic review and meta-analysis. Open Heart. 2015;2:e000163.
5. Doll JA, Hellkamp A, Ho PM, Kontos MC, Whooley MA, Peterson ED, Wang TY. Participation in cardiac rehabilitation programs among older patients after acute myocardial infarction. JAMA Intern Med. 2015;175:1700–2.

6. Colella TJ, Gravely S, Marzolini S, Grace SL, Francis JA, Oh P, Scott LB. Sex bias in referral of women to outpatient cardiac rehabilitation? A meta-analysis. Eur J Prev Cardiol. 2015;22:423–41.
7. De Smedt D, De Bacquer D, De Sutter J, Dallongeville J, Gevaert S, De Backer G, Bruthans J, Kotseva K, Reiner Ž, Tokgözoğlu L, Clays E. The gender gap in risk factor control: effects of age and education on the control of cardiovascular risk factors in male and female coronary patients. The EUROASPIRE IV study by the European Society of Cardiology. Int J Cardiol. 2016;209:284–90.
8. Dallongevillle J, De Bacquer D, Heidrich J, De Backer G, Prugger C, Kotseva K, Montaye M, Amouyel P, EUROASPIRE Study Group. Gender differences in the implementation of cardiovascular prevention measures after an acute coronary event. Heart. 2010;96:1744–9.
9. Hambraeus K, Tydén P, Lindahl B. Time trends and gender differences in prevention guideline adherence and outcome after myocardial infarction: data from the SWEDEHEART registry. Eur J Prev Cardiol. 2016;23:340–8.
10. European Association of Cardiovascular Prevention and Rehabilitation Committee for Science Guidelines, EACPR, Corrà U, Piepoli MF, Carré F, Heuschmann P, Hoffmann U, Verschuren M, Halcox J, Document Reviewers, Giannuzzi P, Saner H, Wood D, Piepoli MF, Corrà U, Benzer W, Bjarnason-Wehrens B, Dendale P, Gaita D, McGee H, Mendes M, Niebauer J, Zwisler AD, Schmid JP. Secondary prevention through cardiac rehabilitation: physical activity counselling and exercise training: key components of the position paper from the cardiac rehabilitation section of the European Association of Cardiovascular Prevention and Rehabilitation. Eur Heart J. 2010;31:1967–74.
11. Kavanagh T, Mertens DJ, Hamm LF, Beyene J, Kennedy J, Corey P, Shephard RJ. Peak oxygen intake and cardiac mortality in women referred for cardiac rehabilitation. J Am Coll Cardiol. 2003;42:2139–43.
12. Kotseva K, Wood D, De Bacquer D, De Backer G, Ryden L, Jennings C, Gyberg V, Amouyel P, Bruthans J, Castro Conde A, Cifkova R, Deckers JW, De Sutter J, Dilic M, Dolzhenko M, Erglis A, Fras Z, Gaita D, Gotcheva N, Goudevenos J, Heuschmann P, Laucevicius A, Lehto S, Lovic D, Miličić D, Moore D, Nicolaides E, Oganov R, Pajak A, Pogosova N, et al. EUROASPIRE IV: A European Society of Cardiology survey on the lifestyle, risk factor and therapeutic management of coronary patients from 24 European countries. Eur J Prev Cardiol. 2016;23(6):636–48.
13. Anand SS, Islam S, Rosengren A, Franzosi MG, Steyn K, Yusufali AH, Keltai M, Diaz R, Rangarajan S, Yusuf S. Risk factors for myocardial infarction in women and men: insights from the INTERHEART study. Eur Heart J. 2008;29:932–40.
14. Vanhees L, Rauch B, Piepoli M, van Buuren F, Takken T, Borjesson M, Bjarnason-Wehrens B, Doherty P, Dugmore D, Halle M, Börjesson M, Bjarnason-Wehrens B, Doherty P, Dugmore D, Halle M, Writing Group, EACPR. Importance of characteristics and modalities of physical activity and exercise in the management of cardiovascular health in individuals with cardiovascular disease (Part III). Eur J Prev Cardiol. 2012;19:1333–56.
15. Piepoli MF, Hoes AW, Agewall S, Albus C, Brotons C, Catapano AL, Cooney MT, Corrà U, Cosyns B, Deaton C, Graham I, Hall MS, Hobbs FDR, Løchen M-L, Löllgen H, Marques-Vidal P, Perk J, Prescott E, Redon J, Richter DJ, Sattar N, Smulders Y, Tiberi M, van der Worp HB, van Dis I , Verschuren WMM. 2016 European Guidelines on cardiovascular disease prevention in clinical practice. Eur Heart J. 2016;37(29):2315–81.
16. Smith SC, Benjamin EJ, Bonow RO, Braun LT, Creager MA, Franklin BA, Gibbons RJ, Grundy SM, Hiratzka LF, Jones DW, Lloyd-Jones DM, Minissian M, Mosca L, Peterson ED, Sacco RL, Spertus J, Stein JH, Taubert KA. AHA/ACCF secondary prevention and risk reduction therapy for patients with coronary and other atherosclerotic vascular disease: 2011 update: a guideline from the American Heart Association and American College of Cardiology Foundation World Heart Federation and the Preventive Cardiovascular Nurses Association. J Am Coll Cardiol. 2011;58:2432–46.
17. Borg G. Psychophysical bases of perceived exertion. Med Sci Sports Exerc. 1982;14(5):377–81.

18. Pischon T, Boeing H, Hoffmann K, Bergmann M, Schulze MB, Overvad K, van der Schouw YT, Spencer E, Moons KGM, Tjønneland A, Halkjaer J, Jensen MK, Stegger J, Clavel-Chapelon F, Boutron-Ruault MC, Chajes V, Linseisen J, Kaaks R, Trichopoulou A, Trichopoulos D, Bamia C, Sieri S, Palli D, Tumino R, Vineis P, Panico S, PHM P, May AM, Bueno-de-Mesquita HB, van Duijnhoven FJB, et al. General and abdominal adiposity and risk of death in Europe. N Engl J Med. 2008;359:2105–20.
19. Coutinho T, Goel K, Corrêa de Sá D, Carter RE, Hodge DO, Kragelund C, Kanaya AM, Zeller M, Park JS, Kober L, Torp-Pedersen C, Cottin Y, Lorgis L, Lee SH, Kim YJ, Thomas R, Roger VL, Somers VK, Lopez-Jimenez F. Combining body mass index with measures of central obesity in the assessment of mortality in subjects with coronary disease: role of 'normal weight central obesity'. J Am Coll Cardiol. 2013;61:553–60.
20. Lemieux S, Prud'homme D, Bouchard C, Tremblay A, Després JP, Pud'homme D, Bouchard C, Tremblay A, Despres JP. Sex differences in the relation of visceral adipose tissue accumulation to total body fatness. Am J Clin Nutr. 1993;58:463–7.
21. Mosca L, Benjamin EJ, Berra K, Bezanson JL, Dolor RJ, Lloyd-Jones DM, Newby LK, Pina IL, Roger VL, Shaw LJ, Zhao D, Beckie TM, Bushnell C, D'Armiento J, Kris-Etherton PM, Fang J, Ganiats TG, Gomes AS, Gracia CR, Haan CK, Jackson EA, Judelson DR, Kelepouris E, Lavie CJ, Moore A, Nussmeier NA, Ofili E, Oparil S, Ouyang P, Pinn VW, et al. Effectiveness-based guidelines for the prevention of cardiovascular disease in women—2011 update: a guideline from the American Heart Association. Circulation. 2011;123:1243–62.
22. Romero-Corral A, Montori VM, Somers VK, Korinek J, Thomas RJ, Allison TG, Mookadam F, Lopez-Jimenez F. Association of bodyweight with total mortality and with cardiovascular events in coronary artery disease: a systematic review of cohort studies. Lancet. 2006;368:666–78.
23. Goel K, Thomas RJ, Squires RW, Coutinho T, Trejo-Gutierrez JF, Somers VK, Miles JM, Lopez-Jimenez F. Combined effect of cardiorespiratory fitness and adiposity on mortality in patients with coronary artery disease. Am Heart J. 2011;161:590–7.
24. Pack QR, Rodriguez-Escudero JP, Thomas RJ, Ades PA, West CP, Somers VK, Lopez-Jimenez F. The prognostic importance of weight loss in coronary artery disease: a systematic review and meta-analysis. Mayo Clin Proc. 2014;89:1368–77.
25. Todaro JF, Shen BJ, Niaura R, Tilkemeier PL, Roberts BH. Do men and women achieve similar benefits from cardiac rehabilitation? J Cardpulm Rehabil. 2004;24:45–51.
26. Osler M, Mårtensson S, Wium-Andersen IK, Prescott E, Andersen PK, Jørgensen TSH, Carlsen K, Wium-Andersen MK, Jørgensen MB. Depression after first hospital admission for acute coronary syndrome: a study of time of onset and impact on survival. Am J Epidemiol. 2016;183:218–26.
27. Rugulies R. Depression as a predictor for coronary heart disease: a review and meta-analysis. Am J Prev Med. 2002;23:51–61.
28. Whooley MA, de Jonge P, Vittinghoff E, Otte C, Moos R, Carney RM, Ali S, Dowray S, Na B, Feldman MD, Schiller NB, Browner WS. Depressive symptoms, health behaviors, and risk of cardiovascular events in patients with coronary heart disease. JAMA. 2008;300:2379–88.
29. Cooney G, Dwan K, Mead G. Exercise for depression. JAMA. 2014;311:2432–3.
30. Lichtman JH, Bigger JT, Blumenthal JA, Kaufmann PG, Lespérance F, Mark DB, Sheps DS, Taylor CB, Froelicher ES. Recommendations for screening, referral, and treatment a science advisory from the American Heart Association Prevention Committee of the Council on Cardiovascular Nursing, Council on Clinical Cardiology, Council on Epidemiology and Prevention, and Interdisciplinary Council on Quality of Care and Outcomes Research: endorsed by the American Psychiatric Association. Circulation. 2008;118(17):1768–75.
31. Celano CM, Millstein RA, Bedoya CA, Healy BC, Roest AM, Huffman JC. Association between anxiety and mortality in patients with coronary artery disease: a meta-analysis. Am Heart J. 2015;170:1105–15.
32. Remes O, Brayne C, van der Linde R, Lafortune L. A systematic review of reviews on the prevalence of anxiety disorders in adult populations. Brain Behav. 2016;6:e00497.

33. Richardson S, Shaffer JA, Falzon L, Krupka D, Davidson KW, Edmondson D. Meta-analysis of perceived stress and its association with incident coronary heart disease. Am J Cardiol. 2012;110:1711–6.
34. Appels A, Höppener P, Mulder P. A questionnaire to assess premonitory symptoms of myocardial infarction. Int J Cardiol. 1987;17:15–24.
35. Frestad D, Prescott E. Vital exhaustion and coronary heart disease Risk: a systematic review and meta-analysis. Psychosom Med. 2017;79(3):260–72.
36. Schnohr P, Marott JL, Kristensen TS, Gyntelberg F, Grønbæk M, Lange P, Jensen MT, Jensen GB, Prescott E. Ranking of psychosocial and traditional risk factors by importance for coronary heart disease: the Copenhagen City Heart Study. Eur Heart J. 2015;36:1385–93.
37. Prescott E, Holst C, Grønbaek M, Schnohr P, Jensen G, Barefoot J, Grønbæk M, Schnohr P, Jensen G, Barefoot J, Grønbaek M, Schnohr P, Jensen G, Barefoot J, Grønbæk M, Schnohr P, Jensen G, Barefoot J. Vital exhaustion as a risk factor for ischaemic heart disease and all-cause mortality in a community sample. a prospective study of 4084 men and 5479 women in the Copenhagen City Heart Study. Int J Epidemiol. 2003;32:990–7.
38. Sherwood A, Blumenthal JA, Trivedi R, Johnson KS, O'Connor CM, Adams KF, Dupree CS, Waugh RA, Bensimhon DR, Gaulden L, Christenson RH, Koch GG, Hinderliter AL. Relationship of depression to death or hospitalization in patients with heart failure. Arch Intern Med. 2007;167:367–73.
39. Blumenthal JA, Smith PJ, Hoffman BM. Opinion and evidence: is exercise a viable treatment for depression? ACSM's Heal Fit J. 2012;16:14–21.
40. Blumenthal JA, Sherwood A, Babyak MA, Watkins LL, Waugh R, Georgiades A, Bacon SL, Hayano J, Coleman RE, Hinderliter A. Effects of exercise and stress management training on markers of cardiovascular risk in patients with ischemic heart disease. J Cardpulm Rehabil. 2005;25:235.
41. Gulliksson M, Burelle G, Vessby B, Lundin L, Toss H, Svardsudd K. Randomized controlled trial of cognitive behavioral therapy vs standard treatment to prevent recurrent cardiovascular events in patients with coronary heart disease. Arch Intern Med. 2014;171:134–40.
42. Orth-Gomer K, Schneiderman N, Wang HX, Walldin C, Blom M, Jernberg T. Stress reduction prolongs life in women with coronary disease: the Stockholm Women's Intervention Trial for Coronary Heart Disease (SWITCHD). Circ Cardiovasc Qual Outcomes. 2009;2:25–32.
43. Taylor RS, Dalal H, Jolly K, Zawada A, Dean SG, Cowie A, Norton RJ. Home-based versus centre-based cardiac rehabilitation. Cochrane Database Syst Rev. 2015;1:CD007130.
44. Mead H, Ramos C, Grantham SC. Drivers of racial and ethnic disparities in cardiac rehabilitation use: patient and provider perspectives. Med Care Res Rev. 2016;73:251–82.
45. Mochari H, Lee JR, Kligfield P, Mosca L. Ethnic differences in barriers and referral to cardiac rehabilitation among women hospitalized with coronary heart disease. Prev Cardiol. 2006;9:8–13.

Chapter 12
Stroke and Cognitive Disorder in Women

Mia von Euler

Abstract Women have a higher prevalence of stroke at an older age compared to men. Atrial fibrillation (AF) and diabetes have a higher mortality and stroke risk in women than in men. Migraine with aura is twice to four times as common in women than in men and doubles the risk of stroke. A previous history of preeclampsia is an independent female-specific risk factor for stroke. The use of hormonal therapy (HT) in menopause also increases stroke risk. Women may have more speech difficulties at onset of stroke, which may delay hospital referral. This chapter updates our knowledge on sex- and gender differences in stroke.

Keywords Atrial fibrillation (AF) • Carotid stenosis • CHA2DS2-VASc risk score • Cognitive decline • Dementia • Depression • Hormone replacement therapy (HRT) • Menopause • Migraine • Migraine with aura • Novel oral anticoagulants (NOACs) • Oral contraceptives • Preeclampsia • Stroke • Thrombectomy • Thrombolysis • Traditional risk factors • Transitory ischemic attack (TIA)

Stroke, Definition and Demographics

Stroke is one of the most common causes of death and acquired functional disability world-wide. Globally 15 million persons suffer a stroke each year of which 5 million people die [1]. Women have stroke at an older age compared to men but also have a longer life expectancy resulting in a higher life-time risk and also a higher prevalence of stroke [1, 2]. For many years the stroke incidence has been rising, but lately it has declined in Western Europe, North America and Australia. There are some indications

M. von Euler, M.D., Ph.D.
Department of Clinical Science and Education, Karolinska Institutet Stroke Research Network, Södersjukhuset, Stockholm, Sweden

Section of Neurology, Department of Internal Medicine, Södersjukhuset, Stockholm, Sweden

Department of Clinical Pharmacology, Karolinska University Hospital, Stockholm, Sweden
e-mail: Mia.Von.Euler@ki.se

A.H.E.M. Maas, C.N. Bairey Merz (eds.), *Manual of Gynecardiology*,
DOI 10.1007/978-3-319-54960-6_12

that the risk of stroke is not declining as much in women as in men [3–6]. In developing countries however, stroke incidence continues to rise [1, 7]. The World Health Organization has defined stroke as a "neurological deficit of cerebrovascular cause that persists beyond 24 hours or is interrupted by death within 24 hours" [8]. If the condition lasts less than 24 h it is called a transitory ischemic attack (TIA) [9]. *Ischemic stroke* is the most common stroke type, accounting for 80–85% of all strokes. The incidence is higher in men than in women except for in the oldest age group (>85 years) where most, but not all, studies show a higher prevalence in women [10–17]. When comparing incidence, prevalence, and outcome of stroke age-adjusted rates may mask important differences between men and women due to age. Around 10% of all strokes in an adult population are *intracerebral hemorrhages*. In adults, most, but not all, studies have reported the incidence of intracerebral hemorrhage to be lower in women [11–17]. Ethnic differences have also been reported with White persons having a lower risk than Afro-American , Hispanic or Asian individuals [16]. *Subarachnoidal hemorrhage (SAH)* is the most uncommon type of stroke, comprising 5% of the stroke population. It is commonly characterized by a sudden onset of severe headache. Important risk factors are familiar preponderance (of cerebral aneurysms), hypertension, smoking and alcohol abuse [18]. The risk of subarachnoidal hemorrhage is estimated to be 1.2 times higher in women compared to men, whereby the gender disparity starts at ages above 55 years [18]. Presence and location of cerebral aneurysms have been suggested as an explanation to the higher prevalence of SAH in older women [19, 20]. In younger persons, the risk is higher in men [18]. In Finland and Eastern Europe however, the overall risk is higher in men which may indicate diversity in risk factors among different populations [18]. A meta-analysis has showed the risk of SAH to be somewhat higher in women using combined oral contraceptives and in postmenopausal women [21] (see Fig. 12.1).

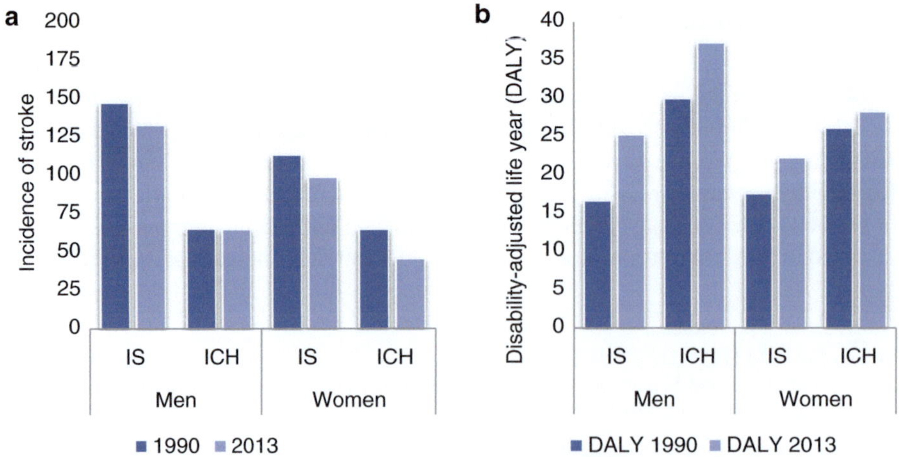

Fig. 12.1 (**a**) The incidence of stroke is higher in men compared to women. The incidence was significantly lower for women in 2013 compared to 1990. As mortality is declining more persons live with a stroke and prevalence has increased. In (**b**) The disability adjusted life year (DALY) is shown and is higher for ICH compared to ischemic stroke with a trend of increasing. Data from the Global burden of disease [24]

Cognitive Disorder, Definition and Demographics

Cognitive impairment is common after stroke and has a great impact on the disability, particularly in the elderly [22]. It has been shown that stroke patients experience an acute decline in global cognition after stroke with a faster course than before [22]. Stroke can lead to dementia but cognitive impairment and dementia itself are also associated with a higher risk of stroke. Stroke rates are threefold higher in individuals with mild dementia and are seven times more likely to occur in persons with severe dementia [23, 24]. Even though there are indications that the incidence of dementia, just as stroke, is declining in developed countries, longer life expectancy has led to an increased prevalence of dementia [25–27]. Dementia is usually divided into Alzheimer disease, for which stroke may precipitate the onset, vascular dementia, usually due to multiple lacunar infarctions, or mixed types [28]. It has been estimated that 5% of the population over 65 years old, and up to 50% by age 90, suffer from dementia [28]. Mild cognitive impairment (MCI) can be the first stage towards dementia and is common in older persons. The prevalence of MCI has been estimated to 10–20% in those above the age of 65 years [29]. Risk increases with age and seems to be lower in women than in men. There are several differential diagnoses such as depression, thyroid disorders, and polypharmacy with adverse events to be considered. Aortic and arterial stiffness and a disturbed cerebral microcirculation have been identified as provoking risk factors [30]. There is no specific treatment for mild cognitive impairment but reducing risk factors for stroke and cardiovascular disease are crucial preventive measures. To minimalize the risk of deterioration of cognitive function regular mental activity and aerobic exercise is recommended, regardless of medical history [29].

Gender Differences in Risk Factors for Stroke

There are a number of risk factors for stroke that are listed in Table 12.1. Many are similar for men and women while some, such as reproductive and hormonal related factors, are unique to women. For some risk factors the risk is higher in women demanding a more intense treatment [31]. Hypertension is an important risk factor for stroke in both men and women [31–33]. In a large meta-analysis including 31 randomized clinical trials (103,268 men and 87,349 women) the effect of blood pressure lowering on reducing the risk of stroke was at least as good in women as in men [34]. Treatment of hypertension and obtaining normal blood pressure is important both in primary and secondary prevention of stroke [32]. Smoking cessation is another of the major behavioral risk modifiers for stroke [32, 33]. Pooled data from meta-analyses found that smoking has a more harmful effect in women compared to men in Western but not in Asian populations [33]. Quitting smoking has comparable beneficial effects in men and women [33] (Tables 12.2, 12.3 and 12.4).

Table 12.1 Primary prevention of stroke/intracranial bleeding

Primary prevention	Ischemic stroke	Intracerebral hemorrhage (ICH)	Subarachnoidal hemorrhage (SAH)
Treat hypertension	X	X	X
No smoking	X	X	X
Avoid alcohol overuse or binge drinking	X	X	X
Treat atrial fibrillation if CHA_2DS_2-Vasc >1	X		
Physical activity	X	X	X
Avoid psychosocial stress	X	X	X
If diabetes mellitus—good metabolic control	X		
Teach FAST or similar	X	X	X

Table 12.2 Acute treatment of stroke/intracranial bleeding

Acute treatment	Ischemic stroke	Intracerebral hemorrhage (ICH)	Subarachnoidal hemorrhage (SAH)
Ambulance transport to hospital	X	X	X
Clinical examination and GCS	X	X	X
NIHSS	X	X	
CT-scan and CT-angio	X	X	X
Thrombolysis if no contraindication	X		
Thrombectomy if large arterial occlusion	X		
Neurosurgery	NA	NA	X

Table 12.3 Secondary prevention after stroke/intracranial bleeding

Secondary prevention			
Secondary preventive treatment	Ischemic stroke	Intracerebral hemorrhage (ICH)	Subarachnoidal hemorrhage (SAH)
Antihypertensives	X	X	X
Antithrombotics	X		
Statins	X		
No smoking	X	X	X
Physical activity	X	X	X
CEA if carotid stenosis within 2 weeks of stroke	X		
No alcohol overuse	X	X	X
Treat depression if needed	X	X	X
Rehabilitation, repeated if needed	X	X	X

Table 12.4 Risk factors for stroke in women compared to men

Risk factor stroke	Sex-specific	Higher risk	More prevalent	Unknown difference
Hypertension			X	
Smoking				X
High age			X	
Atrial fibrillation		X		
Diabetes mellitus		X		
Physical inactivity				X
Migraine with aura			X	
Diet				X
Obesity				X
Metabolic syndrome				X
Depression			X	X
Psychosocial stress			X	X
Pregnancy	X			
Preeclampsia	X			
Gestational diabetes	X			
Oral contraceptive use	X			
HRT	X			

While the number of individuals who smoke and have untreated hypertension is decreasing, the prevalence of obesity is not. In the US 35% of women and 32% of men are currently obese. In many European countries however, obesity and overweight is less common among women compared to men [31, 35, 36]. Avoiding obesity and being physical active lowers the risk for stroke as well as for other manifestations of cardiovascular disease and cognitive impairment. So does a low to moderate alcohol consumption (<1 drink/day in non-pregnant women) and a healthy diet rich in fruit, vegetables, grain and nuts and low in saturated fats [32].

Depression and psychosocial stress are more common in women than in men. In the multinational INTERSTROKE study [31] the increased risk of stroke in persons with self-reported depression and psychosocial stress was 35% in women and 30% in men, after correcting for age. Sex divided analysis was not performed in this study.

Risk Factors with a Higher Risk for Stroke in Women

Atrial fibrillation (AF) is an important risk factor for embolic ischemic stroke. Both prevalence and incidence of AF increases with age and is lower in women compared to men in all age groups [37–39]. The lifetime risk of AF is therefore lower in women [39, 40]. However, women with AF have a higher mortality and intrinsic risk of stroke than men with AF [40, 41], with higher risk of cardiovascular mortality, ischemic cardiac events and heart failure [41]. Estimating the stroke risk using $CHADS_2$-Vasc or $CHADS_2$ should be done in all patients with AF and treatment with anticoagulants encouraged if there are additional stroke risks, such as in women [42]. It should be noted that the novel oral anticoagulants (NOACs) dabigatran, rivaroxaban, and apixaban have been shown to lower the stroke risk similarly to warfarin but with a lower risk of intracranial hemorrhage [43, 44, 45]. To varying degree all these NOACs are excreted through the kidneys, necessitating control of kidney function regularly, particularly in elderly women who in general have a lower kidney function compared to men.

Similarly to AF, diabetes mellitus is also more prevalent in men but it carries a 27% higher risk of stroke in women according to a large meta-analysis [33]. A suggested explanation is that women have more metabolic and vascular disturbances related to their diabetes [33]. Moreover, treatment of diabetes may be less aggressive in women, although improvement has been shown [33, 46].

Migraine and the Risk of Stroke in Women

Migraine is a risk factor of stroke in both men and women, however migraine with aura is twice to four times as common in women and epidemiological studies estimate its prevalence to be around 15% in the female population [47]. Migraine is characterized by a unilateral pulsating headache that may be preceded by focal neurological symptoms such as homonymous visual disturbance, unilateral paraesthesia, numbness or weakness, or speech difficulties. These symptoms, labeled as migraine with aura, may last up to 30 min and occur in almost one third of those suffering migraines. Even though the risk of stroke among persons with migraine is low the risk is more than doubled in persons with migraine accompanied by aura [47]. In smoking women with migraine accompanied by aura the risk of stroke has been shown to be nine times higher than in non-smoking women without migraine with aura. Use of combined oral contraceptives also increases the risk of stroke two- to fourfold in women with migraine accompanied with aura [48]. It has been suggested that premenopausal women with migraine with aura could use progestin-only oral contraceptives, however, the evidence is not fully conclusive yet [48]. Women with migraine headaches with aura should be strongly advised not to smoke and to avoid at least combined oral contraceptives [49]. Triptans, such as sumatriptan, are contraindicated in patients with a previous cerebrovascular disease, as they may induce coronary or cerebrovascular spasm [50]. There is a lack of evidence regarding of the risk of triptan treatment in women having migraine with aura. Considering the elevated risk for stroke it seems sensible to avoid triptan use at least in those who also smoke, use oral contraceptives or have other stroke risk factors.

Female-Specific Risk Factors for Stroke

Use of Hormonal Therapy

A Cochrane analysis from 2015 of hormonal replacement therapy (HRT) and prevention of cardiovascular disease found an increased risk of stroke for women on HRT, applying for both primary and secondary prevention [51]. The relative risk was 1.26 with a calculated number needed to harm (NNH) of 164 patients. Similar results, with an increased risk of ischemic stroke for women with postmenopausal HRT of combined estrogen and progesterone or estrogen therapy alone were found in another meta-analysis [52]. There is some evidence that the timing of HRT may be important and that a lower risk is found if hormonal therapy is started soon after the onset of menopause and continued during a shorter period of time [53]. However, the evidence is not yet conclusive and in women at increased risk of stroke HRT is not recommended.

Use of Oral Contraceptives

The risk of stroke in women using oral contraceptives (OC) seems to be slightly elevated, at least for ischemic stroke. Several meta-analyses have found the risk to be almost doubled if combined OCs are used but no increased risk has been found with progesterone only [54, 55]. A large Danish study found the risk to be somewhat lower [56]. Data on the risk of hemorrhagic stroke are not consistent. An elevated risk for OC us for all stroke types has been reported in women with hypertension who also smoke cigarettes. Older age and migraine are other risk factors to be considered [57, 58]. A Dutch study found that women with other risk factors of cardiovascular disease, such as hypercholesterolemia and obesity, had an increased risk in combination with OC use [59]. In the presence of pro-thrombotic genetic mutations such as factor V Leiden, methyl tetrahydrofolate reductase (resulting in folic acid deficiency), and especially for lupus anticoagulant the risk of stroke has been shown to increase with use of OC [60, 61]. Migraine with aura is a risk for stroke and in women who smoke, OC use should be avoided as the risk of stroke has been shown to be sevenfold higher, although in non-smoking women the adverse risk of OC use is debated [49].

Pregnancy and Stroke

Stroke is very rare in pregnancy but the risk of stroke is elevated, particularly in the last trimester and in the puerperium [31]. This is caused by physiological changes with venous stasis, edema, and a hypercoagulability state due to increased protein C resistance, lower levels of protein S and higher levels of fibrinogen. Preeclampsia/eclampsia and pregnancy-induced hypertension are the most common causes to both ischemic and hemorrhagic stroke in pregnancy and should be well controlled. Labetalol is often used to lower blood pressure, but the evidence for optimal medical treatment is still weak [31]. Based on a 2013 Cochrane analysis nimodipine, diazoxide and ketanserin should be avoided as well as magnesium sulphate, if not required as an anticonvulsant [62]. Evidence for optimal pharmacologic treatment of mild to moderate hypertension during pregnancy is debated [63, 64]. It should be noted that preeclampsia/eclampsia are risk factors of future stroke, with a twofold higher risk compared to women with uncomplicated pregnancies [65]. The risk is particularly high in early-onset preeclampsia where a fivefold increased risk has been reported [31, 65]. A Cochrane review from 2014, including results from 12 trials in 15,730 women, found calcium supplementation of ≥1 g/d to reduce the risk of pre-eclampsia, particularly for women with low calcium diets [66]. The WHO recommends supplementation with calcium for women with low dietary intake [67]. Another preventive measure to lower the risk of preeclampsia can be treatment with a platelet inhibitor. A Cochrane review of 46 trials with preventive use of a platelet inhibitor, mostly low dose aspirin, in 32,891 women at risk for preeclampsia found a relative risk of 0.83 with a number needed to treat (NNT) of 72 in favor of treatment [68].

A clinical problem in pregnant women with stroke is their treatment. It is unknown whether thrombolysis is safe during pregnancy in the postpartum period [31]. Pregnant women have been excluded from all randomized trials and the actual number of affected women is very low. A publication from the US found similar rates of acute stroke reperfusion therapy in women during pregnancy or postpartum vs non-pregnant women, although non-pregnant women were more likely to receive intravenous recombinant tissue plasminogen activator (rt-PA) monotherapy than thrombectomy [69]. The data showed a trend toward increased symptomatic intracranial hemorrhage in pregnancy or thereafter with rt-PA but no cases of major systemic bleeding or in-hospital death occurred. Compared to the non-pregnant women, those who were (recently) pregnant had fewer risk factors for stroke and were younger. In spite of having more severe strokes at onset, they had a similar rate of discharge to home.

Cerebral Venous Thrombosis in Women

A very uncommon cause, about 0.5–1% of all strokes, is when thrombus formation in at least one of the venous sinuses causes a cerebral venous thrombosis. This condition is much more common in women than in men with a predominance of 70–75%. Headache is the predominant symptom, sometimes combined with nausea and psychiatric symptoms. The most common risk factor for cerebral venous thrombosis is pregnancy/puerperium. Other risk factors are dehydration, infections, trauma, oral contraceptives, recent neurosurgical procedures and myeloproliferative neoplasms. The recommended treatment is heparin or low-molecular heparin to dissolve the thrombus followed by oral anticoagulants. At present none of the NOACs have been approved for this indication. The condition can be difficult to diagnose. The prognosis, if treated correctly, has been shown to be good with full recovery in the vast majority of patients [70, 71].

Clinical Setting of Acute Stroke in Women

In clinical practice the primary concern is to identify stroke and to transport the patient as fast as possible to the hospital. The earlier the patients arrive, the higher the chance of treatment success. As women in general are older at the time of an acute stroke than men, they are more dependent on others in their surrounding for contacting emergency medical services. This is not unique to women, but as many elderly women live alone, it is important that the general public is well aware of the signs and symptoms of stroke to ensure correct and immediate help when needed. In some studies it is suggested that women suffer more speaking difficulties in the acute phase of stroke, which complicates the possibility to get help [72–75].

Thrombolysis with rt-PA for acute ischemic stroke has been shown to be as effective in women as in men [76–80]. In pregnant women having an acute ischemic stroke, however, the choice of thrombolysis or not and the safety of mother and child is a difficult question for which good evidence is lacking [31]. Thrombectomy only could then be an alternative in large vessel occlusion. Secondary preventive medication for elevated blood pressure in all strokes and anti-thrombotics and statins in ischemic stroke has good evidence to prevent recurrent stroke or other cardiovascular morbidity in both women and men. However, adherence to guidelines has been shown to be modest in numerous publications. Use of Stroke Unit care has been shown to be equally effective in women and men and effective regardless of age [81]. Adherence for statins seems to be lower in women although treatment is equally effective in prevention of cardiovascular disease in both sexes and for stroke maybe even more pronounced in women [82]. Rehabilitation to regain lost function after stroke is imperative. Even though many women are older, the need of rehabilitation needs to be evaluated and met if possible. After stroke, HRT and oral contraceptives are usually discouraged as the risk of recurrent stroke increases [31].

Diagnostic Pathway in Women with Stroke

Symptoms of stroke depend on which and how large part of the brain is affected by the impaired circulation. Sudden onset of hemiparesis and speech impairment are classical symptoms of stroke that have been used in many campaigns to raise awareness of stroke. There are studies finding that women to have more speech disturbances than men [73], while others find no difference [74]. Altered mental state is more frequently described for women than for men [75, 76]. This can make it more difficult to identify stroke and may delay presentation at hospital. With the availability of more effective treatments of stroke that are highly time dependent identification of stroke and immediate care has become even more important. It has been shown that pre-hospital identification of acute stroke increases the possibility of early acute treatment and better outcomes. The chance of having thrombolysis is higher for patients arriving as "stroke alarms" to the emergency department [77–80]. Very few stroke patients call the emergency services themselves and importantly depend on family or other bystanders for help [74, 76].

Diagnostic evaluation is the same in men and women. Neuroimaging of the brain should be performed as soon as possible in the acute phase to distinguish between ischemic or hemorrhagic stroke. CT-scan is extremely sensitive in detecting hemorrhage. Early after ischemic stroke onset, a CT scan of the brain may appear to be normal. Diffusion weighted MRI is more sensitive in spotting early ischemic changes. If there is a large vessel occlusion, as can be detected by CT or MRI angiography, thrombectomy can be useful. An angiography can also show vascular malformations causing hemorrhagic stroke and is thus indicated regardless of stroke type. Imaging of carotid arteries and detection of AF with ECG or long term ECG-monitoring should also be done to determine a potential cause of stroke and to apply optimal treatment. In both women and men, with significant symptomatic carotid stenosis, suspected of causing an ischemic stroke or TIA, carotid end artery surgery is recommended within 2 weeks of the event [83]. The perioperative risk seems to be comparable in men and women [84]. There is limited data on how to treat asymptomatic carotid stenosis, i.e. a carotid stenosis that had not yet caused a TIA or ischemic stroke [85]. Improvement of "best medical treatment", particularly with the introduction of statins, has made it difficult to rely on results of the old, large asymptomatic carotid stenosis studies. While both men and women with stenosis progression are at increased risk of ipsilateral stroke, the degree of stenosis and presence of irregular plaque surface increases the stroke risk only in men but not in women [86]. For cognitive assessment the Montreal Cognitive Assessment (MoCA) test is easy to administer and is validated in stroke patients with a high sensitivity and specificity [87, 88].

Two Clinical Cases

I. The patient is a non-smoking widowed woman in her early 80s. She has mild cognitive impairment but manages herself with some help from her daughter and daily visits from home care. She used to be an avid walker but feels her balance is a bit impaired and she rarely gets out anymore. She recently had a TIA and although the ECG at the emergency room did not reveal anything abnormal, long term ECG shows several episodes of AF with duration of 1–2 min each. After the TIA she started with an ACE-inhibitor, platelet inhibitor and a statin daily. She tolerates the medication well and it works easy with the new dosing aid her daughter gave her. Her blood pressure is 135/85 mmHg. Electrolytes levels are normal, creatinine is 95 umol/L with a reduced creatinine clearance of 35 mL/min.

There is a strong indication for permanent oral anticoagulant treatment. A mild cognitive impairment is no contraindication, particularly when medication adherence is well with the dosing aid. The platelet inhibitor is exchanged for a NOAC, which can be kept in the dosing aid. Due to her rather low creatinine clearance, the NOAC with the least renal excretion is chosen. Physical activity is important. A walking aid would make her feel more confident and prone to take walks and get out of the house.

II. A 43 year old woman is presented in the emergency room with headache, a dull ache on the left of her neck that has been present since a hiking trip 3 days prior to admission. She has had several episodes of numbness and motor dysfunction in her right arm, combined with some slight speech difficulties during the last 2 days. Her blood pressure is slightly elevated, 150/90 mmHg, normal laboratory measures, no fever and a normal neurological, pulmonal and cardiac status. She uses oral contraceptives in order to regulate the heavy periods she suffered all her life but no other medication. She smokes, a couple of cigarettes a day but has an otherwise healthy lifestyle.

The patient history makes repeated TIAs due to a dissection of the left carotid artery a preliminary diagnosis. Although rare, in younger persons, dissection is the second most common cause of stroke. It may be due to trauma but can also occur without any obvious trauma. The prognosis is good if emboli can be avoided. The diagnosis is made by CAT scan with angiography, MRI with angiography or by ultrasound. Radiology is often used for acute diagnosis, if the healing process is wished to be monitored, ultrasound may be a good alternative avoiding unnecessary radiation.

Treatment for a dissected carotid artery consist of antithrombotic treatment either with anti-platelet therapy or with vitamin K antagonists. There is no evidence at present suggesting the superiority of either [84]. Due to the patient's heavy periods, that likely will increase with vitamin K antagonists and cessation of OC, temporary antithrombotic treatment with a platelet inhibitor is chosen to avoid even heavier menstrual bleeding. Many dissections heal spontaneously over a couple of months. Advised is to monitor the healing of the dissection and if so to consider discontinuation of antithrombotic treatment after a couple of months.

Treatment Advice for TIA/Stroke

Primary Prevention

Primary prevention of stroke includes healthy lifestyle habits such as not smoking and being physical active. As smoking women might be of even higher risk of stroke than their male counterparts this issue should be underscored. Detection and control of hypertension is essential. An important aspect in elderly women is the presence of AF. In a Swedish study screening for AF with intermittent ECG recordings in 75–76 year-old individuals found that 5% of the screened population had untreated AF [37]. As the risk of stroke in women with AF is high and the strokes that results from AF are often extensive this is of great importance. Another group in which preventive measures are exceedingly important are women with previous pre-eclampsia who may be a potential high risk group for stroke [31].

Acute Treatment

Acute treatment of ischemic stroke has changed dramatically recently. The earlier treatment can be started the more effective it is. Thrombolysis with the rt-PA has good results if given within 4.5 h of stroke-onset in patients without contraindications [89, 90]. Studies have also shown the effect in elderly over 80 years [91]. Several studies have shown that women are less often treated than men [92], despite comparable effectiveness of treatment in women as in men [76–78, 93]. The dosage is weight based which might explain why the risk of adverse events such as intracranial hemorrhage is equally common in men and women, occurring in 4–5% of all treated [91] and there are even studies showing trends towards a lower risk [77, 79]. For patients with large artery occlusion strokes thrombolysis is seldom enough to achieve adequate reperfusion. Thrombectomy with stent retrievers have been shown to be very effective in several randomized trials [80]. As with thrombolysis, the earlier after stroke onset the treatment is started, the better prognosis. The chance of a good functional outcome is more than doubled if treatment can be started within 6 h of stroke onset, often after thrombolysis has been given. The importance of 'time' makes it immensely important to be referred to hospital immediately, preferably as a 'stroke alarm' in the ambulance [94–96].

In patients treated with thrombolysis alone or combined thrombolysis/thrombectomy, a control CT-scan should be performed 24 h after treatment to ensure no bleeding complications have occurred. A platelet inhibitor should then be started. In patients without reperfusion treatment, a platelet inhibitor should be started as soon as a CT scan has ruled out an intracerebral hemorrhage. The platelet inhibitor Aspirin has been shown to be very effective in early treatment of ischemic stroke and should not be delayed [97]. In patients with dysphagia rectal administration of acetyl salicylic acid can be used [98].

Treatment in a stroke unit has been shown to increase the chance of better outcomes and all stroke patients, regardless of age or sex, and in the current era all stroke patients should be offered this possibility [99]. There is at present no specific therapeutic treatment of intracerebral hemorrhages in general beside stroke unit care and blood pressure lowering. Lowering elevated blood-pressure in the acute phase to at least 140–160 mmHg has beneficial evidence in both men and women [100].

Secondary Prevention

The risk of recurrent stroke is considerable and it is therefore imperative to provide optimal secondary prevention. Lifestyle parameters such as not smoking, moderate alcohol-use, and regular physical activity are of great importance regardless of stroke type [32]. Adequate antihypertensive treatment and follow up is also required. In ischemic stroke or TIA, when no source of cardiac emboli is present, prolonged anti-platelet therapy is recommended [101–103]. After embolic ischemic stroke or TIA vitamin K antagonists are strongly recommended. Statin use in women for primary prevention has been debated, for secondary prevention however there are strong recommendations [102, 103]. Patients having a significant symptomatic carotid stenosis are recommended to have surgery for this within 2 weeks, regardless of sex and age as long as the patient has at least a couple of years estimated survival [104].

Conclusions

- Women have similar traditional risk factors for stroke as men. However, women also have sex-specific risks connected with pregnancy/puerperium, use of OC and HRT.
- Although AF and diabetes are less prevalent in women, the risk of stroke is higher and preventive treatment needs to be tailored for women.
- In women with multiple risk factors of stroke including hypertension, migraine with aura, smoking and obesity, the risk of stroke is increased with use of combined OC or HRT.
- Acute treatment of ischemic stroke with thrombolysis/thrombectomy is time-dependent and at least as effective in women as in men
- Adherence to medication in secondary prevention should be encouraged more in women to avoid recurrent stroke.

References

1. Arnao V, Acciarresi M, Cittadini E, Caso V. Stroke incidence, prevalence and mortality in women worldwide. Int J Stroke. 2016;11:287–301.
2. Seshadri S, Beiser A, Kelly-Hayes M, Kase CS, Au R, Kannel WB, Wolf PA. The lifetime risk of stroke: estimates from the Framingham study. Stroke. 2006;37:345–50.
3. Kolominsky-Rabas PL, Wiedmann S, Weingärtner M, Liman TG, Endres M, Schwab S, Buchfelder M, Heuschmann PU. Time trends in incidence of pathological and etiological stroke subtypes during 16 years: the Erlangen Stroke Project. Neuroepidemiology. 2015;44(1):24–9.
4. Carandang R, Seshadri S, Beiser A, Kelly-Hayes M, Kase CS, Kannel WB, Wolf PA. Trends in incidence, lifetime risk, severity, and 30-day mortality of stroke over the past 50 years. JAMA. 2006;296:2939–46.

5. Heuschmann PU, Grieve AP, Toschke AM, Rudd AG, Wolfe CD. Ethnic group disparities in 10-year trends in stroke incidence and vascular risk factors: the South London Stroke Register (SLSR). Stroke. 2008;39:2204–10.
6. Wieberdink RG, Ikram MA, Hofman A, Koudstaal PJ, Breteler MM. Trends in stroke incidence rates and stroke risk factors in Rotterdam, the Netherlands from 1990 to 2008. Eur J Epidemiol. 2012;27:287–95.
7. Rosengren A, Giang KW, Lappas G, Jern C, Torén K, Björck L. Twenty-four-year trends in the incidence of ischemic stroke in Sweden from 1987 to 2010. Stroke. 2013;44:2388–93.
8. World Health Organisation. Cerebrovascular disorders (offset publications). Geneva: World Health Organization; 1978. isbn:978-92-4-170043-2.
9. Easton JD, Saver JL, Albers GW, Alberts MJ, Chaturvedi S, Feldmann E, Hatsukami TS, Higashida RT, Johnston SC, Kidwell CS, Lutsep HL, Miller E, Sacco RL, American Heart Association, American Stroke Association Stroke Council, Council on Cardiovascular Surgery and Anesthesia, Council on Cardiovascular Radiology and Intervention, Council on Cardiovascular Nursing, Interdisciplinary Council on Peripheral Vascular Disease. Definition and evaluation of transient ischemic attack: a scientific statement for healthcare professionals from the American Heart Association/American Stroke Association Stroke Council; Council on Cardiovascular Surgery and Anesthesia; Council on Cardiovascular Radiology and Intervention; Council on Cardiovascular Nursing; and the Interdisciplinary Council on Peripheral Vascular Disease. The American Academy of Neurology affirms the value of this statement as an educational tool for neurologists. Stroke. 2009;40:2276–93.
10. Petrea RE, Beiser AS, Seshadri S, Kelly-Hayes M, Kase CS, Wolf PA. Gender differences in stroke incidence and poststroke disability in the Framingham heart study. Stroke. 2009;40:1032–7.
11. Rothwell PM, Coull AJ, Silver LE, Fairhead JF, Giles MF, Lovelock CE, Redgrave JN, Bull LM, Welch SJ, Cuthbertson FC, Binney LE, Gutnikov SA, Anslow P, Banning AP, Mant D, Mehta Z. Population-based study of event-rate, incidence, case fatality, and mortality for all acute vascular events in all arterial territories (Oxford Vascular Study). Lancet. 2005;366:1773–83.
12. Haberman S, Capildeo R, Rose FC. Sex differences in the incidence of cerebrovascular disease. J Epidemiol Community Health. 1981;35:45–50.
13. Nilsson OG, Lindgren A, Ståhl N, Brandt L, Säveland H. Incidence of intracerebral and subarachnoid haemorrhage in southern Sweden. J Neurol Neurosurg Psychiatry. 2000;69:601–7.
14. Jacobs BS, Boden-Albala B, Lin IF, Sacco RL. Stroke in the young in the Northern Manhattan Stroke Study. Stroke. 2002;33:2789–93.
15. Appelros P, Jonsson F, Asplund K, Eriksson M, Glader EL, Asberg KH, Norrving B, Stegmayr B, Terént A, Riks-Stroke Collaboration. Trends in baseline patient characteristics during the years 1995–2008: observations from risk-stroke, the Swedish Stroke Register. Cerebrovasc Dis. 2010;30:114–9.
16. Go AS, Mozaffarian D, Roger VL, et al. Heart disease and stroke statistics – 2013 update: a report from the American Heart Association. Circulation. 2013;127:e6–e245.
17. Mendis S. Prevention and care of stroke in low- and middle-income countries; the need for a public health perspective. Int J Stroke. 2010;5:86–91.
18. de Rooij NK, Linn FH, van der Plas JA, Algra A, Rinkel GJ. Incidence of subarachnoid haemorrhage: a systematic review with emphasis on region, age, gender and time trends. J Neurol Neurosurg Psychiatry. 2007;78:1365–72.
19. Kleindorfer D, Broderick J, Khoury J, Flaherty M, Woo D, Alwell K, Moomaw CJ, Schneider A, Miller R, Shukla R, Kissela B. The unchanging incidence and case-fatality of stroke in the 1990s: a population-based study. Stroke. 2006;37:2473–8.
20. Wardlaw JM, White PM. The detection and management of unruptured intracranial aneurysms. Brain. 2000;123:205–21.
21. Algra AM, Klijn CJ, Helmerhorst FM, Algra A, Rinkel GJ. Female risk factors for subarachnoid hemorrhage: a systematic review. Neurology. 2012;79:1230–6.

22. Levine DA, Galecki AT, Langa KM, Unverzagt FW, Kabeto MU, Giordani B, Wadley VG. Trajectory of cognitive decline after incident stroke. JAMA. 2015;314:41–51.
23. Liebetrau M, Steen B, Skoog I. Stroke in 85-year-olds: prevalence, incidence, risk factors, and relation to mortality and dementia. Stroke. 2003;34:2617–22.
24. Zhu L, Fratiglioni L, Guo Z, Winblad B, Viitanen M. Incidence of stroke in relation to cognitive function and dementia in the Kungsholmen project. Neurology. 2000;54:2103–7.
25. Feigin VL, Krishnamurthi RV, Parmar P, et al. Update on the global burden of ischemic and hemorrhagic stroke in 1990–2013: the GBD 2013 study. Neuroepidemiology. 2015;45:161–76.
26. Wu YT, Fratiglioni L, Matthews FE, et al. Dementia in Western Europe: epidemiological evidence and implications for policy making. Lancet Neurol. 2016;15:116–24.
27. Satizabal CL, Beiser AS, Chouraki V, Chene G, Dufouil C, Seshadri S. Incidence of dementia over three decades in the Framingham Heart Study. N Engl J Med. 2016;374:523–32.
28. Snowdon DA, Greiner LH, Mortimer JA, Riley KP, Greiner PA, Markesbery WR. Brain infarction and the clinical expression of Alzheimer disease. The Nun Study. JAMA. 1997;277:813–7.
29. Langa KM, Levine DA. The diagnosis and management of mild cognitive impairment: a clinical review. JAMA. 2014;312:2551–61.
30. Cooper LL, Woodard T, Sigurdsson S, van Buchem MA, Torjesen AA, Inker LA, Aspelund T, Eiriksdottir G, Harris TB, Gudnason V, Launer LJ, Mitchell GF. Cerebrovascular damage mediates relations between aortic stiffness and memory. Hypertension. 2016;67:176–82.
31. Bushnell C, McCullough LD, Awad IA, Chireau MV, Fedder WN, Furie KL, Howard VJ, Lichtman JH, Lisabeth LD, Piña IL, Reeves MJ, Rexrode KM, Saposnik G, Singh V, Towfighi A, Vaccarino V, Walters MR, American Heart Association Stroke Council, Council on Cardiovascular and Stroke Nursing, Council on Clinical Cardiology, Council on Epidemiology and Prevention, Council for High Blood Pressure Research. Guidelines for the prevention of stroke in women: a statement for healthcare professionals from the American Heart Association/American Stroke Association. Stroke. 2014;45:1545–88.
32. O'Donnell MJ, Xavier D, Liu L, Zhang H, Chin SL, Rao-Melacini P, Rangarajan S, Islam S, Pais P, McQueen MJ, Mondo C, Damasceno A, Lopez-Jaramillo P, Hankey GJ, Dans AL, Yusoff K, Truelsen T, Diener HC, Sacco RL, Ryglewicz D, Czlonkowska A, Weimar C, Wang X, Yusuf S, INTERSTROKE Investigators. Risk factors for ischaemic and intracerebral haemorrhagic stroke in 22 countries (the INTERSTROKE study): a case-control study. Lancet. 2010;376:112–23.
33. Peters SA, Huxley RR, Woodward M. Smoking as a risk factor for stroke in women compared with men: a systematic review and meta-analysis of 81 cohorts, including 3,980,359 individuals and 42,401 strokes. Stroke. 2013;44:2821–8.
34. Turnbull F, Woodward M, Neal B, Barzi F, Ninomiya T, Chalmers J, Perkovic V, Li N, MacMahon S, Blood Pressure Lowering Treatment Trialists' Collaboration. Do men and women respond differently to blood pressure-lowering treatment? Results of prospectively designed overviews of randomized trials. Eur Heart J. 2008;29(21):2669–80.
35. Neovius M, Janson A, Rössner S. Prevalence of obesity in Sweden. Obes Rev. 2006;7:1–3.
36. Giampaoli S, Palmieri L, Donfrancesco C, Lo Noce C, Pilotto L, Vanuzzo D, Osservatorio Epidemiologico Cardiovascolare/Health Examination Survey Research Group. Cardiovascular health in Italy. Ten-year surveillance of cardiovascular diseases and risk factors: Osservatorio Epidemiologico Cardiovascolare/Health Examination Survey 1998-2012. Eur J Prev Cardiol. 2015;22:9–37.
37. Friberg L, Bergfeldt L. Atrial fibrillation prevalence revisited. J Intern Med. 2013;274(5):461–8.
38. Go AS, et al. Prevalence of diagnosed atrial fibrillation in adults: national implications for rhythm management and stroke prevention: the Anticoagulation and Risk Factors in Atrial Fibrillation (ATRIA) study. JAMA. 2001;285:2370–5.
39. Heeringa J, et al. Prevalence, incidence and lifetime risk of atrial fibrillation: the Rotterdam study. Eur Heart J. 2006;27(8):949–53.

40. Michelena HI, Powell BD, Brady PA, Friedman PA, Ezekowitz MD. Lifetime risk for development of atrial fibrillation: the Framingham Heart Study. Circulation. 2004;110:1042–6.
41. Emdin CA, Wong CX, Hsiao AJ, Altman DG, Peters SA, Woodward M, Odutayo AA. Atrial fibrillation as risk factor for cardiovascular disease and death in women compared with men: systematic review and meta-analysis of cohort studies. BMJ. 2016;53:h7013.
42. Kirchhof P, Benussi S, Kotecha D, Ahlsson A, Atar D, Casadei B, Castella M, Diener HC, Heidbuchel H, Hendriks J, Hindricks G, Manolis AS, Oldgren J, Popescu BA, Schotten U, Van Putte B, Vardas P, Agewall S, Camm J, Baron Esquivias G, Budts W, Carerj S, Casselman F, Coca A, De Caterina R, Deftereos S, Dobrev D, Ferro JM, Filippatos G, Fitzsimons D, Gorenek B, Guenoun M, Hohnloser SH, Kolh P, Lip GY, Manolis A, McMurray J, Ponikowski P, Rosenhek R, Ruschitzka F, Savelieva I, Sharma S, Suwalski P, Tamargo JL, Taylor CJ, Van Gelder IC, Voors AA, Windecker S, Zamorano JL, Zeppenfeld K. 2016 ESC guidelines for the management of atrial fibrillation developed in collaboration with EACTS. Eur Heart J. 2016;37(38):2893–962.
43. Conolly SJ, Ezekowitz MD, Yusuf S, et al. Dabigatran versus warfarin in patients with atrial fibrillation. N Engl J Med. 2009;361:1139–51.
44. Patel MR, Mahaffey KW, Garg J, et al. Rivaroxaban versus warfarin in nonvalvular atrial fibrillation. N Engl J Med. 2011;365:883–91.
45. Granger CB, Alexander JH, McMurray JJV, et al. Apixaban versus warfarin in patients with atrial fibrillation. N Engl J Med. 2011;365:981–92.
46. Hendriks SH, van Hateren KJ, Groenier KH, Houweling ST, Maas AH, Kleefstra N, Bilo HJ. Sex differences in the quality of diabetes care in the Netherlands (ZODIAC-45). PLoS One. 2015;10:e0145907.
47. Kurth T, Winter AC, Eliassen AH, Dushkes R, Mukamal KJ, Rimm EB, Willett WC, Manson JE, Rexrode KM. Migraine and risk of cardiovascular disease in women: prospective cohort study. BMJ. 2016;353:i2610.
48. Tepper NK, Whiteman MK, Zapata LB, Marchbanks PA, Curtis KM. Safety of hormonal contraceptives among women with migraine: a systematic review. Contraception. 2016;94(6):630–40.
49. MacClellan LR, Giles W, Cole J, Wozniak M, Stern B, Mitchell BD, Kittner SJ. Probable migraine with visual aura and risk of ischemic stroke: the stroke prevention in young women study. Stroke. 2007;38:2438–45.
50. Brayfield A. Martindale the complete drug reference. 38th ed. New York: Pharmaceutical Press; 2014. isbn:978-0-85711-139-5.
51. Boardman HM, Hartley L, Eisinga A, Main C, Roqué i Figuls M, Bonfill Cosp X, Gabriel Sanchez R, Knight B. Hormone therapy for preventing cardiovascular disease in post-menopausal women. Cochrane Database Syst Rev. 2015;3:CD002229.
52. Nelson HD, Walker M, Zakher B, Mitchell J. Menopausal hormone therapy for the primary prevention of chronic conditions: a systematic review to update the U.S. Preventive Services Task Force recommendations. Ann Intern Med. 2012;157:104–13.
53. Grodstein F, Manson JE, Stampfer MJ, Rexrode K. Postmenopausal hormone therapy and stroke: role of time since menopause and age at initiation of hormone therapy. Arch Intern Med. 2008;168:861–6.
54. Chan W-S, Ray J, Wai EK, Ginsburg S, Hannah ME, Corey PN, Ginsberg JS. Risk of stroke in women exposed to low-dose oral contraceptives: a critical evaluation of the evidence. Arch Intern Med. 2004;164:741–7.
55. Baillargeon JP, McClish DK, Essah PA, Nestler JE. Association between the current use of low-dose oral contraceptives and cardiovascular arterial disease: a meta-analysis. J Clin Endocrinol Metab. 2005;90:3863–70.
56. Lidegaard Ø, Løkkegaard E, Jensen A, Skovlund CW, Keiding N. Thrombotic stroke and myocardial infarction with hormonal contraception. N Engl J Med. 2012;366(24):2257–66.
57. WHO Collaborative Study of Cardiovascular Disease and Steroid Hormone Contraception. Ischaemic stroke and combined oral contraceptives: results of an international, multicenter, case-control study. Lancet. 1996;348:498–505.

58. WHO Collaborative Study of Cardiovascular Disease and Steroid Hormone Contraception. Haemorrhagic stroke, overall stroke risk, and combined oral contraceptives: results of an international, multicenter, case-control study. Lancet. 1996;348:505–10.
59. Kemmeren JM, Tanis BC, van den Bosch MA, Bollen EL, Helmerhorst FM, van der Graaf Y, Rosendaal FR, Algra A. Risk of arterial thrombosis in relation to oral contraceptives (RATIO) study: oral contraceptives and the risk of ischemic stroke. Stroke. 2002;33:1202–8.
60. Slooter AJ, Rosendaal FR, Tanis BC, Kemmeren JM, van der Graaf Y, Algra A. Prothrombotic conditions, oral contraceptives, and the risk of ischemic stroke. J Thromb Haemost. 2005;3:1213–7.
61. Urbanus RT, Siegerink B, Roest M, Rosendaal FR, de Groot PG, Algra A. Antiphospholipid antibodies and risk of myocardial infarction and ischaemic stroke in young women in the RATIO study: a case-control study. Lancet Neurol. 2009;8:998–1005.
62. Duley L, Meher S, Jones L. Drugs for treatment of very high blood pressure during pregnancy. Cochrane Database Syst Rev. 2013;7:CD001449.
63. Abalos E, Duley L, Steyn DW. Antihypertensive drug therapy for mild to moderate hypertension during pregnancy. Cochrane Database Syst Rev. 2014;2:CD002252.
64. European Society of Gynecology (ESG), Association for European Paediatric Cardiology (AEPC), German Society for Gender Medicine (DGesGM), Regitz-Zagrosek V, Blomstrom Lundqvist C, Borghi C, Cifkova R, Ferreira R, Foidart JM, Gibbs JS, Gohlke-Baerwolf C, Gorenek B, Iung B, Kirby M, Maas AH, Morais J, Nihoyannopoulos P, Pieper PG, Presbitero P, Roos-Hesselink JW, Schaufelberger M, Seeland U, Torracca L, ESC Committee for Practice Guidelines. ESC guidelines on the management of cardiovascular diseases during pregnancy: the Task Force on the Management of Cardiovascular Diseases during pregnancy of the European Society of Cardiology (ESC). Eur Heart J. 2011;32: 3147–97.
65. McDonald SD, Malinowski A, Zhou Q, Yusuf S, Devereaux PJ. Cardiovascular sequelae of preeclampsia/eclampsia: a systematic review and meta-analyses. Am Heart J. 2008;156:918–30.
66. Hofmeyr GJ, Lawrie TA, Atallah AN, Duley L, Torloni MR. Calcium supplementation during pregnancy for preventing hypertensive disorders and related problems. Cochrane Database Syst Rev. 2014;6:CD001059.
67. WHO Recommendations. http://www.who.int/elena/titles/calcium_pregnancy/en/. Accessed 31 Jul 2016.
68. Duley L, Henderson-Smart DJ, Meher S, King JF. Antiplatelet agents for preventing pre-eclampsia and its complications. Cochrane Database Syst Rev. 2007;2:CD004659.
69. Leffert LR, Clancy CR, Bateman BT, Cox M, Schulte PJ, Smith EE, Fonarow GC, Kuklina EV, George MG, Schwamm LH. Treatment patterns and short-term outcomes in ischemic stroke in pregnancy or postpartum period. Am J Obstet Gynecol. 2016;214:723.e1–11.
70. Dentali F, Poli D, Scoditti U, Di Minno MN, De Stefano V, Siragusa S, Kostal M, Palareti G, Sartori MT, Grandone E, Vedovati MC, Ageno W, CErebral VEin Thrombosis International Study Investigators, Falanga A, Lerede T, Bianchi M, Testa S, Witt D, McCool K, Bucherini E, Grifoni E, Coalizzo D, Benedetti R, Marietta M, Sessa M, Guaschino C, di Minno G, Tufano A, Barbar S, Malato A, Pini M, Castellini P, Barco S, Barone M, Paciaroni M, Alberti A, Agnelli G, Giorgi Pierfranceschi M, Dulicek P, Silingardi M, Federica L, Ghirarduzzi A, Tiraferri E, di Lazzaro V, Rossi E, Ciminello A, Pasca S, Barillari G, Rezoagli E, Galli M, Squizzato A, Tosetto A. Long-term outcomes of patients with cerebral vein thrombosis: a multicenter study. J Thromb Haemost. 2012;10:1297–302.
71. Ferro JM, Canhão P, Stam J, Bousser MG, Barinagarrementeria F, ISCVT Investigators. Prognosis of cerebral vein and dural sinus thrombosis: results of the International Study on Cerebral Vein and Dural Sinus Thrombosis (ISCVT). Stroke. 2004;35:664–70.
72. Berglund A, Svensson L, Wahlgren N, von Euler M, HASTA Collaborators. Face arm speech time test use in the prehospital setting, better in the ambulance than in the emergency medical communication center. Cerebrovasc Dis. 2014;37:212–6.

73. Mochari-Greenberger H, Xian Y, Hellkamp AS, Schulte PJ, Bhatt DL, Fonarow GC, Saver JL, Reeves MJ, Schwamm LH, Smith EE. Racial/ethnic and sex differences in emergency medical services transport among hospitalized US stroke patients: analysis of the national get with the guidelines-stroke registry. J Am Heart Assoc. 2015;4:e002099.
74. Berglund A, von Euler M, Schenck-Gustafsson K, Castrén M, Bohm K. Identification of stroke during the emergency call: a descriptive study of callers' presentation of stroke. BMJ Open. 2015;5:e007661.
75. Lisabeth LD, Brown DL, Hughes R, Majersik JJ, Morgenstern LB. Acute stroke symptoms: comparing women and men. Stroke. 2009;40:2031–6.
76. Kent DM, Price LL, Ringleb P, Hill MD, Selker HP. Sex-based differences in response to recombinant tissue plasminogen activator in acute ischemic stroke: a pooled analysis of randomized clinical trials. Stroke. 2005;36:62–5.
77. Nathanson D, Patrone C, Nyström T, von Euler M. Sex, diastolic blood pressure, and outcome after thrombolysis for ischemic stroke. Stroke Res Treat. 2014;2014:747458.
78. Hill MD, Kent DM, Hinchey J, Rowley H, Buchan AM, Wechsler LR, Higashida RT, Fischbein NJ, Dillon WP, Gent M, Firszt CM, Schulz GA, Furlan AJ, PROACT-2 Investigators. Sex-based differences in the effect of intra-arterial treatment of stroke: analysis of the PROACT-2 study. Stroke. 2006;37:2322–5.
79. Meseguer E, Mazighi M, Labreuche J, Arnaiz C, Cabrejo L, Slaoui T, Guidoux C, Olivot JM, Abboud H, Lapergue B, Raphaeli G, Klein IF, Lavallée PC, Amarenco P. Outcomes of intravenous recombinant tissue plasminogen activator therapy according to gender: a clinical registry study and systematic review. Stroke. 2009;40:2104–10.
80. Goyal M, Menon BK, van Zwam WH, Dippel DW, Mitchell PJ, Demchuk AM, Dávalos A, Majoie CB, van der Lugt A, de Miquel MA, Donnan GA, Roos YB, Bonafe A, Jahan R, Diener HC, van den Berg LA, Levy EI, Berkhemer OA, Pereira VM, Rempel J, Millán M, Davis SM, Roy D, Thornton J, Román LS, Ribó M, Beumer D, Stouch B, Brown S, Campbell BC, van Oostenbrugge RJ, Saver JL, Hill MD, Jovin TG, HERMES Collaborators. Endovascular thrombectomy after large-vessel ischaemic stroke: a meta-analysis of individual patient data from five randomised trials. Lancet. 2016;387:1723–31.
81. Stroke Unit Trialists' Collaboration. Organised inpatient (stroke unit) care for stroke. Cochrane Database Syst Rev. 2007;4:CD000197.
82. Hsue PY, Bittner VA, Betteridge J, Fayyad R, Laskey R, Wenger NK, Waters DD. Impact of female sex on lipid lowering, clinical outcomes, and adverse effects in atorvastatin trials. Am J Cardiol. 2015;115:447–53.
83. Hedayati N, Humphries MD, Zhou W. Gender and outcomes of carotid artery interventions. Vasc Endovasc Surg. 2014;48:99–105.
84. Luebke T, Brunkwall J. Meta-analysis and meta-regression analysis of the associations between sex and the operative outcomes of carotid endarterectomy. BMC Cardiovasc Disord. 2015;15:32.
85. De Rango P, Brown MM, Leys D, Howard VJ, Moore WS, Paciaroni M, Ringleb P, Rockman C, Caso V. Management of carotid stenosis in women: consensus document. Neurology. 2013;80:2258–68.
86. Buratti L, Balestrini S, Avitabile E, Altamura C, Vernieri F, Viticchi G, Falsetti L, Provinciali L, Silvestrini M. Sex-associated differences in the modulation of vascular risk in patients with asymptomatic carotid stenosis. J Cereb Blood Flow Metab. 2015;35(4):684–8.
87. Nasreddine ZS, Phillips NA, Bedirian V, Charbonneau S, Whitehead V, Collin I, Cummings JL, Chertkow H. The Montreal cognitive assessment, MoCa: a brief screening tool for mild cognitive impairment. J Am Geriatr Soc. 2005;53:695–9.
88. Lin JS, O'Connor E, Rossom RC, Perdue LA, Burda BU, Thompson M, Eckstrom E. Screening for cognitive impairment in older adults: a systematic review for the U.S. preventive services task force. Ann Intern Med. 2013;159(9):601–12.
89. Wardlaw JM, Murray V, Berge E, del Zoppo GJ. Thrombolysis for acute ischaemic stroke. Cochrane Database Syst Rev. 2014;7:CD000213.

90. Emberson J, Lees KR, Blackwell L, Albers G, et al. Effect of treatment delay, age, and stroke severity on the effects of intravenous thrombolysis with alteplase for acute ischaemic stroke: a meta-analysis of individual patient data from randomised trials. Lancet. 2014;384: 1929–35.
91. IST-3 Collaborative Group, Sandercock P, Wardlaw JM, Lindley RI, Dennis M, Cohen G, et al. The benefits and harms of intravenous thrombolysis with recombinant tissue plasminogen activator within 6 h of acute ischaemic stroke (the third international stroke trial [IST-3]): a randomised controlled trial. Lancet. 2012;379:2352–63.
92. Reeves M, Bhatt A, Jajou P, Brown M, Lisabeth L. Sex differences in the use of intravenous rt-PA thrombolysis treatment for acute ischemic stroke: a meta-analysis. Stroke. 2009;40:1743–9.
93. Shobha N, Sylaja PN, Kapral MK, Fang J, Hill MD, Investigators of the Registry of the Canadian Stroke Network. Differences in stroke outcome based on sex. Neurology. 2010;74:767–71.
94. Nagaraja N, Bhattacharya P, Mada F, Salowich-Palm L, Hinton S, Millis S, et al. Gender based differences in acute stroke care in Michigan hospitals. J Neurol Sci. 2012;314: 88–91.
95. Berglund A, Svensson L, Sjöstrand C, von Arbin M, von Euler M, Wahlgren N, HASTA Collaborators, Engerström L, Höjeberg B, Käll TB, Mjörnheim S, Engqvist A. Higher prehospital priority level of stroke improves thrombolysis frequency and time to stroke unit: the Hyper Acute STroke Alarm (HASTA) study. Stroke. 2012;43:2666–70.
96. Puolakka T, Väyrynen T, Häppölä O, Soinne L, Kuisma M, Lindsberg PJ. Sequential analysis of pretreatment delays in stroke thrombolysis. Acad Emerg Med. 2010;17:965–9.
97. Rothwell PM, Algra A, Chen Z, Diener HC, Norrving B, Mehta Z. Effects of aspirin on risk and severity of early recurrent stroke after transient ischaemic attack and ischaemic stroke: time-course analysis of randomised trials. Lancet. 2016;388:365–75.
98. Sandercock PA, Counsell C, Tseng MC, Cecconi E. Oral antiplatelet therapy for acute ischaemic stroke. Cochrane Database Syst Rev. 2014;3:CD000029.
99. Stroke Unit Trialists' Collaboration. Organised inpatient (stroke unit) care for stroke. Cochrane Database Syst Rev. 2013;9:CD000197.
100. Tsivgoulis G, Katsanos AH, Butcher KS, Boviatsis E, Triantafyllou N, Rizos I, Alexandrov AV. Intensive blood pressure reduction in acute intracerebral hemorrhage: a meta-analysis. Neurology. 2014;83:1523–9. Erratum in: Neurology. 2015;84:2466
101. Hart RG, Pearce LA, Aguilar MI. Meta-analysis: antithrombotic therapy to prevent stroke in patients who have nonvalvular atrial fibrillation. Ann Intern Med. 2007;146:857–67.
102. European Stroke Organisation (ESO) Executive Committee, ESO Writing Committee. Guidelines for management of ischaemic stroke and transient ischaemic attack 2008. Cerebrovasc Dis. 2008;25:457–507.
103. Furie KL, Kasner SE, Adams RJ, Albers GW, Bush RL, Fagan SC, Halperin JL, Johnston SC, Katzan I, Kernan WN, Mitchell PH, Ovbiagele B, Palesch YY, Sacco RL, Schwamm LH, Wassertheil-Smoller S, Turan TN, Wentworth D, American Heart Association Stroke Council, Council on Cardiovascular Nursing, Council on Clinical Cardiology, and Interdisciplinary Council on Quality of Care and Outcomes Research. Guidelines for the prevention of stroke in patients with stroke or transient ischemic attack: a guideline for healthcare professionals from the American heart association/American stroke association. Stroke. 2011;42:227–76.
104. Howard G, Roubin GS, Jansen O, Hendrikse J, Halliday A, Fraedrich G, Eckstein HH, Calvet D, Bulbulia R, Bonati LH, Becquemin JP, Algra A, Brown MM, Ringleb PA, Brott TG, Mas JL, Carotid Stenting Trialists' Collaboration. Association between age and risk of stroke or death from carotid endarterectomy and carotid stenting: a meta-analysis of pooled patient data from four randomised trials. Lancet. 2016;387:1305–11.

Chapter 13
Sex and Gender Differences in Psychosocial Risk Factors for Ischemic Heart Disease

Paula M.C. Mommersteeg, Jos W.M.G. Widdershoven, and Willem Johan Kop

Abstract Women have more depression and anxiety than men, which are associated with an increased risk of mortality in ischemic heart disease (IHD). Psychosocial factors are related to inflammation and an autonomic nervous system imbalance. Younger (premenopausal) women have a stronger effect for psychosocial factors and IHD outcomes than older women. Social norms and status, gender roles and expectations also contribute to health status in individuals with IHD. It may be difficult to distinguish cardiac symptoms from anxiety or a panic attack. Specific interventions are needed to reduce (chronic) psychosocial stress in women.

Keywords Anger • Anxiety • Autonomic dysfunction • Depression • Gender roles • Heart rate variability (HRV) • Inflammation • Ischemic heart disease (IHD) • Loneliness • Panic attack • Psychosocial factors • Psychological distress • Socioeconomic status • Stress • Type D personality

Introduction

Women are more likely than men to report psychological complaints, including depression, anxiety, and general distress [1–4]. Differences in prevalence of psychological distress between men and women emerge in mid-puberty and women show a consistently higher prevalence of elevated distress up until menopause and differences in decline in older adulthood [3, 4]. The prevalence in depression and anxiety

P.M.C. Mommersteeg, Ph.D. (✉) • W.J. Kop, Ph.D.
Department of Medical and Clinical Psychology, Center of Research on Psychology in Somatic Diseases (CoRPS), Tilburg University, Tilburg, The Netherlands
e-mail: P.M.C.Mommersteeg@uvt.nl; W.J.Kop@uvt.nl

J.W.M.G. Widdershoven, M.D., Ph.D.
Department of Medical and Clinical Psychology, Center of Research on Psychology in Somatic Diseases (CoRPS), Tilburg University, Tilburg, The Netherlands

Department of Cardiology, Elisabeth-Tweesteden Hospital, Tilburg, The Netherlands
e-mail: j.widdershoven@etz.nl

A.H.E.M. Maas, C.N. Bairey Merz (eds.), *Manual of Gynecardiology*,
DOI 10.1007/978-3-319-54960-6_13

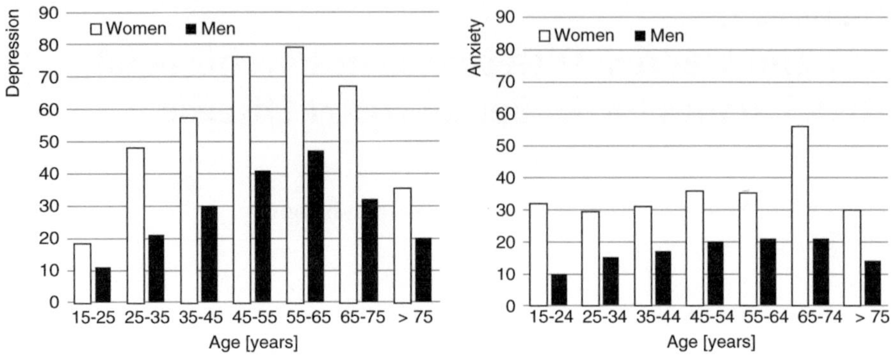

Fig. 13.1 Number of people with either depression (**a**) or anxiety (**b**) per 1000 persons. Data obtained via CBS Statline (2011), representing Dutch physician registries in 2011 [5]

over the lifecycle stratified by sex are displayed in Fig. 13.1. Panel (a) and (b) show the number of women and men presenting to a physician with depression (a) or anxiety (b) in the Netherlands in 2011 [5]. The nearly doubled prevalence of depression and anxiety in women compared to men along the lifecycle is apparent, as well as the decline in older adulthood for women as well as men (Fig. 13.1).

Both depression and anxiety are associated with an increased risk of mortality in individuals with ischemic heart disease (IHD) [6–9]. In patients with an acute coronary syndrome (ACS), depression is a risk factor for poor prognosis including all-cause mortality, cardiac mortality, and nonfatal cardiac events [10]. Other psychosocial factors that have been associated with an elevated risk of IHD include anger/hostility, (low) social support, Type D personality, (low) socioeconomic status, and general psychological distress related to family, work, or care giving [11–14]. These psychosocial factors have been found to be related to the development, prevalence, and progression of coronary artery disease (CAD) [15]. For example, the INTERHEART study examined modifiable risk factor differences in over 13,000 cases with a history of acute MI and over 11,000 controls. They found that the presence of psychosocial risk factors was related to a 32.5% attributable risk for an acute coronary syndrome (ACS), which was on par with the risk of smoking, and exceeding risk for other adverse lifestyle factors and cardiac risk factors [16]. Moreover, anger or being emotional upset was significantly more prevalent in the hour before an acute ACS [17]. Low socioeconomic status predicted cardiovascular mortality in men, and social support appears to be protective for men, but not for women [18]. A recent meta-analysis on social support and loneliness predicted mortality consistent across men and women [19].

The difference between biological sex and the psychological correlates of "gender" is important in the understanding of psychological and social risk factors for cardiovascular disease. In this respect, gender reflects social norms, roles and expectations for women and men, rather than biological sex per se. Gender may be more important than sex in driving adverse cardiovascular risk factors [20] and the prediction of cardiovascular outcomes [21]. Pelletier and colleagues have examined a gender-related score, operationalized by seven items, which was associated with adverse outcomes in a prospective cohort of men and women younger than 55 years after an acute coronary syndrome [21].

Psychosocial risk factors have been suggested by the joint guideline of the European Society of Cardiology (ESC) to become incorporated in clinical practice and research as they may add to the individual risk profile of the patient [22, 23]. A 15 item psychosocial screening inventory based on these ESG guidelines has been validated in patients who underwent percutaneous coronary intervention (PCI). The screening inventory showed good feasibility and was of predictive value for 1-year angina and cardiopulmonary symptoms [24].

To summarize, women on average report more depression and anxiety over the lifespan, and psychosocial factors, including but not limited to depression and anxiety, are related to cardiovascular disease development and progression. In order to understand if and how sex and psychosocial factors are related IHD risk, sex differences in CAD and related conditions of IHD are discussed in the next section.

Coronary Artery Disease in Women; Ischemic Heart Disease and Coronary Microvascular Dysfunction

The term "ischemic heart disease" (IHD) is preferable over CAD when describing heart disease in women [25]. With IHD the importance of myocardial ischemia is implied without requiring involvement of significant obstructive *narrowing* of the epicardial coronary arteries [26]. This is consistent with the relatively higher prevalence of non-obstructive CAD (NOCAD) in women combined with the comparable levels of myocardial ischemia [25]. Moreover, approximately half of the women with chest pain do *not* have significant CAD as measured by coronary angiography (i.e., <50% luminal narrowing of a coronary artery), whereas chest pain in the absence of significant CAD has been found to be less prevalent in men (10–20%) [27–29]. It is therefore remarkable that premenopausal women who have had an acute coronary syndrome (ACS) have a greater incidence of adverse outcomes compared to men, despite having less obstructive CAD [25].

Ischemic heart disease can include microvascular ischemia, which is characterized by abnormal vascular function in "resistance vessels" of the heart, i.e., the microvasculature [30, 31]. This condition can co-exist with endothelial dysfunction in the epicardial coronary arteries. Endothelial dysfunction involves poor function of the lining cells of the coronary vessels (i.e., the endothelium) and is common at all stages of CAD. Endothelial dysfunction can result in transient vasoconstriction and subsequent myocardial ischemia, and can be present in vessels *without* luminal narrowing. Endothelial dysfunction may therefore explain why significant obstructive CAD (i.e., luminal narrowing >50%) is often not detected in women with cardiac symptoms and why non-obstructive CAD (NOCAD) is not necessarily benign. In this context it is relevant to consider coronary microvascular dysfunction (CMD).

This is discussed extensively in Chap. 4 and in short CMD is characterized by: (1) inducible myocardial ischemia as documented by ECG changes, transient wall motion abnormalities, or perfusion defects on cardiac imaging following exercise or pharmacological provocation tests; (2) a history of chest pain or other cardiac symptoms; and (3) normal or minimally narrowed coronary arteries (<50% luminal stenosis) at angiography [30, 32–34]. It is possible that CMD involves both epicardial coronary dysfunction as well as microvasculature dysfunction. Both pathophysiological processes may lead to reduced blood flow and cause myocardial ischemia and symptoms that can be qualitatively different from obstructive CAD [35, 36]. These conditions require further investigation as the differential diagnosis is complicated and treatment options are not well defined.

Case I: A Woman with Coronary Microvascular Dysfunction (CMD)
A 55-year old perimenopausal woman was referred to our outpatient clinic from another hospital for a second opinion because of non-typical cardiac symptoms 1 year after an ST-elevation myocardial infarction (STEMI) and a recurrent STEMI. Several months following the recurrent infarction she experienced chest pain located at the left hemi thorax and behind the sternum. These complaints lasted for several hours with an intermittent sharp sensation. Sometimes her symptoms started at the distal upper extremities and also occurred after exercise. Often work-stress preceded the symptoms and sublingual nitrates were effective but resulted in severe headaches. She was exhausted after work and the complaints made her insecure about her physical condition. Apart from migraine as a teenager and hypercholesterolemia her past medical history was negative for cardiac or other medical conditions. The electrocardiogram at rest showed repolarization abnormalities in the inferolateral region and echocardiography revealed nonsignificant mitral incompetence. No evidence was found for epicardial coronary artery narrowing at coronary angiography. These findings resulted in a diagnosis of microvascular cardiac dysfunction, predominantly triggered by stress. Initially prescribed beta-adrenergic blocking agents were discontinued because of side effects and replaced by long-acting calcium antagonist which resulted in improvements of her complaints.

Sex Differences in Psychological Factors Associated with Ischemic Heart Disease

Women diagnosed with IHD report poorer health status when compared to men [37, 38]. A poor health status has been found to be a predictor for adverse prognosis [39, 40]. However, sex differences related to health status, depression, or anxiety-associated risk of IHD remain under-investigated [41]. The increased prevalence of depression in women is observed in patients with IHD, with a higher frequency in women (19%) compared to men (12%) [42]. Some evidence suggests that depression is only associated with future IHD-related mortality in men but not in women, whereas depression predicts IHD incidence in both men and women [43]. However, sex differences are not consistently found across studies. In the INTERHEART study significant sex differences for ACS risk were present for work stress; non-significant for women, but significant for men, and locus of control with more protective effects in women, but no sex differences in risk were observed for stress at home, financial stress, stressful life events, or feeling depressed [44]. The Women's Ischemia Syndrome Evaluation (WISE) study showed that in women with suspected IHD depression predicted hospitalization as well as mortality [45]. Similar findings were observed in other large epidemiological cohorts in women, such as The Stockholm Female Coronary Angiography Study, showing that women with high stress levels related to work or family challenges develop narrowing of the coronary arteries [46]. Smolderen and colleagues showed that women below 60 years of age with a history of depression were more likely to be admitted for an ACS compared to men [47]. Moreover, recovery after an ACS is worse in young and middle-aged patients who report higher stress at baseline. Higher stress levels were present in women, which partially explained their worse recovery [48]. In patients with IHD, after adjustment for potential confounding factors, depressive symptoms predicted presence of obstructive CAD, as well as follow-up major adverse cardiac events (MACE), and death in women below 55 years, but not in men or women over the age of 55 years [49]. In relatively young women after an ACS, vital exhaustion (an episode of extreme tiredness, demoralization and increased irritability) was associated to accelerated coronary atherosclerosis progression [50]. Low and colleagues reviewed 67 reports on sex differences in psychosocial risk factors for CAD incidence or recurrence. Results indicated that depression, anxiety disorders, and stress related to family issues are associated with an elevated IHD risk among women, whereas the associations of general anxiety, work-related stress and hostility are less clearly associated with IHD in women compared to men [14].

Doyle and colleagues performed a systematic review and individual patient data meta-analysis of sex differences in depression and subsequent prognosis of people with an ACS [51]. The prevalence of depression was higher in women compared to men, and depression was associated with all-cause mortality and cardiac events. Interestingly, the association of depression with all-cause mortality was higher in men (HR 1.38, 95%CI 1.30–1.47), compared to women (HR 1.22, 95%CI 1.14–1.31), which was confirmed by a significant interaction between sex and depression [51]. Similar findings were observed for the presence of depression in people reporting angina pectoris in both Western and non-Western populations; depression was more prevalent in both men and women who reported angina pectoris, but this association was stronger in men [52]. Still, these findings represent IHD conditions which are more prevalent in men. More attention is needed for IHD conditions including non-obstructive CAD, which is more present in women, and age stratified findings.

In summary, psychosocial risk factors are more prevalent among women compared to men both in the general population as well as in individuals with

IHD. Psychosocial risk factors are associated with adverse cardiac outcomes in both men and women. Risk for psychosocial distress and cardiac outcomes appear to be stronger for men, and for younger women with depression or anxiety. This trajectory of elevated psychosocial across the life cycle is in contrast with the relatively low risk of obstructive CAD in women during this time period. This discrepancy may be explained in part by difference in the clinical phenotypes of IHD in women versus men (with predominance of CMD in younger and middle-aged women) and/or the unique presentation of cardiac symptoms in women with IHD.

Psychosocial Factors in Ischemic Heart Disease: Role of Estrogens and Inflammation

A number of biological mechanisms have been suggested and are considered to be associated with psychosocial factors on the one hand, and adverse cardiac outcomes on the other, including neuroendocrine dysfunction, autonomic control, endothelial dysfunction, and inflammation [10, 53, 54], for a detailed review see reference [55]. In addition, the prevalence of depressive symptoms and anxiety across the lifecycle in women may suggest an effect of sex hormones on mood. During reproductive years depressive symptoms have been related to cyclic changes in sex-steroid hormones during the menstrual cycle, infertility treatment, during pregnancy or after delivery (e.g. post-partum depression) [56–58]. In the perimenopausal phase estrogen levels decline and fluctuate substantially and after menopause estrogen is no longer produced by the ovaries but in smaller amounts by the adrenal glands and in fat tissue. The fluctuating levels of estrogens over the lifecycle suggests a 'window of vulnerability' for depression and mood states. Moreover, the fluctuating and declining estrogen levels in perimenopause and thereafter makes estrogen a plausible contributing factor to ageing in the development of atherosclerosis.

Psychosocial factors have consistently been related to inflammation in IHD [13, 59–61], and sex differences have been observed in levels of biomarkers, such as high sensitive C-reactive protein (CRP) and other inflammatory cytokines [62, 63]. This is supported by clinical-observational and epidemiological investigations [64–66]. The predictive value of inflammatory markers such as CRP, interleukin 6 (IL-6), and tumor necrosis factor alpha (TNF-α) for IHD development and prognosis are well established [62, 67–69]. Estrogens inhibit local production of pro-inflammatory markers such as CRP by decreasing IL-6 secretion [69]. Consistent with these immune system-related effects of estrogens, postmenopausal women have increased circulating levels of pro-inflammatory cytokines IL-6 and TNF-α, and an increased response of the body to these cytokines [70]. Although estrogens levels can affect endothelial function [71], inflammation plays a key role in endothelial dysfunction. Endothelial dysfunction has been related to depressive symptoms [72].

Case II: A Woman with Chest Pain and Anxiety

A 42-year-old woman presented to the outpatient department of cardiology with complaints of chest pain since 4 weeks. These complaints occurred during exercise and at rest. She was a non-smoker with slightly elevated cholesterol levels and her family was known with heart disease. She was on aspirin and oral nitrates as prescribed by her general practitioner. Physical examination and an electrocardiogram at rest were normal. An exercise test was inconclusive because of insufficient workload. Because of suspected coronary artery spasm, a calcium antagonist was added to the medication and she was followed up in the outpatient clinic. Two years later a coronary angiogram was performed because of recurrences of chest pain and this study showed normal coronary arteries. However, drug therapy was continued and during the subsequent years she visited the outpatient clinic and the emergency department frequently with complaints of chest pain accompanied by radiation to the jaws, perspiring, heavy feeling of palpitations and dizziness. There was a minor positive effect of sublingual nitrates. A dobutamine stress echo was normal. During the following years a nuclear study showed no abnormalities, a repeated angiogram was normal and an acetylcholine provocation test showed normal endothelial function. Gastrointestinal and pulmonary abnormalities were excluded. A careful history taken at the outpatient department, unfortunately more than 10 years after the initial presentation, showed the complete atypical presentation of the complaints that were related to stress and accompanied by numbness and tingling of both arms, agitation, shortness of breath and fear of dying.

Referral to a medical psychologist and cognitive behavioural therapy (CBT) treatment resulted in marked improvement and the ability for the patient to handle her complaints. It was concluded that this patient was treated for many years for suspected coronary spasm or possible cardiac microvascular disease but in fact she suffered from anxiety and panic attacks that were successfully treated with CBT. Although this long treatment is exceptional it is not uncommon in daily practice that patients with anxiety and panic attacks are misdiagnosed as cardiac patients and treated accordingly. This approach to treatment is partly due to the focus of the patient and the health professional on physical explanations for (cardiac) symptoms. It is of importance for doctors to reassure that there are serious complaints in these patients but also to exclude a physical origin. Gradually the focus may need to shift from physical to psychological explanations for persistent symptoms.

Chest Pain, Cardiac Symptoms and Differentiation from Panic Disorder

Symptoms of chest pain are associated with IHD in men with relatively good sensitivity and specificity, but in women these symptoms are less sensitive/specific [35, 73]. The most common ACS symptoms in women are shortness of breath, weakness, and fatigue in addition to chest pain [35, 73]. Other reported symptoms which are more prevalent in women compared to men include, nausea, vomiting, numbness in hands, back, neck or jaw pain, dizziness, palpitations, chest discomfort, sense of dread, anxiety, or cold sweat [74]. One of the consequences of these different symptom profiles in women is that the patient as well as physicians and other health care providers have to differentiate their interpretations of these symptoms from other conditions such as anxiety, psychological distress, and acute panic disorder. These "competing interpretations" may result in delayed and often missed diagnosis of IHD and lack of initiation of necessary clinical interventions [25, 35, 75–77]. One of the major challenges is to be able to differentiate between cardiac symptoms and complaints that accompany anxiety or a panic attack. Another major challenge is the correct diagnosis of symptoms of IHD that are not characterized by chest discomfort (e.g., dyspnea, fatigue, pain in regions other than the chest and/or radiation to arms or jaw).

A panic attack by definition is a period of intense fear, which develops suddenly. Symptoms of a panic attack largely resemble symptoms of angina pectoris or even a myocardial infarction. Figure 13.2 shows a Venn-diagram for symptoms of a panic attack and angina, and the overlap between both entities. The majority of symptoms overlap, which makes it challenging to distinguish angina from a panic attack in the emergency department and other clinical settings. The meta-analysis by Huffman and Pollack showed that five factors were predictive of panic disorder among persons who present with chest pain: the absence of obstructive CAD, atypical quality of chest pain, female sex, younger age (mean age 45 years), and a high level of self-reported anxiety [78].

Irrespective of 'hard' cardiac outcomes, the presence of chest pain and other cardiac symptoms are important, since patients with NOCAD continue to report chest pain [79], limiting their physical activity, and they continue to have hospital readmissions [80]. From a health perspective, the increased health care utilization, follow-up visits and laboratory testing are costly and demanding to patients and their families. Recurrent chest pain does not necessarily lead to mental health care

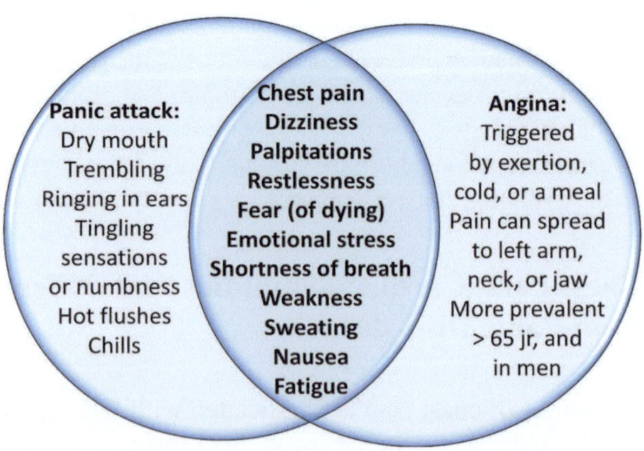

Fig. 13.2 Venn diagram of overlapping and distinctive symptoms of a panic attack and angina pectoris

referral [80]. Still, the presence of panic disorder is not harmless; patients with panic disorder have a 47% increased risk of developing IHD, a 36% increased ACS risk, and a 40% increased risk for MACE [81] compared to individuals without panic disorder. Moreover, both anxiety, mental stress, and a panic attack are associated with coronary vasoconstriction and reversible myocardial perfusion defects indicative of myocardial ischemia [82–86], which have found to be more prevalent in women compared to men [87]. Thus, a bidirectional relationship can be assumed; both stress and panic can cause ischemia, and vice versa ischemia can cause a panic attack. The possibility of an ACS, or coronary ischemia causing a panic attack, is suggested via increased catecholamine levels (noradrenaline and adrenaline), a decreased heart rate variability (HRV), or cerebral CO_2 levels secondary to an increase in lactate as a consequence of ischemia [80].

These findings indicate that although chest pain is prevalent in both angina and panic disorder, the latter can occur with typical angina. Even if a panic disorder is recognized, this does not exclude the possibility of co-occurring CAD [80]. Screening tools to date are not adequate for the differential diagnosis of cardiac chest pain versus chest pain that is part of a panic attack. It is possible that clinical benefits will result from the validation study of a 4-item Panic Screening Score instrument for use in the emergency department [88].

Mechanisms of Chest Pain and Anxiety; Heart Rate Variability

An autonomic nervous system imbalance can be a vital part of the missing link in the association between sex differences in cardiac symptoms, psychosocial distress, and pathophysiological functioning in IHD. Heart rate is regulated by the autonomic nervous system, the parasympathetic branch acting as a brake, via the neurotransmitter acetylcholine, while activation of the sympathetic nerves, releasing noradrenaline, accelerates heart rate. The vagus nerve transmits signals from the brain to the heart to regulate heart rate, but at the same time 80% of the vagus nerve comprises *sensory* (afferent) nerves, informing the brain about the heart and other peripheral organs [89]. Via the vagus nerve autonomic functioning is balanced in a dynamic way to respond to internal and environmental demands, which can be examined noninvasively by heart rate variability (HRV). HRV is the irregularity of consecutive heart beat intervals [90–92]. High HRV represents more variation in interbeat intervals, indicating a more variable and healthy heart rate regulation. A disturbance in autonomic balance, reflected in a reduced HRV suggests a decreased parasympathetic inhibition.

Examining HRV is intriguing for several reasons. There are many studies confirming the relevance of examining HRV in relation to chest pain [93–98], sex differences [90, 99], CAD [90, 91, 100], inflammation [61, 101–103], microvascular and endothelial functioning [104–107], and psychosocial factors [95, 108–112], though inconsistent findings have been reported [113, 114]. Few studies have *combined* these elements: more chest pain and lower HRV was observed in women who report panic attacks [97], and a reduced parasympathetic tone was observed in patients with cardiac symptoms and inducible ischemia but without clinically significant CAD [115, 116]. Differences in vagal nerve activation between men and women suggest sex-related variations in sensory properties of this pathway and/or central perception and interpretation of internal and external signals, resulting in increased perceived chest pain and subsequent feelings of anxiety. It remains to be investigated if and how autonomic dysregulation plays a role in cardiac symptom perception, and sex differences in mood associated with IHD.

Case III: A Woman with Chronic Stress and a Reduced Ejection Fraction

The patient is a woman in her late 40s who presents with chronic recurrent chest pain that tends to be more frequent and severe during periods of psychological distress. She also has occasional complaints of dizziness and sustained low energy levels. These complaints have been present for approximately 7 years. When the patient was more symptomatic, echocardiography revealed evidence for moderate reduced left ventricular function (ejection fraction (EF) 40%). Repeated coronary angiography provided no evidence for significant epicardial CAD. The patient has premature hypertension but no other CVD risk factors. Other co-morbidities include fibromyalgia and chronic pain. The patient also has a history of early-life physical abuse and is diagnosed with post-traumatic stress disorder (PTSD).

The patient complains about stress-related chest pain. The ECG is normal with an intermediate axis and signs of non-specific inferolateral repolarization abnormalities. Her hypertension appears well controlled with beta-adrenergic blockade and an angiotensin-II receptor blocker. Currently, she is unemployed and is under substantial pressure to find other work.

Repeated echocardiograms over the past 7 years show that her ejection fraction is markedly lower during episodes of psychological distress (ranging between 35% and 45%) compared to periods when she feels less tense (EF approximately 50%). This pattern of fluctuating symptoms and parallel changes in cardiac pump function are consistent with stress-induced myocardial dysfunction that could reflect myocardial ischemia related to CMD [117]. It remains to be elucidated whether this chronic form of PTSD-related CMD has pathophysiologic similarities with the more acute Takotsubo syndrome.

Treatment Options of Stress-Related Ischemic Heart Disease

Interventions for patients with IHD typically take place in the context of cardiac rehabilitation (CR) following ACS or revascularization with either PCI or CABG. Cardiac rehabilitation involves modules to enhance physical exercise, medical management of blood pressure and lipids, and lifestyle counseling on diet and smoking cessation (see Chap. 10). Evidence suggests that CR reduces cardiac mortality, hospitalization and improves quality of life [118]. Moreover, exercise-based cardiac rehabilitation interventions results in reduced risk for cardiovascular mortality, hospitalization and improved health related quality of life, but not in improvements in the risk of ACS or coronary intervention or total mortality [119].

Stress reduction, e.g. a stress management training, is not routinely incorporated in the CR program [118], but psychological interventions are often added to a subset of patients with psychosocial problems. Cardiac rehabilitation is not offered yet to IHD patients with CMD who do not have clinical significant CAD. However, CR provides a very useful existing framework that can be adapted to better meet the needs of IHD patients with CMD, particularly those with high levels of psychosocial burden. A recent randomized controlled trial that integrated a stress-management training as an additional part of CR showed significant reductions in stress immediately after treatment, and showed improvement in clinical outcomes [118]. Considering treatment options aimed at reducing psychosocial stress, a recent Cochrane systematic review showed that psychological and pharmacological interventions have small to moderate effects on reducing depression and anxiety, but not on reduction in mortality or cardiac events. However, the number of studies is still relatively small and design characteristics have been heterogeneous [120, 121]. A recent review showed that behavioral change interventions reduced the risk of mortality, but not IHD events [122]. A meta-analysis of collaborative care interventions showed that there are small effects for a reduction in depression, depression remission, anxiety and mental quality of life, but no long-term reduction in MACE [123]. The Cochrane review by Kisely and colleagues concluded that there is a modest to moderate benefit for psychological interventions in reducing non-specific chest pain in patients with normal coronary anatomy [124]. However, there was strong heterogeneity between the findings. More studies on psychological interventions exceeding a period of 12 months are warranted [124].

There is also a need to consider the usefulness of sex-specific CR strategies. Psychological intervention trials in IHD patients indicate that women benefit less than men. Orth-Gomer and colleagues propose to compose same-sex intervention groups on stress management training [125], and for scientists to report more sex-specified outcomes in studies [126]. Screening for high-risk patients may be an important first step to optimize long-term clinical outcomes in IHD. The risk for adverse outcomes stratified for gender or other diversity groups can be observed and reported, e.g. by using the ESC screener for psychosocial factors [23]. Another route that needs to be taken is to incorporate a panic screening instrument in the emergency department to investigate unexplained panic attacks and chest pain, which may improve more appropriate referral [88]. Practical suggestions on how to proceed to study female-specific cardiovascular health and disease are provided by Ouyang and colleagues [127]. The Society for Women's Health Research compiled an inventory for the study of women and CV health across the lifespan, and provides practical recommendations for clinical scientists, including a significant role for the study of psychosocial variables [127].

Conclusions

- Sex differences in psychosocial factors are associated with IHD progression and poor prognosis.
- A stronger effect for psychosocial factors and IHD outcomes is observed in younger (premenopausal) women compared to older women.
- Women report more atypical cardiac chest pain symptoms, and the overlap between ACS and panic disorder or acute anxiety does not exclude IHD in women.
- Specific interventions are needed to reduce (chronic) psychosocial stress in women.

References

1. WHO. The global burden of disease: 2004 update. WHO Library Cataloguing-in-Publication Data. Geneva: World Health Organization, Informatics DoHSa; 2008.
2. Ferrari AJ, Somerville AJ, Baxter AJ, Norman R, Patten SB, Vos T, et al. Global variation in the prevalence and incidence of major depressive disorder: a systematic review of the epidemiological literature. Psychol Med. 2012:1–11.
3. Faravelli C, Alessandra Scarpato M, Castellini G, Lo Sauro C. Gender differences in depression and anxiety: the role of age. Psychiatry Res. 2013;210(3):1301–3.
4. Ferrari AJ, Charlson FJ, Norman RE, Flaxman AD, Patten SB, Vos T, et al. The epidemiological modelling of major depressive disorder: application for the Global Burden of Disease Study 2010. PLoS One. 2013;8(7):e69637.
5. Statline C. Huisarts geregistreerde diagnose van depressie en angst volgens de International Classification of Primary Care [Physician registered diagnosis of depression and anxiety according to the International Classification of Primary Care]. The Hague/Heerlen: Central Bureau of Statistics; 2011. http://statline.cbs.nl/. Accessed 01 Jun 2016.
6. Roest AM, Martens EJ, Denollet J, de Jonge P. Prognostic association of anxiety post myocardial infarction with mortality and new cardiac events: a meta-analysis. Psychosom Med. 2010;72(6):563–9.
7. Frasure-Smith N, Lesperance F. Depression and anxiety as predictors of 2-year cardiac events in patients with stable coronary artery disease. Arch Gen Psychiatry. 2008;65(1):62–71.
8. Nicholson A, Kuper H, Hemingway H. Depression as an aetiologic and prognostic factor in coronary heart disease: a meta-analysis of 6362 events among 146 538 participants in 54 observational studies. Eur Heart J. 2006;27(23):2763–74.
9. van Melle JP, de Jonge P, Spijkerman TA, Tijssen JG, Ormel J, van Veldhuisen DJ, et al. Prognostic association of depression following myocardial infarction with mortality and cardiovascular events: a meta-analysis. Psychosom Med. 2004;66(6):814–22.
10. Lichtman JH, Froelicher ES, Blumenthal JA, Carney RM, Doering LV, Frasure-Smith N, et al. Depression as a risk factor for poor prognosis among patients with acute coronary syndrome: systematic review and recommendations: a scientific statement from the American Heart Association. Circulation. 2014;129(12):1350–69.
11. Dimsdale JE. Psychological stress and cardiovascular disease. J Am Coll Cardiol. 2008;51(13):1237–46.
12. Suls J, Bunde J. Anger, anxiety, and depression as risk factors for cardiovascular disease: the problems and implications of overlapping affective dispositions. Psychol Bull. 2005;131(2):260–300.
13. Everson-Rose SA, Lewis TT. Psychosocial factors and cardiovascular diseases. Annu Rev Public Health. 2005;26:469–500.

14. Low CA, Thurston RC, Matthews KA. Psychosocial factors in the development of heart disease in women: current research and future directions. Psychosom Med. 2010;72(9):842–54.
15. Strike PC, Steptoe A. Psychosocial factors in the development of coronary artery disease. Prog Cardiovasc Dis. 2004;46(4):337–47.
16. Yusuf S, Hawken S, Ounpuu S, Dans T, Avezum A, Lanas F, et al. Effect of potentially modifiable risk factors associated with myocardial infarction in 52 countries (the INTERHEART study): case-control study. Lancet. 2004;364(9438):937–52.
17. Smyth A, O'Donnell M, Lamelas P, Teo K, Rangarajan S, Yusuf S. Physical activity and anger or emotional upset as triggers of acute myocardial infarction. The INTERHEART study. Circulation. 2016;134(15):1059–67.
18. Stringhini S, Berkman L, Dugravot A, Ferrie JE, Marmot M, Kivimaki M, et al. Socioeconomic status, structural and functional measures of social support, and mortality: the British Whitehall II Cohort Study, 1985–2009. Am J Epidemiol. 2012;175(12):1275–83.
19. Holt-Lunstad J, Smith TB, Baker M, Harris T, Stephenson D. Loneliness and social isolation as risk factors for mortality: a meta-analytic review. Perspect Psychol Sci. 2015;10(2):227–37.
20. Schiebinger L. Scientific research must take gender into account. Nature. 2014;507(7490):9.
21. Pelletier R, Khan NA, Cox J, Daskalopoulou SS, Eisenberg MJ, Bacon SL, et al. Sex versus gender-related characteristics: which predicts outcome after acute coronary syndrome in the young? J Am Coll Cardiol. 2016;67(2):127–35.
22. Perk J, De Backer G, Gohlke H, Graham I, Reiner Z, Verschuren M, et al. European guidelines on cardiovascular disease prevention in clinical practice (version 2012). The Fifth Joint Task Force of the European Society of Cardiology and other societies on cardiovascular disease prevention in clinical practice (constituted by representatives of nine societies and by invited experts). Eur Heart J. 2012;33(13):1635–701.
23. Piepoli MF, Hoes AW, Agewall S, Albus C, Brotons C, Catapano AL, et al. 2016 European guidelines on cardiovascular disease prevention in clinical practice. Eur J Prev Cardiol. 2016;23(11):np1–np96.
24. Van Montfort EV, Denollet J, Widdershoven J, Kupper N. Validity of the European society of cardiology's psychosocial screening interview in patients with coronary heart disease—the THORESCI study. Psychosom Med. 2016. DOI: 10.1097/PSY.0000000000000433.
25. Vaccarino V, Badimon L, Corti R, de Wit C, Dorobantu M, Manfrini O, et al. Presentation, management, and outcomes of ischaemic heart disease in women. Nat Rev Cardiol. 2013;10(9):508–18.
26. Regitz-Zagrosek V, Oertelt-Prigione S, Prescott E, Franconi F, Gerdts E, Foryst-Ludwig A, et al. Gender in cardiovascular diseases: impact on clinical manifestations, management, and outcomes. Eur Heart J. 2016;37(1):24–34.
27. Shaw JA, Kingwell BA, Walton AS, Cameron JD, Pillay P, Gatzka CD, et al. Determinants of coronary artery compliance in subjects with and without angiographic coronary artery disease. J Am Coll Cardiol. 2002;39(10):1637–43.
28. Jespersen L, Hvelplund A, Abildstrom SZ, Pedersen F, Galatius S, Madsen JK, et al. Stable angina pectoris with no obstructive coronary artery disease is associated with increased risks of major adverse cardiovascular events. Eur Heart J. 2012;33(6):734–44.
29. Sedlak TL, Lee M, Izadnegahdar M, Merz CN, Gao M, Humphries KH. Sex differences in clinical outcomes in patients with stable angina and no obstructive coronary artery disease. Am Heart J. 2013;166(1):38–44.
30. Camici PG, Crea F. Coronary microvascular dysfunction. N Engl J Med. 2007;356(8):830–40.
31. Crea F, Camici PG, Bairey Merz CN. Coronary microvascular dysfunction: an update. Eur Heart J. 2014;35(17):1101–11.
32. Kemp Jr HG, Vokonas PS, Cohn PF, Gorlin R. The anginal syndrome associated with normal coronary arteriograms. Report of a six year experience. Am J Med. 1973;54(6):735–42.
33. Arthur HM, Campbell P, Harvey PJ, McGillion M, Oh P, Woodburn E, et al. Women, cardiac syndrome X, and microvascular heart disease. Can J Cardiol. 2012;28(2 Suppl):S42–9.

34. Sara JD, Widmer RJ, Matsuzawa Y, Lennon RJ, Lerman LO, Lerman A. Prevalence of coronary microvascular dysfunction among patients with chest pain and nonobstructive coronary artery disease. JACC Cardiovasc Interv. 2015;8(11):1445–53.
35. Bairey Merz CN, Shaw LJ, Reis SE, Bittner V, Kelsey SF, Olson M, et al. Insights from the NHLBI-Sponsored Women's Ischemia Syndrome Evaluation (WISE) Study: Part II: gender differences in presentation, diagnosis, and outcome with regard to gender-based pathophysiology of atherosclerosis and macrovascular and microvascular coronary disease. J Am Coll Cardiol. 2006;47(3 Suppl):S21–9.
36. Panting JR, Gatehouse PD, Yang GZ, Grothues F, Firmin DN, Collins P, et al. Abnormal subendocardial perfusion in cardiac syndrome X detected by cardiovascular magnetic resonance imaging. N Engl J Med. 2002;346(25):1948–53.
37. Mehta LS, Beckie TM, DeVon HA, Grines CL, Krumholz HM, Johnson MN, et al. Acute myocardial infarction in women: a scientific statement from the American Heart Association. Circulation. 2016;133(9):916–47.
38. Dreyer RP, Smolderen KG, Strait KM, Beltrame JF, Lichtman JH, Lorenze NP, et al. Gender differences in pre-event health status of young patients with acute myocardial infarction: a VIRGO study analysis. Eur Heart J Acute Cardiovasc Care. 2016;5(1):43–54.
39. Mastenbroek MH, Versteeg H, Zijlstra W, Meine M, Spertus JA, Pedersen SS. Disease-specific health status as a predictor of mortality in patients with heart failure: a systematic literature review and meta-analysis of prospective cohort studies. Eur J Heart Fail. 2014;16(4):384–93.
40. Mommersteeg PMC, Denollet J, Spertus JA, Pedersen SS. Health status as a risk factor in cardiovascular disease: a systematic review of current evidence. Am Heart J. 2009;157(2):208–18.
41. Moller-Leimkuhler AM. Women with coronary artery disease and depression: a neglected risk group. World J Biol Psychiatry. 2008;9(2):92–101.
42. Shanmugasegaram S, Russell KL, Kovacs AH, Stewart DE, Grace SL. Gender and sex differences in prevalence of major depression in coronary artery disease patients: a meta-analysis. Maturitas. 2012;73(4):305–11.
43. Ferketich AK, Schwartzbaum JA, Frid DJ, Moeschberger ML. Depression as an antecedent to heart disease among women and men in the NHANES I study. National Health and Nutrition Examination Survey. Arch Intern Med. 2000;160(9):1261–8.
44. Rosengren A, Hawken S, Ounpuu S, Sliwa K, Zubaid M, Almahmeed WA, et al. Association of psychosocial risk factors with risk of acute myocardial infarction in 11119 cases and 13648 controls from 52 countries (the INTERHEART study): case-control study. Lancet. 2004;364(9438):953–62.
45. Rutledge T, Reis SE, Olson M, Owens J, Kelsey SF, Pepine CJ, et al. Depression is associated with cardiac symptoms, mortality risk, and hospitalization among women with suspected coronary disease: the NHLBI-sponsored WISE study. Psychosom Med. 2006;68(2):217–23.
46. Wang HX, Leineweber C, Kirkeeide R, Svane B, Schenck-Gustafsson K, Theorell T, et al. Psychosocial stress and atherosclerosis: family and work stress accelerate progression of coronary disease in women. The Stockholm Female Coronary Angiography Study. J Intern Med. 2007;261(3):245–54.
47. Smolderen KG, Strait KM, Dreyer RP, D'Onofrio G, Zhou S, Lichtman JH, et al. Depressive symptoms in younger women and men with acute myocardial infarction: insights from the VIRGO study. J Am Heart Assoc. 2015;4(4):e001424.
48. Xu X, Bao H, Strait K, Spertus JA, Lichtman JH, D'Onofrio G, et al. Sex differences in perceived stress and early recovery in young and middle-aged patients with acute myocardial infarction. Circulation. 2015;131(7):614–23.
49. Shah AJ, Ghasemzadeh N, Zaragoza-Macias E, Patel R, Eapen DJ, Neeland IJ, et al. Sex and age differences in the association of depression with obstructive coronary artery disease and adverse cardiovascular events. J Am Heart Assoc. 2014;3(3):e000741.
50. Zimmermann-Viehoff F, Wang HX, Kirkeeide R, Schneiderman N, Erdur L, Deter HC, et al. Women's exhaustion and coronary artery atherosclerosis progression: The Stockholm Female Coronary Angiography Study. Psychosom Med. 2013;75(5):478–85.

51. Doyle F, McGee H, Conroy R, Conradi HJ, Meijer A, Steeds R, et al. Systematic review and individual patient data meta-analysis of sex differences in depression and prognosis in persons with myocardial infarction: a MINDMAPS Study. Psychosom Med. 2015;77(4):419–28.
52. Loerbroks A, Bosch JA, Mommersteeg PMC, Herr RM, Angerer P, Li J. The association of depression and angina pectoris across 47 countries: findings from the 2002 World Health Survey. Eur J Epidemiol. 2014;29(7):507–15.
53. Möller-Leimkühler AM. Higher comorbidity of depression and cardiovascular disease in women: a biopsychosocial perspective. World J Biol Psychiatry. 2010;11(8):922–33.
54. Kop WJ, Mommersteeg PMC. Psychoneuroimmunological processes in coronary artery disease and heart failure. In: Kusnecov AW, Anisman H, editors. The Wiley-Blackwell handbook of psychoneuroimmunology. 1st ed. Hoboken: Wiley; 2013.
55. Kop WJ, Mommersteeg PMC. Psychoneuroimmunological pathways and sex differences in coronary artery disease: the role of inflammation and estrogen. In: Orth-Gomér K, Schneiderman N, Vaccarino V, Deter H-C, editors. Psychosocial stress and cardiovascular disease in women concepts, findings, future perspectives. New York: Springer; 2015. p. 129–49.
56. Soares CN. Depression in peri- and postmenopausal women: prevalence, pathophysiology and pharmacological management. Drugs Aging. 2013;30(9):677–85.
57. Douma SL, Husband C, O'Donnell ME, Barwin BN, Woodend AK. Estrogen-related mood disorders: reproductive life cycle factors. Adv Nurs Sci. 2005;28(4):364–75.
58. Williams KE, Marsh WK, Rasgon NL. Mood disorders and fertility in women: a critical review of the literature and implications for future research. Hum Reprod Update. 2007;13(6):607–16.
59. Dantzer R. Cytokine-induced sickness behavior: mechanisms and implications. Ann N Y Acad Sci. 2001;933(1):222–34.
60. De Jonge P, Rosmalen JG, Kema IP, Doornbos B, van Melle JP, Pouwer F, et al. Psychophysiological biomarkers explaining the association between depression and prognosis in coronary artery patients: a critical review of the literature. Neurosci Biobehav Rev. 2010;35(1):84–90.
61. Gidron Y, Kupper N, Kwaijtaal M, Winter J, Denollet J. Vagus-brain communication in atherosclerosis-related inflammation: a neuroimmunomodulation perspective of CAD. Atherosclerosis. 2007;195(2):e1–9.
62. Danesh J, Collins R, Peto R. Chronic infections and coronary heart disease: is there a link? Lancet. 1997;350(9075):430–6.
63. Agushi E, Xhyheri B, Bugiardini R. Sex differences in biomarkers for predicting cardiovascular and coronary events. Curr Vasc Pharmacol. 2013;11(5):785–94.
64. Liuzzo G, Biasucci LM, Gallimore JR, Grillo RL, Rebuzzi AG, Pepys MB, et al. The prognostic value of C-reactive protein and serum amyloid a protein in severe unstable angina. N Engl J Med. 1994;331(7):417–24.
65. Kuller LH, Tracy RP, Shaten J, Meilahn EN. Relation of C-reactive protein and coronary heart disease in the MRFIT nested case-control study. Multiple risk factor intervention trial. Am J Epidemiol. 1996;144(6):537–47.
66. Ridker PM, Cushman M, Stampfer MJ, Tracy RP, Hennekens CH. Inflammation, aspirin, and the risk of cardiovascular disease in apparently healthy men. N Engl J Med. 1997;336(14):973–9.
67. Lavie CJ, Milani RV, Verma A, O'Keefe JH. C-reactive protein and cardiovascular diseases-is it ready for primetime? Am J Med Sci. 2009;338(6):486–92.
68. Danesh J, Wheeler JG, Hirschfield GM, Eda S, Eiriksdottir G, Rumley A, et al. C-reactive protein and other circulating markers of inflammation in the prediction of coronary heart disease. N Engl J Med. 2004;350(14):1387–97.
69. Cossette E, Cloutier I, Tardif K, DonPierre G, Tanguay JF. Estradiol inhibits vascular endothelial cells pro-inflammatory activation induced by C-reactive protein. Mol Cell Biochem. 2013;373(1–2):137–47.
70. Gameiro CM, Romao F, Castelo-Branco C. Menopause and aging: changes in the immune system—a review. Maturitas. 2010;67(4):316–20.

71. Knowlton AA, Lee AR. Estrogen and the cardiovascular system. Pharmacol Ther. 2012;135(1):54–70.
72. van Sloten TT, Schram MT, Adriaanse MC, Dekker JM, Nijpels G, Teerlink T, et al. Endothelial dysfunction is associated with a greater depressive symptom score in a general elderly population: the Hoorn Study. Psychol Med. 2013;44(7):1403–16.
73. McSweeney JC, Cody M, O'Sullivan P, Elberson K, Moser DK, Garvin BJ. Women's early warning symptoms of acute myocardial infarction. Circulation. 2003;108(21):2619–23.
74. DeVon HA, Pettey CM, Vuckovic KM, Koenig MD, McSweeney JC. A review of the literature on cardiac symptoms in older and younger women. J Obstet Gynecol Neonatal Nurs. 2016;45(3):426–37.
75. Madsen R, Birkelund R. Women's experiences during myocardial infarction: systematic review and meta-ethnography. J Clin Nurs. 2016;25(5–6):599–609.
76. Chiaramonte GR, Friend R. Medical students' and residents' gender bias in the diagnosis, treatment, and interpretation of coronary heart disease symptoms. Health Psychol. 2006;25(3):255–66.
77. Roger VL, Farkouh ME, Weston SA, Reeder GS, Jacobsen SJ, Zinsmeister AR, et al. Sex differences in evaluation and outcome of unstable angina. JAMA. 2000;283(5):646–52.
78. Huffman JC, Pollack MH. Predicting panic disorder among patients with chest pain: an analysis of the literature. Psychosomatics. 2003;44(3):222–36.
79. Mommersteeg PMC, Widdershoven JW, Aarnoudse W, Denollet J. Personality subtypes and chest pain in patients with nonobstructive coronary artery disease from the TweeSteden Mild Stenosis Study: mediating effect of anxiety and depression. Eur J Pain. 2016;20(3):427–37.
80. Katerndahl DA. Chest pain and its importance in patients with panic disorder: an updated literature review. Prim Care Companion J Clin Psychiatry. 2008;10(5):376–83.
81. Tully PJ, Turnbull DA, Beltrame J, Horowitz J, Cosh S, Baumeister H, et al. Panic disorder and incident coronary heart disease: a systematic review and meta-regression in 1 131 612 persons and 58 111 cardiac events. Psychol Med. 2015:1–12.
82. Fleet R, Lesperance F, Arsenault A, Gregoire J, Lavoie K, Laurin C, et al. Myocardial perfusion study of panic attacks in patients with coronary artery disease. Am J Cardiol. 2005;96(8):1064–8.
83. Arrighi JA, Burg M, Cohen IS, Soufer R. Simultaneous assessment of myocardial perfusion and function during mental stress in patients with chronic coronary artery disease. J Nucl Cardiol. 2003;10(3):267–74.
84. Kim CK, Bartholomew BA, Mastin ST, Taasan VC, Carson KM, Sheps DS. Detection and reproducibility of mental stress-induced myocardial ischemia with Tc-99m sestamibi SPECT in normal and coronary artery disease populations. J Nucl Cardiol. 2003;10(1):56–62.
85. Ronel J, Mehilli J, Ladwig KH, Blattler H, Oversohl N, Byrne RA, et al. Effects of verbal suggestion on coronary arteries: results of a randomized controlled experimental investigation during coronary angiography. Am Heart J. 2011;162(3):507–11.
86. Vermeltfoort IA, Raijmakers PG, Odekerken DA, Kuijper AF, Zwijnenburg A, Teule GJ. Association between anxiety disorder and the extent of ischemia observed in cardiac syndrome X. J Nucl Cardiol. 2009;16(3):405–10.
87. Paine NJ, Bacon SL, Pelletier R, Arsenault A, Diodati JG, Lavoie KL. Do women with anxiety or depression have higher rates of myocardial ischemia during exercise testing than men? Circ Cardiovasc Qual Outcomes. 2016;9(2 Suppl. 1):S53–61.
88. Foldes-Busque G, Denis I, Poitras J, Fleet RP, Archambault P, Dionne CE. A prospective cohort study to refine and validate the panic screening score for identifying panic attacks associated with unexplained chest pain in the emergency department. BMJ Open. 2013;3(10):e003877.
89. Berthoud HR, Neuhuber WL. Functional and chemical anatomy of the afferent vagal system. Auton Neurosci. 2000;85(1–3):1–17.
90. Xhyheri B, Manfrini O, Mazzolini M, Pizzi C, Bugiardini R. Heart rate variability today. Prog Cardiovasc Dis. 2012;55(3):321–31.
91. Thayer JF, Yamamoto SS, Brosschot JF. The relationship of autonomic imbalance, heart rate variability and cardiovascular disease risk factors. Int J Cardiol. 2010;141(2):122–31.

92. Reyes del Paso GA, Langewitz W, Mulder LJ, van Roon A, Duschek S. The utility of low frequency heart rate variability as an index of sympathetic cardiac tone: a review with emphasis on a reanalysis of previous studies. Psychophysiology. 2013;50(5):477–87.
93. Ong ME, Goh K, Fook-Chong S, Haaland B, Wai KL, Koh ZX, et al. Heart rate variability risk score for prediction of acute cardiac complications in ED patients with chest pain. Am J Emerg Med. 2013;31(8):1201–7.
94. Kahan T, Forslund L, Held C, Bjorkander I, Billing E, Eriksson SV, et al. Risk prediction in stable angina pectoris. Eur J Clin Investig. 2013;43(2):141–51.
95. Steptoe A, Molloy GJ, Messerli-Burgy N, Wikman A, Randall G, Perkins-Porras L, et al. Fear of dying and inflammation following acute coronary syndrome. Eur Heart J. 2011;32(19):2405–11.
96. Lanza GA, Cianflone D, Rebuzzi AG, Angeloni G, Sestito A, Ciriello G, et al. Prognostic value of ventricular arrhythmias and heart rate variability in patients with unstable angina. Heart. 2006;92(8):1055–63.
97. Smoller JW, Pollack MH, Wassertheil-Smoller S, Brunner R, Curb D, Torner J, et al. Panic attacks, daily life ischemia, and chest pain in postmenopausal women. Psychosom Med. 2006;68(6):824–32.
98. Miwa K, Igawa A, Miyagi Y, Nakagawa K, Inoue H. Alterations of autonomic nervous activity preceding nocturnal variant angina: sympathetic augmentation with parasympathetic impairment. Am Heart J. 1998;135(5 Pt 1):762–71.
99. Liu CC, Kuo TB, Yang CC. Effects of estrogen on gender-related autonomic differences in humans. Am J Physiol Heart Circ Physiol. 2003;285(5):H2188–93.
100. Pivatelli FC, Dos Santos MA, Fernandes GB, Gatti M, de Abreu LC, Valenti VE, et al. Sensitivity, specificity and predictive values of linear and nonlinear indices of heart rate variability in stable angina patients. Int Arch Med. 2012;5(1):31.
101. Haensel A, Mills PJ, Nelesen RA, Ziegler MG, Dimsdale JE. The relationship between heart rate variability and inflammatory markers in cardiovascular diseases. Psychoneuroendocrinology. 2008;33(10):1305–12.
102. Thayer JF, Loerbroks A, Sternberg EM. Inflammation and cardiorespiratory control: the role of the vagus nerve. Respir Physiol Neurobiol. 2011;178(3):387–94.
103. Huston JM, Tracey KJ. The pulse of inflammation: heart rate variability, the cholinergic anti-inflammatory pathway and implications for therapy. J Intern Med. 2011;269(1):45–53.
104. Egashira K, Inou T, Hirooka Y, Yamada A, Maruoka Y, Kai H, et al. Impaired coronary blood flow response to acetylcholine in patients with coronary risk factors and proximal atherosclerotic lesions. J Clin Investig. 1993;91(1):29–37.
105. Ong P, Athanasiadis A, Borgulya G, Mahrholdt H, Kaski JC, Sechtem U. High prevalence of a pathological response to acetylcholine testing in patients with stable angina pectoris and unobstructed coronary arteries. The ACOVA Study (Abnormal COronary VAsomotion in patients with stable angina and unobstructed coronary arteries). J Am Coll Cardiol. 2012;59(7):655–62.
106. Yeung AC, Vekshtein VI, Krantz DS, Vita JA, Ryan Jr TJ, Ganz P, et al. The effect of atherosclerosis on the vasomotor response of coronary arteries to mental stress. N Engl J Med. 1991;325(22):1551–6.
107. Stillman AN, Moser DJ, Fiedorowicz J, Robinson HM, Haynes WG. Association of anxiety with resistance vessel dysfunction in human atherosclerosis. Psychosom Med. 2013;75(6):537–44.
108. Alvares GA, Quintana DS, Kemp AH, Van Zwieten A, Balleine BW, Hickie IB, et al. Reduced heart rate variability in social anxiety disorder: associations with gender and symptom severity. PLoS One. 2013;8(7):e70468.
109. Fanselow MS. Fear and anxiety take a double hit from vagal nerve stimulation. Biol Psychiatry. 2013;73(11):1043–4.
110. Ahs F, Sollers 3rd JJ, Furmark T, Fredrikson M, Thayer JF. High-frequency heart rate variability and cortico-striatal activity in men and women with social phobia. NeuroImage. 2009;47(3):815–20.

111. Friedman BH, Thayer JF. Autonomic balance revisited: panic anxiety and heart rate variability. J Psychosom Res. 1998;44(1):133–51.
112. Zimmermann-Viehoff F, Orth-Gomer K, Wang HX, Deter HC, Merswolken M, Ghadiyali Z, et al. Depressive symptoms and heart rate variability in younger women after an acute coronary event. Eur J Cardiovasc Prev Rehabil. 2010;17(5):509–13.
113. Penninx BW, Milaneschi Y, Lamers F, Vogelzangs N. Understanding the somatic consequences of depression: biological mechanisms and the role of depression symptom profile. BMC Med. 2013;11:129.
114. Licht CM, de Geus EJ, van Dyck R, Penninx BW. Association between anxiety disorders and heart rate variability in the Netherlands Study of Depression and Anxiety (NESDA). Psychosom Med. 2009;71(5):508–18.
115. Gulli G, Cemin R, Pancera P, Menegatti G, Vassanelli C, Cevese A. Evidence of parasympathetic impairment in some patients with cardiac syndrome X. Cardiovasc Res. 2001;52(2):208–16.
116. Adamopoulos S, Rosano GM, Ponikowski P, Cerquetani E, Piepoli M, Panagiota F, et al. Impaired baroreflex sensitivity and sympathovagal balance in syndrome X. Am J Cardiol. 1998;82(7):862–8.
117. Spoladore R, Fisicaro A, Faccini A, Camici PG. Coronary microvascular dysfunction in primary cardiomyopathies. Heart. 2014;100(10):806–13.
118. Blumenthal JA, Sherwood A, Smith PJ, Watkins L, Mabe S, Kraus WE, et al. Enhancing cardiac rehabilitation with stress management training: a randomized, clinical efficacy trial. Circulation. 2016;133(14):1341–50.
119. Anderson L, Oldridge N, Thompson DR, Zwisler AD, Rees K, Martin N, et al. Exercise-based cardiac rehabilitation for coronary heart disease: cochrane systematic review and meta-analysis. J Am Coll Cardiol. 2016;67(1):1–12.
120. Whalley B, Rees K, Davies P, Bennett P, Ebrahim S, Liu Z, et al. Psychological interventions for coronary heart disease. Cochrane Database Syst Rev. 2011;8:CD002902.
121. Baumeister H, Hutter N, Bengel J. Psychological and pharmacological interventions for depression in patients with coronary artery disease. Cochrane Database Syst Rev. 2011;9:CD008012.
122. Goodwin L, Ostuzzi G, Khan N, Hotopf MH, Moss-Morris R. Can we identify the active ingredients of behaviour change interventions for coronary heart disease patients? A systematic review and meta-analysis. PLoS One. 2016;11(4):e0153271.
123. Tully PJ, Baumeister H. Collaborative care for comorbid depression and coronary heart disease: a systematic review and meta-analysis of randomised controlled trials. BMJ Open. 2015;5(12):e009128.
124. Kisely SR, Campbell LA, Yelland MJ, Paydar A. Psychological interventions for symptomatic management of non-specific chest pain in patients with normal coronary anatomy. Cochrane Database Syst Rev. 2012;13(6):CD004101.
125. Orth-Gomer K, Schneiderman N, Wang HX, Walldin C, Blom M, Jernberg T. Stress reduction prolongs life in women with coronary disease: the Stockholm Women's Intervention Trial for Coronary Heart Disease (SWITCHD). Circ Cardiovasc Qual Outcomes. 2009;2(1):25–32.
126. Orth-Gomer K, Deter HC. Sex and gender issues in cardiovascular research. Psychosom Med. 2015;77(9):1067–8.
127. Ouyang P, Wenger NK, Taylor D, Rich-Edwards JW, Steiner M, Shaw LJ, et al. Strategies and methods to study female-specific cardiovascular health and disease: a guide for clinical scientists. Biol Sex Differ. 2016;7:19.

Chapter 14
Pharmacotherapy in Women

Karin Schenck-Gustafsson and Mia von Euler

Abstract Pharmacokinetic properties such as absorption, distribution, metabolism, and elimination of drugs often differ between men and women and change over lifetime. Women experience more adverse events and side-effects of medications than men. Hormonal changes during the menstrual cycle usually have limited effect on the pharmacokinetics of drugs, except for drugs that interfere with QT-interval. It is debated whether there is a systematic difference in compliance to medication in women compared to men. Drug interactions and drug safety during pregnancy are discussed.

Keywords Anti-arrhythmic drugs • Beta-blockers • CYP3A4 inhibitors • Drug interactions • Drug safety • Estrogen • Glomerular filtration rate (GFR) • Medication adherence • Menopause • Pharmacodynamics • Pharmacokinetics • Pregnancy • QT-interval • Sex-hormones • Side-effects • Statins • Torsade de Pointes (TdP)

Introduction

Pharmacotherapy is the most common treatment used in health care [1]. During their life span, women in general use more drugs than men, not only because of (contraceptive) hormonal treatments [2]. Even when the nature of the treatment effect is similar in men and women, there are different factors that needs to be taken into consideration when treating women. Pharmacokinetic properties such as

K. Schenck-Gustafsson (✉)
Department of Medicine, Cardiac Unit, Center of Gender Medicine, Karolinska Institutet, Karolinska University Hospital, Stockholm, Sweden
e-mail: Karin.Schenck-Gustafsson@ki.se

M. von Euler
Karolinska Institutet Stroke Research Network, Södersjukhuset, Stockholm, Sweden

Department of Clinical Science and Education, Karolinska Institutet, Södersjukhuset, Stockholm, Sweden

Department of Clinical Pharmacology, Karolinska University Hospital, Stockholm, Sweden
e-mail: Mia.Von.Euler@ki.se

A.H.E.M. Maas, C.N. Bairey Merz (eds.), *Manual of Gynecardiology*,
DOI 10.1007/978-3-319-54960-6_14

absorption, distribution, metabolism, and elimination of drugs quite often differ between men and women which might be clinically significant [3]. Over the course of life and particularly during pregnancy and hormonal therapy, pharmacokinetic variables change, affecting therapeutic effectivity and interactions [4]. Whereas pharmacokinetic differences are rather common, pharmacodynamics properties are usually less distinct between the sexes. However, they may differ between men and women, but also change with ageing [5–15].

The risk of adverse events of drugs differs between the sexes [16, 17]. Overall, women experience more adverse events and side-effects than men. Other major risk factors for adverse events at old age are also more commonly present in women, including polypharmacy [16–19]. Even though women in general use more drugs than men they may be undertreated for several indications [20]. Also, overuse or inadequate use of drugs often occur [21].

Sex-Differences in Pharmacokinetics and Pharmacodynamics

In general, women have a lower body weight than men. Usually this is accounted for in pharmacokinetic studies where weight adjustments are made. However, in adults dosing is not as often corrected for weight which may result in too high doses in women [6, 7]. The absorption of drugs taken orally depends on the drug's chemical and physical properties, physiologic factors such as the pH in the ventricle, motility in the gastrointestinal tract, gut transit time, first passage metabolism, blood flow at site of absorption, and interaction with other drugs and food. The transit time in the gastrointestinal tract is affected by sex hormones resulting in a considerably longer transit time in women [7, 10, 22].

The most common enzymes involved in drug metabolism are cytochrome P450 (CYP) isoenzymes, uridindiphosphat glucuronyl transferases (UGT) and N-acetyl transferases (NAT). Activity of these enzymes varies with sex, ethnicity and other genetic factors. Women have a lower activity in CYP1A2, CYP2E1 and UGT compared to men whereas the activity in CYP3A4, CYP2A6 and CYP2B6 is higher. Pregnancy or use of oral contraceptives and hormone replacement therapy may also affect their activity (Table 14.1). P-glycoproteins (Pgp) are membrane-bound proteins transporting drugs which may affect absorption and renal clearance of some substances. Many CYP3A4 substrates are also Pgp substrates. While CYP3A4 activity in general is higher in women Pgp activity is lower and therefore sex differences in drug metabolism can be affected into both directions which may explain contradictory findings [6, 7].

Transdermal absorption seems to be similar between men and women [12]. There are studies describing lower delivery of *inhaled aerosol drugs* such as ribavirin and cyclosporine in women compared with men [12]. In a study on inhalation technique in asthma or COPD patients using metered dose inhalers (33 men, 26 women) the majority of participants had an incorrect inhalation technique. This was more pronounced in women, regardless of age, and only 4% of women compared to 43% of men had a correct inhalation technique [23].

Table 14.1 Described activity on different metabolic pathways in women compared to men and the effect of hormonal changes with use of combined oral contraceptives, hormonal replacement therapy (HRT) or by pregnancy [55, 56]

	Women relative to men	Oral contraceptives	HRT	Pregnancy
CYP1A2	↓	↓	↑	↓
CYP2A6	↑	↑	↑	
CYP2B6	↑	↓		?
CYP2C9	=			↑
CYP2C19	[a]	↓		↓
CYP2D6	=			↑
CYP2E1	↓			?
CYP3A4	↑			↑
Pgp	↓			
NAT2	=			(↓)[b]
UGT	↓	↑		↑
Renal elimination	↓			↑

[a]There are reported sex differences in various ethnic groups but in these studies the use of oral contraceptives is unknown
[b]Slight decrease during the first trimester

Women have more body fat than men while the latter have more total body water [6, 7]. Therefore, the distribution volume of lipophilic drugs is higher in women whereas this is lower for hydrophilic drugs [24]. A smaller distribution volume implies that the drug is delivered at higher concentration [24]. Alcohol, for example, is a hydrophilic substance with a smaller distribution volume in women compared to men. This is one of the main reasons why women achieve higher alcohol concentrations while drinking the same amount as men [25].

Clearance measures the elimination of a drug in relation to the plasma concentration. Elimination includes metabolism and excretion. Clearance can also be used to compare the kidney capacity to eliminate various substances. Women have in general a lower renal clearance compared to men because women's glomerular filtration rate (GFR) is lower. There is also some evidence for women having less transport proteins such as P-glycoproteins (Pgp) which could add to lower elimination rates in women. Drugs with renal excretion depend on kidney function. Creatinine is used as a measure of renal function. The substance is formed in muscles through non-enzymatic dehydration of muscle creatinine while cystatin C, another marker of renal function, is a small protein that is formed in almost all cells in the body. Creatinine is excreted through glomerular filtration, tubular secretion, and extrarenal in the colon. Excretion of creatinine is lower in persons with small muscle mass, diet low in proteins, at older age and in women. To get an estimate of renal function assessment of glomerular filtration rate (eGFR) is usually sufficient, for which various formulas such as Cockroft-Gault, MDRD or CKD-EPI can be used. Creatinine value, weight, age, sex, and sometimes ethnicity need to be known. Female sex induces a correction factor of 0.75–0.85 as women have lower renal excretion compared to men [24, 26, 27].

Pregnancy, Contraceptive Use and Female Sex-Hormones

During pregnancy the distribution volume changes due to an expansion of total body water and an increase in renal plasma flow and glomerular filtration. Its clinical relevance varies as organ blood flow is redistributed, drug-binding proteins change as well as circulating sex-hormones. For some drugs such as lamotrigine, an anti-epileptic drug, repeated adaptations in dosing are required during pregnancy, for others such as carbamazepine no change in dosing is needed [7, 12, 13, 28].

Use of oral contraceptives can affect the pharmacokinetics of many drugs, with for instance a higher clearance for benzodiazepines, phenytoin, and cyclosporine and a lower clearance for other drugs such as corticosteroids, amitriptyline and caffeine. Both estrogens and progestins undergo intestinal absorption and hepatic metabolism during enterohepatic recycling [14].

Hormonal changes during the menstrual cycle usually have limited effect on the pharmacokinetics of drugs. An exception is for drugs which induce QT prolongation (Table 14.2). This especially accounts for the ovulatory phase of the menstrual cycle. Whether this is due to pharmacokinetic or pharmacodynamic hormone-induced changes is unclear [15].

Concerning other drugs, such as corticosteroids, women are more sensitive to cortisol suppression than men which may lead to an enhanced sensitivity during treatment with corticosteroids. There are several other hormonal systems showing differences between men and women, for example the renin angiotensin system (RAS). Estrogens increase the availability of angiotensinogen and plasma levels of angiotensin II, but decrease renin and ACE activities and the expression of angiotensin receptor 1, whereas androgens upregulate the RAS system [8]. There are also indications that women have a greater cardiac-specific sympathetic activation than men [29], whereas they are less responsive to sympathetic vasoconstrictor activity [30]. This may be due to an increase in β2-adrenoreceptor sensitivity [31], and a higher β2-adrenoreceptor density in lymphocytes [32]. Estrogens and progesterone

Table 14.2 Examples of drugs that either have a risk of TdP or a prolonged QT interval. This may increase the risk for TdP, or TdP under certain conditions such as overdose, drug-drug interactions or when administered to patients with congenital long-QT syndrome [54]

Amiodarone	Escitalopram	Granisetron	Olanzapine	Sorafenib
Amitriptyline	Famotidine	Haloperidol	Promethazine	Sotalol
Apomorphine	Felbamate	Hydrochlorothiazide	Quetiapine	Tacrolimus
Ciprofloxacin	Fingolimod	Ketoconazole	Quinidine	Tamoxifen
Citalopram	Flecainide	Levofloxacin	Risperidone	Tolterodine
Clarithromycin	Fluconazole	Lithium	Ritonavir	Trimethoprim-Sulfa
Clomipramine	Fluoxetine	Metronidazole	Saquinavir	Vardenafil
Disopyramide	Furosemide	Mirabegron	Sertraline	Venlafaxine
Dronedarone	Fosphenytoin	Mirtazapine	Sevoflurane	Voriconazole
Erythromycin	Galantamine	Norfloxacin	Solifenacin	Ziprasidone

inhibit the cardiac expression of β1-adrenoceptors and reduce β-adrenergic-mediated stimulation exerting a cardio-protective effect. Thus, gender-specific differences in the pharmacodynamics of β- blockers might be expected [33, 34]. However, meta-analyses of the big clinical trials have not shown sex-differences in outcomes [35].

Most pharmacotherapeutic studies include both men and women, although in many therapeutic areas relevant sex analyses are not performed and presented. For example Weinberg et al. found that of 150 published randomized controlled trials (RCTs) on treatment for depression, 15% did not report the number of women included in the study and 50% did not analyze outcomes by gender [36]. This is also true for many studies of cardiovascular treatment in the areas of ischemic heart disease, dyslipidemia, hypertension, heart failure and atrial fibrillation. Sex-distribution is often skewed as upper age limits exclude more women than men. Thus, there is still much to learn about sex-differences in pharmacodynamics. The Food and Drug Administration (FDA) and National Institutes of Health (NIH) as well as the Canadian Institutes of Health Research (CIHR) have recently released recommendations for improvement [37].

Adverse Drug Reactions in Women

An Adverse Drug Reaction (ADR) is defined as all undesired effects of a drug in general, women report more ADRs than men and the causes of this are still debated [16, 17]. One explanation is that doses are not weight-adjusted resulting in more women than men being treated with too high doses. Another reason might be that women seek more health care and use more medications. According to Swedish data 70% of all Swedish women, compared to 59% of all men, were dispensed at least one prescription during a year [2]. The risk of experience an ADR increases with the number of medications used. Also, the risk of interactions and a higher risk of an ADR increase with number of medications, which could be another cause for more ADRs in women than men.

Most of reported ADRs are probably dose-dependent and can be explained by the mode of action of drugs, but differences in anatomy, pathophysiology, symptoms, sex-hormones and pharmacogenetics may also play a role.

Some examples of more frequent occurring ADRs in women are the following:

1. Sensitive skin and skin eruptions [38, 39].
2. Adverse ventricular tachycardia's type Torsade de Pointes (TdP) during administration of certain drugs and/or electrolyte disorders and other conditions that prolong cardiac repolarization, see Table 14.2 [40–42]. Especially some cardiovascular drugs might induce this life-threatening ADR [43–47]. The pathophysiological basis of TdP ventricular tachycardia is unclear but may be related to the longer QT duration on ECGs in adult women compared to men. Women are also more prone to drug interactions [48].

3. Persistent cough, as a side effect of angiotensin-converting enzyme (ACE) inhibitors, which occurs more often in women than in men [49]. In some studies the effect of the polymorphism in the angiotensin I converting enzyme gene has been found to be sex-specific, having a protective effect in men while increasing the risk in women. Another side effect of ACE- inhibitors is angioedema. Although a genome-wide association analysis did not find any genetic variant with a large effect sizes, a previous study reported a sex-dependent association of a polymorphism in the X-prolyl aminopeptidase P 2. When treating a patient with ACE-induced cough it is recommended to switch to angiotensin-II antagonists whereafter this side-effect mostly disappears. In some cases the cough is misinterpreted as a deterioration of heart failure for which the patient is given an higher dose of ACE-inhibitor leading to even more cough.
4. Statin induced myopathy has been considered to be more common in women than men [50]. A meta-analysis of nine studies concluded that a polymorphism in the solute carrier organic anion transporter family member 1B1 (*SLCO1B1*) gene is associated with an increased risk for statin-related myopathy, especially in individuals receiving simvastatin [51], but in this study and other genetic studies a female preponderance has not been confirmed [52]. Another argument for the increased susceptibility for side effects of statins in women is their interaction with CYP3A4 inhibitors [53].
5. Drug induced liver injury has been shown to be more common in women [18, 19].

Gender Difference in Adherence to Medication

Patient compliance depends on many factors: perceived seriousness of the treated condition, financial costs, adverse events or perceived risk of adverse events, age of the patient, length of treatment, goal of treatment (prevention, curative, symptomatic), and socioeconomic factors such as age and sex. Studies show varying results of compliance to pharmacological treatment depending on geographic/cultural setting and the type of treatment that was studied. It is debated whether there is a systematic difference in compliance in women compared to men: some studies show higher adherence in men, while other show better adherence in women [21]. In a review of 51 studies covering 19 different disease categories, 771 individual factor items were identified related to non-adherence to chronic therapies of which most were determinants of implementation, and only 47 were related to persistence with medication [54]. Factors with an unambiguous effect on adherence were further grouped into 8 clusters of socio-economic-related factors, 6 of health care team and system related factors, 6 of condition related factors, 6 of therapy related factors, and 14 of patient related factors. The lack of standardized definitions and poor measurement methods however have resulted in many inconsistencies [54]. Despite, some studies show that patient-related factors such as older age, female gender, higher income, and higher education have positive, if rather small, effect on adherence to therapy [55]. Medication non-adherence is therefore affected by multiple determinants. The prediction of non-adherence in the individual patients is difficult however and suitable measurement and multifaceted interventions may be the most effective answer towards unsatisfactory adherence. The limited number of publications assessing determinants of persistence with medication, and lack of those providing determinants of adherence to short-term treatment, are areas where future research is needed. In general, a well-informed motivated patient who has been involved in the decision of treatment which is also affordable are key-factors that increase drug compliance.

Drug Treatment During Pregnancy

The need of medication during pregnancy is rather common. Pregnant women suffer chronic diseases as well as acute disease and pregnancy complications may require treatment. There are several concerns with drug treatment during pregnancy, related to the unborn child such as the risk of a teratogenic effect of the drug, exposure of the fetus to the drug and withdrawal syndromes in the fetus after delivery. There are also concerns about treatment of pregnant women in relation to their increased plasma volume, higher renal clearance and liver enzyme activity. While there is a wish of keeping the fetus' exposure of the drug as low as possible the pharmacokinetic changes due to pregnancy might also require increased doses to maintain the desired effect in the pregnant woman. To avoid over- or under-treatment, it is important to reconsider appropriate dosing during pregnancy as this may change throughout pregnancy and post-partum [13, 14, 28].

Some drugs, such as vitamin K-antagonists, valproic acid, and isoretinoine should be avoided in pregnant women as well as in women who may become pregnant, as the risk of teratogenic complications is high. Other drugs such as ACE inhibitors and angiotensin-II antagonists are more harmful during the second and third trimester due to their pharmacologic effect on the fetus. To which level the fetus is exposed to a drug depends on the dose and subsequent maternal concentration, if the drug passes over the placenta or not, and if so to what extent. Also, the ability of the fetus to metabolize the drug affects the drug exposure [28, 56]. In efforts to limit drug exposure of the fetus, it is important to remember that untreated conditions in the mother may be even more harmful to both mother and child. As low adherence to prescribed medication is a problem and has been reported in large populations of pregnant women it is important to discuss the need of treatment during and after pregnancy [57]. The website www.safefetus.com provides actual information on drug safety during pregnancy.

Gender Differences in Drug Interactions

Drug-drug interaction is common and the more drugs a person uses, the higher the risk of interactions. These are usually divided into pharmacokinetic and pharmacodynamic interactions. Pharmacokinetic interactions are due to absorption, distribution, metabolism or excretion of the drug which are being affected by the interacting drug. An example of pharmacokinetic interaction is induction of CYP3A4 by St John's Wort (*Hypericum perforatum*), promoting an increased metabolism and thus lowering effect of oral contraceptives and antiepileptic drugs like carbamazepine or oxcarbazepine. The pharmacodynamic interactions depend on modes of action of the interacting drugs. An example of this is the QT prolongation and increased risk of TdP following co-administration of ciprofloxacin, citalopram or hydeoxizine with amiodarone. As adult women have longer QT intervals, particularly during the ovulation phase of the menstrual cycle but also with increasing age, this risk is especially important for women [15, 42].

To prevent drug interactions it is recommended to:

- Assess weight and creatinine values (and estimate creatinine clearance) when prescribing or using drugs with renal excretion.
- Perform pharmacogenetic analysis in selected cases.
- Measure blood or serum concentrations of the drug, when using drugs with a narrow therapeutic window or with high propensity to interact with other drugs.
- Measure blood or serum concentrations of drugs in specific conditions, such as during pregnancy, cardiac failure or hypoalbuminemia.

Clinical Cases

Case I: Digitalis in an Elderly Woman

Patient history: the patient was an 80 year old woman with atrial fibrillation (AF) and systolic heart failure. She attended the GP station because of extreme nausea, difficulties in reading, and diarrhea.

Physical examination and laboratory: Weight 50 kg, height 168 cm, s-creatinine 80 mmol/L, K^+ 3.2, Na 122 mmol/L.

Medication: digoxin 0.25 mg × 1, furosemide retard 60 mg × 1, candesartan 8 mg × 1, bisoprolol 5 mg × 1 and medication for RA, diabetes mellitus and hypothyroidism.

ECG: atrial fibrillation, 100 beats per min, BP 150/95 mmHg.

Diagnosis: the serum digoxin levels were measured and showed a concentration of 1.4 ng/L (intoxication considered at concentrations >2 ng/mL (>2.6 nmol/L). A diagnosis of digitalis intoxication was made in spite of having concentration within the recommended interval. Digoxin medication was stopped and her bisoprolol dosage was increased to 5 mg twice daily for heart rate control.

Discussion: Digitalis has a very steep dose-concentration relationship and a small change in kidney function, such as in elderly patients with heart failure. This can increase the serum concentration and provoke rapid intoxication. Recent reviews have recommended concentrations <1.0 ng/mL (<1.3 nmol/L) to avoid intoxication in the elderly. Also, in many countries like Sweden the recom-mended dose interval has recently been changed into a smaller range (in Sweden 0.9–1.2 nmol/L).

Case II: Enalapril in a Female Patient with Systolic Heart Failure

Patient history: The patient was a 55 year old woman with a newly diagnosed systolic heart failure due to a dilated cardiomyopathy. She was recently discharged from the hospital and attended the GP station because of severe cough, particularly during the night. This was so severe that her sleep was impaired. She had no fever and no other signs of upper airways infection, BP 105/85 mmHg. Resting ECG: atrial fibrillation with rate 90/min, (unchanged).

Medication: warfarin, enalapril 10 mg 1 × 1, spironolactone 25 mg 1 × 1, metoprolol 25 mg 1 × 1, furosemide retard 20 mg 1 × 1.

Diagnosis: The GP increased the enalapril dose to 20 mg daily and increased the furosemide to 40 mg daily.

After 4 weeks the patient returned with more cough and complete exhaustion because of insomnia.

Enalapril was changed into the angiotensin-II antagonist candesartan and after a couple of weeks the patient's cough disappeared.

Discussion: persistent cough is a rather common adverse reaction to ACE inhibitors, which occurs more often in women than in men.

Case III: Woman with Slightly Impaired Renal Function Which Can Be Deleterious

Patient history: A 60-year-old woman was presenting at the emergency department (ER) one morning with somnolence, stiff neck, and weak extremities. Glasgow coma scale (GCS) was 12. The week before arrival at the ER she had had gastroenteritis with diarrhea and subsequent dehydration. The previous night she had developed nausea, vomiting, and a severe headache. In the morning she was unable to speak or stand up. Her past medical history included hypertension and recurrent herpes meningitis with radiculitis and neuropathy for more than 10 years.

Medication: valacyclovir 6 g daily, amitriptyline 50 mg × 1, enalapril 10 mg 1 × 1, venlafaxine 1 × 2, gabapentin 600 mg × 3, metoprolol 100 mg 1 × 1, baclofen 30 mg daily, methenamine 1 g 1 × 3, furosemide 80 mg 1 × 1 and montelukast and salmeterol/fluticasone inhalations.

Diagnosis: Several differential diagnoses were considered primarily subarachnoidal haemorrhage, or acute meningitis/encephalitis. A CT scan was performed immediately and turned out to be normal. Intravenous treatment with ampicillin, betamethasone, cefotaxime, and 700 mg of acyclovir was started on the suspicion of bacterial meningitis or encephalitis. A spinal tap showed four erythrocytes and one mononuclear cell. Her leucocyte count was 6.9×10^9 ($4.0–6.0 \times 10^9$), CRP 14 mg/L (<10 mg/L), plasma creatinine count was 185 μmol/L (reference value 45–84 μmol/L). Four months earlier the creatinine had been 85 μmol/L. She also had a bladder paresis with retention of >1000 mL of urine. Other blood tests were normal. EEG showed slow waves and signs of metabolic disturbances. Thus, subarachnoidal haemorrhage and bacterial meningitis could be ruled out although Herpes encephalitis or a Tick Borne Encephalitis could not be excluded. The Infectious Diseases consultant suggested that only the IV-acyclovir treatment should be continued. As she had been treated with valacyclovir for a long time and her renal function was impaired, analyses of acyclovir and its metabolite CMMG were performed in blood, CSF, and urine. All these were markedly elevated and consequently she was diagnosis with aciclovir-induced neuropsychiatric symptoms (AINS). This is a dreaded condition due to intoxication with the metabolite CMMG and if moderate, as in this case, forced diuresis with fluids and furosemide is usually sufficient. In severe cases with hypoxia, coma and need for mechanical ventilation acute hemodialysis is usually warranted. In this case the forced diuresis was sufficient. Later in the afternoon, on the same day she arrived somnolent in an ambulance to hospital, she was sitting in a hospital bed, chatting with her family and solving a cross word puzzle. In patients where the intoxication is not detected, the outcome can be fatal.

Discussion: This case shows the importance of renal function surveillance for drugs that are excreted by the kidneys and that have toxic potentials if overdosed. Particularly in (elderly) women, renal function needs to be considered with fast changes due to dehydration by a rather benign gastroenteritis for example. Acyclovir is metabolised by alcohol dehydrogenase which is metabolised to the main metabolite CMMG. Women have lower alcohol dehydrogenase activity in the gastrointestinal system making them more vulnerable to intoxication. Normally, Acyclovir is considered a safe drug with few adverse effects but if kidney function deteriorates, the risk of accumulation of the metabolite is high if the dose is not corrected.

Medical Treatment Advice in Women
(www.janusinfo.se/In-English)

When prescribing a drug it is advisable to check if there are known sex-differences and if dosing or adverse effects should be adjusted in women. Fertile women needing chronic treatment of drugs that are potentially teratogenic are recommended to avoid or, if this is not feasible, to be informed on the potential risks. The website www.janusinfo.se/In-English [58] has information on sex- and gender differences for more than 200 drugs registered on the website, which is continuously expanding and up-dated. There is also information on pregnancy and lactation which can also be found in the PDR or basic pharmacological handbooks. For drugs that are excreted by the kidneys, always calculate an eGFR. As women have fewer muscle mass than men creatinine values may be deceiving. Therapeutic drug monitoring, measuring plasma concentrations, is also an option for some drugs. There are several websites that have information on drugs that induce QT prolongation, such as the web site https://crediblemeds.org/ [59].

Conclusions

- Pharmacokinetic sex-differences are usually of limited clinical relevance, particularly if corrected for weight and renal function. However, dosing is often not weight adjusted and it needs to be remembered that renal function changes over time.
- Always make an estimation of glomerular filtration rate when using drugs that are excreted by the kidneys, particularly in elderly women.
- Use of drugs during pregnancy sometimes needs dose adjustment as pharmacokinetics change during the pregnancy.
- QT prolongation is more common in women and the risk of cumulative adverse effects of different drugs with QT-prolongation properties and potassium disturbance needs to be considered.

References

1. Socialstyrelsen. Statistik om läkemedel år 2015 (Drug Statistics, Swedish Board of Health and Welfare). http://www.socialstyrelsen.se/publikationer2016/2016-4-4. Accessed 31 Jul 2016.
2. Loikas D, Wettermark B, von Euler M, Bergman U, Schenck-Gustafsson K. Differences in drug utilisation between men and women: a cross-sectional analysis of all dispensed drugs in Sweden. BMJ Open. 2013;3(5):e002378.
3. Mattison D, Mattison FA. Drug disposition and effect. In: Handbook of clinical gender medicine. Basel: Karger Medical and Scientific Publishers; 2012. p. 473–9.
4. Koren G. Sex dependent pharmacokinetics and bioequivalence—time for a change. J Popul Ther Clin Pharmacol. 2013;20:e358–61.
5. Anderson GD. Gender differences in pharmacological response. Int Rev Neurobiol. 2008;83:1–10.
6. Anderson GD. Sex and racial differences in pharmacological response: where is the evidence? Pharmacogenetics, pharmacokinetics, and pharmacodynamics. J Women's Health. 2005;14:19–29.
7. Franconi F, Campesi I. Pharmacogenomics, pharmacokinetics and pharmacodynamics: interaction with biological differences between men and women. Br J Pharmacol. 2014;171:580–94.
8. Fischer M, Baessler A, Schunkert H. Renin angiotensin system and gender differences in the cardiovascular system. Cardiovasc Res. 2002;53:672–7.
9. Hutson WR, Roehrkasse RL, Wald A. Influence of gender and menopause on gastric emptying and motility. Gastroenterology. 1989;96:11–7.
10. Mearadji B, Penning C, Vu MK, van der Schaar PJ, van Petersen AS, Kamerling IM, Masclee AA. Influence of gender on proximal gastric motor and sensory function. Am J Gastroenterol. 2001;96:2066–73.
11. Sadik R, Abrahamsson H, Stotzer PO. Gender differences in gut transit shown with a newly developed radiological procedure. Scand J Gastroenterol. 2003;38:36–42.
12. Schwartz JB. The influence of sex on pharmacokinetics. Clin Pharmacokinet. 2003;42:107–21.
13. Singer AJ, Brandt LJ. Pathophysiology of the gastrointestinal tract during pregnancy. Am J Gastroenterol. 1991;86:1695–712.
14. Spoletini I, Vitale C, Malorni WMC, Rosano GM. Sex differences in drug effects: interaction with sex hormones in adult life. Sex and gender differences in pharmacology. In: Regitz-Zagrosek W, editor. Handbook of experimental pharmacology, vol. 214. Berlin: Springer; 2012. p. 91–105.
15. Rodriguez I, Kilborn MJ, Liu XK, Pezzullo JC, Woosley RL. Drug-induced QT prolongation in women during the menstrual cycle. JAMA. 2001;285:1322–6.
16. Lazarou J, Pomeranz BH, Corey PN. Incidence of adverse drug reactions in hospitalized patients: a meta-analysis of prospective studies. JAMA. 1998;279:1200–5.

17. von Euler M, Eliasson E, Öhlén G, Bergman U. Adverse drug reactions causing hospitalization can be monitored from computerized medical records and thereby indicate the quality of drug utilization. Pharmacoepidemiol Drug Saf. 2006;15:179–84.
18. Leise MD, Poterucha JJ, Talwalkar JA. Drug-induced liver injury. Mayo Clin Proc. 2014;89:95–106.
19. Amacher DE. Female gender as a susceptibility factor for drug-induced liver injury. Hum Exp Toxicol. 2014;33:928–39.
20. Melloni C, Berger JS, Wang TY, Gunes F, Stebbins A, Pieper KS, Dolor RJ, Douglas PS, Mark DB, Newby LK. Representation of women in randomized clinical trials of cardiovascular disease prevention. Circ Cardiovasc Qual Outcomes. 2010;3:135–42.
21. Eriksson I, Bergman U, Vlahovic-Palcevski V, von Euler M. Drug utilization studies across patient and prescriber characteristics. In: Elseviers M, Wettermark B, Birna Almarsdóttir A, Andersen M, Benko R, Bennie M, Eriksson I, Godman B, Krska J, Poluzzi E, Taxis K, Vlahovic-Palcevski V, Vander Stichele R, editors. Drug utilization research: methods and applications. Hoboken: Wiley; 2016.
22. Stephen M, Wiggins HS, Englyst HN. The effect of age, sex and level of intake of dietary fibre from wheat on large-bowel function in thirty healthy subjects. Br J Nutr. 1986;56:349–61.
23. Goodman DE, Israel E, Rosenberg M, Johnston R, Weiss ST, Drazen JM. The influence of age, diagnosis, and gender on proper use of metered-dose inhalers. Am J Respir Crit Care Med. 1994;150:1256–61.
24. Atkinson AJ, Anernathy DR, Daniels CE, Dedrick RL, Markey SP, editors. Principles of clinical pharmacology. 2nd ed. San Diego: Academic/Elsevier; 2007.
25. Frezza M, di Padova C, Pozzato G, Terpin M, Baraona E, Lieber CS. High blood alcohol levels in women. The role of decreased gastric alcohol dehydrogenase activity and first-pass metabolism. N Engl J Med. 1990;322:95–9.
26. SBU. Skattning av njurfunktion: en systematisk litteraturöversikt. Rapport nr: 214. Mölnlycke: Elanders; 2013. ISBN: 978-91-85413-53-9.
27. Skoglund P. Farmakokinetiska grundbegrepp. Apoteket AB. Marknads-/Försäljningsstöd; 2001.
28. Pieper PG. Use of medication for cardiovascular disease during pregnancy. Nat Rev Cardiol. 2015;12:718–29.
29. Mitoff PR, Gam D, Ivanov J, Al-hesayen A, Azevedo ER, Newton GE, Parker JD, Mak S. Cardiac-specific sympathetic activation in men and women with and without heart failure. Heart. 2011;97:382–7.
30. Momen A, Gao Z, Cohen A, Khan T, Leuenberger UA, Sinoway LI. Coronary vasoconstrictor responses are attenuated in young women as compared with age-matched men. J Physiol. 2010;588:4007–16.
31. Kneale BJ, Chowienczyk PJ, Brett SE, Coltart DJ, Ritter JM. Gender differences in sensitivity to adrenergic agonists of forearm resistance vasculature. J Am Coll Cardiol. 2000;36:1233.
32. Wheeldon NM, Newnham DM, Coutie WJ, Peters JA, McDevitt DG, Lipworth BJ. Influence of sex-steroid hormones on the regulation of lymphocyte beta 2-adrenoceptors during the menstrual cycle. Br J Clin Pharmacol. 1994;37:583–8.
33. Kam KW, Qi JS, Chen M, Wong TM. Estrogen reduces cardiac injury and expression of beta1-adrenoceptor upon ischemic insult in the rat heart. J Pharmacol Exp Ther. 2004;309:8–15.
34. Thawornkaiwong A, Preawnim S, Wattanapermpool J. Upregulation of β1-adrenergic receptors in ovariectomized rat hearts. Life Sci. 2003;72:1813–24.
35. Kotecha D, Manzano L, Krum H, et al. Effect of age and sex on efficacy and tolerability of β-blockers in patients with heart failure with reduced ejection fraction: individual patient data meta-analysis. BMJ. 2016;353:i18.
36. Weinberger AH, McKee SA, Mazure CM. Inclusion of women and gender-specific analyses in randomized clinical trials of treatments for depression. J Womens Health (Larchmt). 2010;19:1727–32.
37. Tannenbaum C, Schwarz JM, Clayton JA, de Vries GJ, Sullivan C. Evaluating sex as a biological variable in preclinical research: the devil in the details. Biol Sex Differ. 2016;7:13. doi:10.1186/s13293-016-0066-x.

38. Ward KE, Archambault R, Mersfelder TL. Severe adverse skin reactions to nonsteroidal anti-inflammatory drugs: a review of the literature. Am J Health Syst Pharm. 2010;67:206–13.
39. Willis CM, Shaw S, De Lacharrière O, Baverel M, Reiche L, Jourdain R, Bastien P, Wilkinson JD. Sensitive skin: an epidemiological study. Br J Dermatol. 2001;145:258–63.
40. Moss AJ. The QT interval and Torsade de pointes. Drug Saf. 1999;21(Suppl. 1):5–10.
41. Taylor CJ, Hodgkinson J, Hobbs FD. Rhythm control agents and adverse events in patients with atrial fibrillation. Int J Clin Pract. 2010;64:1069–75.
42. Roden DM. Drug-induced prolongation of the QT interval. N Engl J Med. 2004;350:1013–22.
43. Makkar RR, Fromm BS, Steinman RT, Meissner MD, Lehmann MH. Female gender as a risk factor for Torsades de pointes associated with cardiovascular drugs. JAMA. 1993;270:2590–7.
44. Fitzgerald PT, Ackerman MJ. Drug-induced torsades de pointes: the evolving role of pharmacogenetics. Heart Rhythm. 2005;2:S30–7.
45. Lehmann MH, Hardy S, Archibald D, MacNeil DJ. QTc prolongation with d,l-sotalol in women versus men. Am J Cardiol. 1999;83:354–9.
46. Schenck-Gustafsson K, Dahlqvist R. Pharmacokinetics of digoxin in patients subjected to the quinidine-digoxin interaction. Br J Clin Pharmacol. 1981;11(2):181–6.
47. Reinoehl J, Frankovich D, Machado C, Kawasaki R, Baga JJ, Pires LA, et al. Probucol associated tachyarrhythmic events and QT prolongation: importance of gender. Am Heart J. 1996;131:1184–91.
48. Lim HE, Pak HN, Ahn JC, Song WH, Kim YH. Torsade de pointes induced by short-term oral amiodarone therapy. Europace. 2006;8:1051–3.
49. Os I, Bratland B, Dahlof B, Gisholt K, Syvertsen JO, Tretli S. Female sex as an important determinant of lisinopril-induced cough. Lancet. 1992;339:372.
50. Pasternak RC, Smith Jr SC, Bairey-Merz CN, Grundy SM, Cleeman JI, Lenfant C. ACC/AHA/NHLBI clinical advisory on the use and safety of statins. Circulation. 2002;106:1024–8.
51. Hou Q, Li S, Li L, Li Y, Sun X, Tian H. Association between SLCO1B1 gene T521C, polymorphism and statin-related myopathy risk: a meta-analysis of case-control studies. Medicine (Baltimore). 2015;94(37):e1268.
52. Luzum JA, Kitzmiller JP, Isackson PJ, Ma C, Medina MW, Dauki AM, et al. GATM polymorphism associated with the risk for statin-induced myopathy does not replicate in case-control analysis of 715 dyslipidemic individuals. Cell Metab. 2015;21:622–7.
53. Rosano GM, Lewis B, Agewall S, Wassmann S, Vitale C, Schmidt H, et al. Gender differences in the effect of cardiovascular drugs: a position document of the working group on pharmacology and drug therapy of the ESC. Eur Heart J. 2015;36:2677–80.
54. Kardas P, Lewek P, Matyjaszczyk M. Determinants of patient adherence: a review of systematic reviews. Front Pharmacol. 2013;4:1–16.
55. DiMatteo MR. Variations in patients' adherence to medical recommendations: a quantitative review of 50 years of research. Med Care. 2004;42:200–9.
56. Regitz-Zagrosek V, Blomstrom Lundqvist C, Borghi C, Cifkova R, Ferreira R, Foidart J-M, Gibbs JSR, Gohlke-Baerwolf C, Gorenek B, Iung B, Kirby MC, Maas AHEM, Morais J, Nihoyannopoulos P, Pieper PG, Presbitero P, Roos-Hesselink JW, Schaufelberger M, Seeland U, Torracca L. ESC guidelines on the management of cardiovascular diseases during pregnancy. Eur Heart J. 2011;32:3147–97.
57. Lupattelli A, Spigset O, Björnsdóttir I, Hämeen-Anttila K, Mårdby AC, Panchaud A, Juraski RG, Rudolf G, Odalovic M, Drozd M, Twigg MJ, Juch H, Moretti ME, Kennedy D, Rieutord A, Zagorodnikova K, Passier A, Nordeng H. Patterns and factors associated with low adherence to psychotropic medications during pregnancy—a cross-sectional, multinational web-based study. Depress Anxiety. 2015;32:426–36.
58. www.janusinfo.se/In-English.
59. https://crediblemeds.org/.

Chapter 15
The Critically Ill Female Patient

Susanna Price and Shahana Uddin

Abstract Differential outcomes are present among female and male patients with critical illness, related to co-morbidity, immune response, pharmacology and the underlying physiological response to intensive care and its complications. Women are more susceptible to the effects of neuromuscular blockade, opioid receptor agonists, and beta adrenergic agents and they are more likely to develop Torsade de pointes and liver dysfunction in response to pharmacological agents. Elderly female patients with basal septal hypertrophy may respond to dobutamine by developing worsening of diastolic dysfunction and increasing left-ventricular outflow tract obstruction. There are important differences in post-traumatic stress disorder (PTSD) between genders, with women at risk for markedly worse psychological outcomes after critical illness.

Keywords Beta-blockers • Critical illness • Diastolic dysfunction • Dobutamine • Estrogen • Extracorporeal cardiac support • Immune response • Immunomodulation • Inflammation • Intensive care • Pharmacokinetics • Post-traumatic stress disorder (PTSD) • Pregnancy • Sex-hormones • Sepsis • Torsade de pointes (TdP) • Trauma

Introduction

Management of critically ill patients with cardiovascular disease (CVD) has moved from the domain of single organ cardiac dysfunction, to an increasingly elderly patient population with numerous co-morbidities and ever more severe derangement of cardiovascular physiology. In this rapidly developing specialty, there is an increasing emphasis on understanding the pathophysiological processes that drive critical illness in order to deliver personalised evidence-based medicine thereby improving patient outcomes. It is in this context that there has recently been

S. Price, M.D., Ph.D. (✉)
Consultant Cardiologist and Intensivist, Royal Brompton Hospital, Imperial College, London, UK
e-mail: S.Price@rbht.nhs.uk

S. Uddin, M.D., Ph.D.
Consultant Intensivist, Anaesthetist and Major Trauma, King's College Hospital, London, UK
e-mail: shahanauddin@nhs.net

A.H.E.M. Maas, C.N. Bairey Merz (eds.), *Manual of Gynecardiology*,
DOI 10.1007/978-3-319-54960-6_15

increased interest in the influence of sex and gender on disease development and survival in critical illness. Although gender differences in the assessment and management of acute coronary syndromes are relatively well-appreciated, the importance of such differences in patients with other life-threatening cardiovascular conditions are not so well understood. This accounts in particular for critical care, where the prognosis depends not only on the primary cardiovascular diagnosis, but to a large extent on the severity of other organ involvement and the patient response to critical illness. This chapter will outline some of emerging evidence regarding the potential challenges of managing the critically ill female patient with CVD, as well as some of the relevant practical considerations for the management of such patients.

Gender Differences in Critical Illness Outcomes

Observational studies have demonstrated gender differences in outcomes of critical illness. The heterogeneous nature of the studies makes interpretation challenging, however, it appears that women have a higher mortality than men, in particular in the context of some CVD, and that female gender may be protective for other conditions. The presence of disparities in presentation, diagnosis, comorbidities, critical care admission, intervention and decision-making probably all contribute to the heterogeneity of findings (Table 15.1). Numerous biologically plausible hypotheses have been generated relating to differential outcomes comparing male and female patients, in particular relating to the immune response to critical illness, however, other factors must be considered including pharmacology (including genetic differences in response to drugs) and the underlying physiological response to intensive care and its complications.

Physical and Pharmacological Differences

Physical differences between male and female patients largely do not affect their management in the cardiac intensive care unit except relating to physical size. Other than basic critical care considerations regarding airway and ventilatory management (endotracheal tube/tracheostomy size, ideal body weight tidal volumes) and drug dosage, there is little that is not encompassed in general critical care management, however some areas warrant specific consideration. First, women who meet nutritional goals have a lower hazard ratio of dying on the intensive care compared with men, but this benefit is lost if they meet their energy target but fail to reach their protein target (possibly due to the smaller total protein stores in women). Second, the anatomical and physiological differences between genders (including body weight, composition, GI motility, liver metabolism and glomerular filtration rate) significantly alter pharmacokinetics and dynamics of drugs, including absorption, distribution, metabolism and elimination. Women are more susceptible to the effects of neuromuscular blockade, opioid receptor agonists, and beta adrenergic agents, as well as having a variable but attenuated response to pressor agents under conditions

Table 15.1 Sex and gender differences in outcomes of critical illness

Study	Study type	Aim	Main findings	Dates	Patients	Additional findings
Romo et al. [1]	Retrospective analysis mixed medical and surgical ICU	Evaluate difference in mortality between genders and between medical and surgical ICUs	Women had a higher mortality than men	1983	4420 admissions	Worse outcome especially in women >50 years
				1995 (2 × 12 month periods studied)	–1587 female	
					–2833 male	
			–15% vs. 13%; OR 1.18 (95% CI 1.02–1.38; P < 0.05)			There is an interaction with gender with length of ICU stay—the difference in outcome less apparent after longer LOS OR of 1.54 (95% CI, 1.25–1.89) overall and an OR of 0.95 (95% CI, 0.92–0.98) for each day of increase in LOS
	Belgian ICUs		Worse survival in women with cardiovascular diseases			
			–23% vs. 12%; OR, 2.07; (95% CI 1.50–2.87; P < 0.001)			
Sathianathan et al. [2]	Retrospective single centre study: Australian ICU	Identify factors associated with survival on comatose survivors of arrest	Male gender improved survival to hospital discharge	20 years 1993–2012	582 patients	Median ICU LOS 3 days and hospital LOS 5
					62% male	
						Shockable rhythm and shorter time to ROSC associated with survival to discharge
Samuelsson et al. [3]	Observational study—Registry date (multicentre)	? women of premenopausal age have better outcome	No survival advantage in pre-menopausal women	4 years 2008–2012	127,254 episodes	Presumed menopause at median age 45 years—arbitrary cut-off
					57% male	
	Swedish ICU		No difference in 30 day mortality in women whether <45> years		43% female	
			Better outcome in men >45 years			

(continued)

Table 15.1 (continued)

Study	Study type	Aim	Main findings	Dates	Patients	Additional findings
Morrison et al. [4]	Registry data Observational study	To study the relationship between gender and outcomes in non traumatic out of hospital cardiac arrest (OHCA)	Lower survival in women	Dec 2005–May 2007	14,690 patients	Cohort to study effect of female reproductive hormones
			unadjusted OR 0.69, 95% CI: 0.60, 0.77		36.4% women	
	North American and Canadian ICUs		With adjustment for Utstein predictors → women 15–45 years better survival to discharge (OR 1.66–95% CI 1.04–2.64)		64.2% men	Women more likely to achieve ROSC pre-hospital
Tao et al. [5]	Meta analysis	Influence of sex on outcomes in trauma patients	Protective effect of female gender on outcomes (mortality, LOS and fatal complications)	Upto 2013	Pooled data—19 studies 100,566 men 39,762 women	
Mahmood et al. [6]	Observational retrospective study in American ICUs	Assess the association of gender with	Overall Survival advantage for younger women	Jan 2004–December 2008	261,255 pts	ICU mortality 7.2% men and 7.9% women
					144,254 men (55.2%)	
		1. ICU mortality	Worse outcome women post-CABG		117,001women (44.8%)	Pts <50 years—women had reduced ICU mortality vs. men: OR 0.83 (95% CI 0.79–0.91)—adjusted for physiology score, ethnicity, co-morbid conditions, pre-ICU LOS, pre-ICU location and hospital teaching status
		2. Active therapies	Better outcome after COPD			
		3. Outcomes in disease subgroups				No difference amongst >50 years
						No difference in sepsis, ACS, trauma

Pietropaoli et al. [7]	Retrospective database cohort	Hypothesis—hospital mortality is higher in men compared to women with sepsis or septic shock requiring ICU	Hospital mortality higher in women	2003–2006	18,757 pts	Disparity in delivery and processes of care
					10,055 men (54%)	
	Multi centre—98 ICUs in 71 US hospitals and four Canadian/Brazilian units		OR = 1.11 95% CI 1.04–1.19 p = 0.002		8702 women (46%)	Equal number of organ dysfunction between genders
						No difference if >or< 50 years
Quenot et al. [8]	Prospective multicentre	Evaluate prognostic factors associated with 28 days mortality in septic shock	Same mortality men and women	Nov 2009–March 2011	1495 shocked	
					63.9% male	
	French units				36.1% female	
Raine et al. [9]	ICNARC registry data	Comparison of case mix and outcomes of male and female patients admitted to ICUs	No difference in admission and mortality in cardiac arrhythmia, COPD, asthma, self poisoning, seizures. Some inequity in AMI and neurological bleeding	3 years	46,587	Demonstration of horizontal and vertical inequity in ICU
	91 UK units					
Vincent et al. [10]	Multi centre observational cohort	To define the incidence and characteristics of critically ill patients in Europe	Female gender independent risk factor for mortality	2 weeks	3147 patients	Numerous additional substudies published
	198 European ICUs			May 2002		

CU intensive care unit, *LOS* length of stay, *APACHE* acute physiology and chronic health evaluation, *CABG* coronary artery bypass graft, *COPD* chronic obstructive pulmonary disease, *ACS* acute coronary syndrome, *ARDS* adult respiratory distress syndrome, *ROSC* return of spontaneous circulation of stress. The potential response to beta adrenergic agents on cardiovascular function should also be carefully considered prior to institution of therapy. In particular, elderly female patients with basal septal hypertrophy may respond to dobutamine by developing worsening abnormalities of diastolic dysfunction and significantly increasing left-ventricular outflow tract obstruction. The condition should be suspected in case of deteriorating cardiac output in the presence of escalating inotropic support, and is readily confirmed using echocardiography. Treatment comprises cessation of beta adrenergic agents, volume and pressor resuscitation, and timely re-introduction of beta blocking agents (where right ventricular function allows).

Differences also include susceptibility to adverse drug effects, with women more likely to develop, for example, Torsade de pointes and liver dysfunction in response to pharmacological agents. Gender differences additionally exist in relevant responses to recreational drugs. Here, the interplay between alcohol consumption and gender, and effects on coagulation may be particularly important in patients receiving extracorporeal cardiac support. In terms of prescription drugs, it is estimated that around 21% women in USA receive hormonal treatment, however it is unknown how this affects critical care outcomes and response to therapies.

Clinical decision-making in critical care is clearly affected in pregnancy, and on occasion, urgent/emergency decisions will be required in the face of life-threatening illness. In addition to the usual considerations relating to pharmacology and physiology, clinicians must work within a (sometimes emergently convened) multidisciplinary team in order to optimise decision-making for both patients (clinical case).

Gender Differences in the Response to Critical Illness

There is increasing recognition that there are gender-specific differences in response to acute illness, particularly in trauma, sepsis and following resuscitation from cardiac arrest. Sex-hormones have been shown to influence inflammatory cell lines, endothelial cells and the inflammatory cascade, to the extent that hormone therapy has been considered a potential therapeutic strategy in response to critical illness in some scenarios, including short-term androgen receptor antagonists in male trauma patients. Experimental pre-clinical studies using animal models suggest that oestradiol and the pro-oestrus states are pro-inflammatory and associated with improved survival after trauma and in sepsis, whereas testosterone and the pro-androgenic states are anti-inflammatory and associated with immune suppression and reduced survival. Whether these differences confer benefit to the individual patient remain unclear. Indeed, observational clinical studies in in sepsis, burns and trauma have demonstrated less clear differential outcomes.

The response to trauma is probably the most primitive of human survival mechanisms in the face of acute injury. The immediate metabolic responses to trauma (including thoracic/aortic trauma) are affected by age and severity of injury, and also gender. Although the relative responses within the affected multi-organ systems are complex and diverse, the majority of studies have shown female gender to be protective. Sex-hormone levels post-trauma have shown correlation between oestrogen/

progesterone and tumour necrosis factor-a (TNFa) immediately after injury. High oestradiol levels are associated with increased mortality, and serum oestradiol is a marker of injury severity and predictor of death in critically injured patients, regardless of gender. However, whether oestradiol plays a causal role in outcomes remains unclear. Prospective studies have confirmed additional gender differences in response to trauma, with female patients responding to increasing severity of injury with increased serum insulin-like growth factor-1 (ILGF-1) and little change in transthyretin concentrations early after injury, but in in men, both ILGF-1 and transthyretin concentrations decrease with increasing injury severity. Whether these differing patterns of response to injury could provide potential therapeutic targets in the future demands further investigation.

The commonest cause of mortality in intensive care is sepsis. Current understanding of sepsis and associated inflammatory syndromes suggests that morbidity/mortality may result from an excessively vigorous or imbalanced immune response between pro- and anti-inflammatory pathways. Numerous animal (murine) models have demonstrated gender differences in response to microbial or endotoxin challenges. Whether the gender difference in response to sepsis in these models is associated with distinct sexually dimorphic immune responses remains uncertain. Consistent with the central role of the immune response in determining survival from sepsis, gender-specific immune responses appear to confer gender-specific benefits (or not) from attempts at immunomodulation. More recent studies have made significant progress in addressing the potential contribution of gender differences to differences in the inflammatory response. Toll-like receptors (TLRs) are members of the pattern recognition receptors (PRR), detecting nucleic acids (Pattern-associated Molecular Patterns—PAMPs) from invading pathogens and triggering cytokine release during inflammation and infection, and also potentially during associated tissue damage. Interleukin-1 receptor associated kinase-1 (IRAK-1) a constituent member of the TLR signalling cascade, resides on the X-chromosome and plays a central role in the TLR-2 and 4-induced activation of nuclear factor NFkB, a critical event in the transcriptional regulation of many pro-inflammatory mediators. The IRAK-1 protein has multiple haplotypes, with a less common variation being found to be associated with worse outcomes in septic patients, and IRAK1 polymorphism therefore a potential mechanism responsible for gender-based outcome differences in response to injury. The IRAK-1 variant has been shown to be associated with poor clinical outcome, with a sixfold greater risk of multi-organ failure, and fivefold increase in mortality. Here outcomes were overall worse in males, but were 'dose-dependent' in women. Given these findings it is unsurprising that a gender-specific/biased response to an immune-based phenomenon (such as sepsis/inflammatory response) might exist, and that the complex cellular and humoral immunity responses to critical care may also differ between the two sexes. These fundamental differences in immune response make it even more challenging to determine the relevant contributions of endogenous patient factors, treatment differences, the patient response to interventions or acute changes in sex hormone levels in outcomes from critical illness. This is further compounded by most clinical studies being limited by their retrospective design, lack of any information on hormonal status, and the usual difficulty in controlling the other variables in clinical critical care studies.

Intensive Care of the Critically Ill Cardiac Patient: Ethical Considerations

Critical care medicine relates to the assessment and management of patients with acute life-threatening conditions, either on a specialised intensive care unit, or at any point throughout the patient pathway. The demand for critical care services (and beds) is increasing, and in parallel is the demand for cardiovascular critical care. However, the supply is not unlimited. Where a patient requires admission to a specialist unit (ICU or CICU) this should usually be determined by the needs of the patient. Despite this, under certain circumstances patients may find themselves denied critical care admission and there is some evidence that the female patient population differ significantly in terms of critical care utilisation, although these findings vary between countries. Systematic denial of critical care admission (horizontal inequity) and application of intensive care interventions (vertical inequity) are recognised challenges in the provision of equitable and high quality critical care. In terms of acute cardiovascular disease, considering acute myocardial infarction, arrhythmia and ventricular failure, equity of admission to intensive care together with ongoing treatment have been specifically studied. Indeed, both horizontal and vertical inequity exist in patients requiring intensive care with acute myocardial infarction, but what is less well understood is why. By contrast, there seems to be gender bias against male patients admitted to intensive care with left ventricular failure, but again, the causes remain unknown. There is, however, evidence that elderly patients (in particular female elderly patients) may be denied intensive care admission on grounds of perceived futility. A challenge to this perception has been raised in more recent studies that demonstrate that although outcomes are less good in elderly patients, they benefit the most from intensive care, and should not be systematically denied admission to intensive care on the basis of age alone. Finally, where patients survive critical care admission, there are important differences in post-traumatic stress disorder (PTSD) between genders, with women at risk for markedly worse psychological outcomes after critical illness, independent of illness severity, with female gender as an independent predictor of worse quality of life, psychological morbidity and rates of PTSD.

Summary

The changing face of cardiac intensive care provides a major challenge to deliverers of healthcare across the World. Rapidly developing technological advances of intensive care, improving understanding of the pathophysiological processes that accompany critical illness (and its treatment), appreciation of the importance of iatrogenic injury, together with the requirement for multidisciplinary team working all combine to provide the clinician with a set of unique diagnostic and management challenges. Certainly there are some practical aspects of managing critically ill female cardiovascular patients that warrant consideration, however, the differing pathophysiological responses of female patients in critical illness are only just beginning to be explored. Here the gender-specific differences in cellular, molecular and hormonal response to critical illness may prove to be an important future avenue to explore in attempts to improve outcome in these most acutely unwell patients.

Clinical Case

A 23 year-old woman (36 weeks pregnant, gravida 1, para 0) presented to her local hospital complaining of epigastric pain and breathlessness. She took no regular medication and had an uneventful pregnancy. On examination she was breathless at rest, pulse 80 beats per minute, of reduced stroke volume and with multiple premature beats. Her jugular venous pressure was not elevated. Heart sounds were normal, with an added third heart sound. Blood pressure was 90/60 mmHg. Her chest was clear and she had minimal pitting oedema. Lab investigations: white cell count 16.5, platelets 236, urea and electrolytes, liver function tests, clotting studies and lactate were all normal. ECG showed sinus rhythm with occasional ventricular extrasystoles. CTG: foetal heart rate 160 bpm with good foetal movements. An echocardiogram was performed, and showed a dilated left ventricle (6.5 mm diastole) and reduced LV ejection fraction 12%, with mild mitral regurgitation.

Her blood pressure was falling progressively (65/48 mmHg) with rising lactate, and therefore dobutamine was commenced (10 μg/kg/min), with subsequent addition of adrenaline (0.02 μg/kg/min). Despite this, she continued to deteriorate (INTERMACS 1) and an emergency multidisciplinary team (cardiac surgeon, cardiologist, obstetrician, cardiac intensivist, cardiac anaesthetist specialised in high risk obstetric delivery, neonatologist) was convened in order to plan her ongoing management.

Priorities were to save the life of the mother and deliver a live infant and therefore a plan was made for urgent Caesarean section combined with institution of cardiac (veno-arterial) extracorporeal membrane oxygenation (VA-ECMO). Steroids were administered to the mother whilst the team (n = 24) convened, comprising in addition, three sets of nursing staff (anaesthetic, neonatal, obstetric) perfusionists, and surgical strategy was planned: general anaesthesia (+transoesophageal echocardiography), four quadrant draping (chest/abdomen/pelvis/groin), surgical exposure and securing of right common femoral vein and artery, Pfannenstiel incision and delivery of infant, haemostasis and closure of abdominal wound, full heparinisation, cannulation for ECMO and institution of VA-ECMO support.

The patient was commenced on bromocriptine, and after 6 days was weaned from ECMO (after treatment with ACE-inhibitors and Levosimendan). She was discharged 2 weeks after intensive care admission.

Learning Points

1. Epigastric pain and breathlessness are common in the healthy pregnant woman but must be investigated, in particular where disproportionate and associated with abnormal clinical signs
2. Patients with peri-partum cardiomyopathy (PPCM) can deteriorate rapidly—anticipation of deterioration and prompt referral to specialist services are vital
3. Multi-disciplinary team working, even in urgent/emergent cases is required for optimal patient outcome

References

1. Romo H, Amaral AC, Vincent JL. Effect of patient sex on ICU survival. Arch Intern Med. 2004;164(1):61–5.
2. Sathianathan K, Tiruvoipati R, Vij S. Prognostic factors associated with hospital survival in comatose survivors of cardiac arrest. World J Crit Care Med. 2016;5(1):103–10.
3. Samuelsson C, Sjöberg F, Karlström G, Nolin T, Walther SM. Gender differences in outcome and use of resources do exist in Swedish intensive care. Crit Care. 2015;19:129.
4. Morrison LJ, Schmicker RH, Weisfeldt ML, Bigham BL, Berg RA, Topjian AA, Abramson BL, Atkins DL, Egan D, Sopko G, Rac VE. Effect of gender on outcome of out of hospital cardiac arrest in the resuscitation outcomes consortium. Resuscitation. 2016;100:76–81.
5. Liu T, et al. The influence of sex on outcomes in trauma patients: a meta-analysis. Am J Surg. 2015;210:911–21.
6. Mahmood K, Eldeirawi K, Wahidi MM. Association of gender with outcomes in critically ill patients. Crit Care. 2012;16(3):R92.
7. Pietropaoli AP, et al. Gender differences in mortality in patients with severe sepsis and septic shock. Gend Med. 2010;7(5):422–37.
8. Quenot J-P, et al. The epidemiology of septic shock in French ICUs: the prospective multicentre cohort EPISS study. Crit Care. 2013;17(2):R65.
9. Raine R, et al. Influence of patient gender on admission to intensive care. J Epidimiol Comm Health. 2002;56(6):418–23.
10. Vincent JL, et al. Sepsis in European ICUs: results of the SOAP study. Crit Care Med. 2006;34(2):344–53.

Further Reading

1. Campesi I, et al. Sex and gender aspects in anesthetics and pain medication. Handb Exp Pharmacol. 2012;(214):265–78. doi: 10.1007/978-3-642-30,726-3_13.
2. El-Eraky H, et al. Effects of sex on the pharmacokinetic and pharmacodynamic properties of quinidine. Br J Clin Pharmacol. 2003;56, 198–204.
3. Spoerke N, et al. Effects of ethanol intoxication and gender on blood coagulation. J Trauma. 2010;68:1106–11.
4. Gilliver SC. Sex steroids as inflammatory regulators. J Steroid Biochem Mol Biol. 2010;120:105-15.

5. Wichman MW, et al. Gender differences: improved immune function in females as opposed to decreased immune function in males following haemorrhagic shock. Surg Forum 1995;46:758–9.
6. Fiorentino DF, et al. IL-10 inhibits cytokine production by activated macrophages. J Immunol. 1991;147:3815–22.
7. Raine R, et al. Influence of patient gender on admission to intensive care. J Epidemiol Community Health 2002;56:418–23.
8. Fowler R, et al. Sex and age based differences in the delivery and outcomes of critical care. CMAJ. 2007;177(12):1513–19.
9. Sharma RK, et al. Male-female patient differences in the association between end-of-life discussions and receipt of intensive care near death. Cancer. 2015;121(16):2814–20.
10. Vezzani A, et al. Gender disparities in the intensive care unit. Ital J Gender Specific Med. 2016;2(1):22–7.
11. Sethuraman KN, et al. Gender specific issues in traumatic injury and resuscitation: consensus-based recommendations for future research. Acad Emerg Med. 2014;21(12):1386–94.

Index

A.H.E.M. Maas, C.N. Bairey Merz (eds.), *Manual of Gynecardiology*,
DOI 10.1007/978-3-319-54960-6

D

E

MIX
Papier aus verantwortungsvollen Quellen
Paper from responsible sources
FSC® C105338

If you have any concerns about our products,
you can contact us on
ProductSafety@springernature.com

In case Publisher is established outside the EU,
the EU authorized representative is:
Springer Nature Customer Service Center GmbH
Europaplatz 3, 69115 Heidelberg, Germany

Printed by Libri Plureos GmbH
in Hamburg, Germany